Advances in
Preschool
Psychopharmacology

Advances in
Preschool
Psychopharmacology

Editors

Joan L. Luby, M.D.
Washington University School of Medicine
St. Louis, Missouri
and
Mark A. Riddle, M.D.
Johns Hopkins University School of Medicine
Baltimore, Maryland

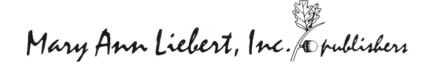

ISBN: 978-1-934854-03-7

Copyright ©2009 by Mary Ann Liebert, Inc., 140 Huguenot Street, 3rd Floor, New Rochelle, NY 10801-5215. www.liebertpub.com

The chapters in this book were previously published in the *Journal of Child and Adolescent Psychopharmacology.*

All papers, comments, opinions, findings, conclusions, or recommendations in *Advances in Preschool Psychopharmacology* are those of the author(s) and do not constitute opinions, findings, conclusions, or recommendations of the Publisher, the Editors, and the editorial staff.

Printed in the United States of America.

Contents

Preface

The question of if, when, and how to prescribe psychopharmacologic agents to preschool children has become an increasingly pressing and contentious public health issue over the last decade. Several converging factors may be contributing to the dramatic increases in psychotropic prescribing to young children that have been reported. These include the availability of promising new psychopharmacologic agents, decreased access and availability of age appropriate psychotherapies, as well as the possibility of accelerated expectations for socially adaptive behavior even earlier in life.

Psychiatrists and other physicians treating preschool aged children face the significant challenge of balancing concerns about risk to the developing brain, off-label prescribing and the absence of sufficient empirical data to fully inform treatment decisions, and perhaps most importantly the need to ameliorate the significant symptoms and impairments that preschool patients with serious mental disorders may manifest. Further complicating this picture, emerging developmental data suggest that treatment of symptoms during this rapid phase of development appears to be of critical importance and may even be a window of opportunity.

The unavailability of developmentally appropriate psychotherapies and the lack of resources to pay for these treatments when indicated and available, either as primary or adjunctive treatment, is another limiting factor. Further, it is clear that some very serious Axis 1 disorders presenting in the preschool period such as attention-deficit/hyperactivity disorder (ADHD) require medication in addition to psychotherapeutic treatment as has been elucidated by the Preschoolers with Attention-Deficit/Hyperactivity Disorder Treatment Study (PATS) outlined in this book. Unfortunately, for the majority of preschool disorders, the dearth of empirical research in this area contributes to the challenge for clinicians. Despite the significant progress in understanding the nosology of preschool mental disorders that has been made over the last decade, new initiatives to embark on the necessary controlled investigations in these young populations have yet to be launched. The lack of support for these studies may be due to the significant social controversy, and related risk, that surrounds the issue.

This book provides an up-to-date collection of psychopharmacologic treatment studies and related case descriptions of serious mental disorders in preschool children. Despite some gaps in the database, this collection demonstrates significant progress in several areas including the treatment of ADHD and autistic spectrum disorders. In other areas, the available studies do provide some needed direction to clinicians that will inform decisions about when to treat and how to monitor adverse effects in young children when psychopharmacologic therapy appears to be clearly indicated based on the nature or severity of symptoms. While the collection of papers also serves as a testament to the need for further research, it provides an up-to-date account of the state of the empirical database on preschool psychopharmacology at this juncture and, therefore, provides an important clinical tool.

Joan L. Luby, M.D.
Mark A. Riddle, M.D.

Contributors

Howard B. Abikoff, Ph.D., New York University Child Study Center, New York, New York

Bruno J. Anthony, Ph.D., Department of Pediatrics, Center for Child and Human Development, Georgetown University, Washington, D.C

L. Eugene Arnold, M.D., Nisonger Center, Ohio State University, Columbus, Ohio

Ayşe Avci, M.D., Department of Child and Adolescent Psychiatry, Cukurova University, Adana, Turkey

William R. Beardslee, M.D., Psychopharmacology Program, Department of Psychiatry, Children's Hospital Boston and Harvard Medical School, Boston, Massachusetts

Andy C. Belden, Ph.D., Department of Psychiatry, Washington University School of Medicine, St. Louis, Missouri

Michael Berant, M.D., Child Cardiology Department, Schneider Children's Hospital, Petach Tikva, Israel; and Sackler Faculty of Medicine, Tel Aviv University, Tel Aviv, Israel

Patricia Biggins, B.A., New York State Psychiatric Institute/ Columbia University, New York, New York[1]

Kristine Bolhofner, B.S., Department of Psychiatry, Washington University School of Medicine, St. Louis, Missouri

Roy Boorady, M.D., New York University Child Study Center, New York, New York

Gonca Celik, M.D., Department of Child and Adolescent Psychiatry, Cukurova University, Adana, Turkey

Shirley Z. Chuang, M.S., Formerly at New York State Psychiatric Institute/ Columbia University, New York, New York

Charles Cunningham, Ph.D., McMaster University, Hamilton, Ontario, Canada

Mark Davies, M.P.H., New York State Psychiatric Institute/ Columbia University, New York, New York[2]

David R. DeMaso, M.D., Psychopharmacology Program, Department of Psychiatry, Children's Hospital Boston and Harvard Medical School, Boston, Massachusetts

Rasim S. Diler, M.D., Department of Child Psychiatry, Western Psychiatric Institute and Clinic, Pittsburgh, Pennsylvania

Alice Dodds, B.A., Psychopharmacology Program, Department of Psychiatry, Children's Hospital Boston and Harvard Medical School, Boston, Massachusetts[3]

Lori Evans, Ph.D., New York University Child Study Center, New York, New York

Prudence Fisher, Ph.D., New York State Psychiatric Institute/ Columbia University, New York, New York

James F. Gardner, Sc.M., Department of Pharmaceutical Health Services Research, School of Pharmacy, University of Maryland, Baltimore, Maryland

Barbara Geller, M.D., Department of Psychiatry, Washington University School of Medicine, St. Louis, Missouri

---

[1]Current affiliation: Enrolled in a doctoral program at Ferkauf Graduate School of Psychology, Clinical PsyD Program, Yeshiva University, Bronx, New York
[2]Retired
[3]Current affiliation: New York University Child Study Center, New York, New York

Jaswinder K. Ghuman, M.D., Department of Psychiatry, University of Arizona, Tucson, Arizona

Joseph Gonzalez-Heydrich, M.D., Psychopharmacology Program, Department of Psychiatry, Children's Hospital Boston and Harvard Medical School, Boston, Massachusetts

Deborah Grady, Ph.D., Department of Biological Chemistry, University of California, Irvine, Irvine, California

Laurence L. Greenhill, M.D., New York State Psychiatric Institute/ Columbia University, New York, New York

S. Sonia Gugga, M.S., New York State Psychiatric Institute/ Columbia University, New York, New York

Suneel Gupta, Ph.D., ALZA Corporation, Mountainview, California[4]

Kristina K. Hardy, Ph.D., Duke University Medical Center, Durham, North Carolina

Amy Heffelfinger, Ph.D., Department of Neurology, Medical College of Wisconsin, Milwaukee, Wisconsin

Lori A. Hines, R.N., Department of Psychiatry, Section of Child and Adolescent Psychiatry, Indiana University School of Medicine, James Whitcomb Riley Hospital for Children, Indianapolis, Indiana

Audrey Kapelinski, LCSW, University of California, Irvine, Irvine, California

Elizabeth Kastelic, M.D., Johns Hopkins University, Baltimore, Maryland

Scott H. Kollins, Ph.D., Duke University Medical Center, Durham, North Carolina

James J. Korelitz, Ph.D., Westat, Rockville, Maryland

Lisa A. Kotler, M.D., New York State Psychiatric Institute/ Columbia University, New York, New York[5]

Christopher J. Kratochvil, M.D., University of Nebraska Medical Center, Omaha, Nebraska

Ann M. Lagges, Ph.D., Department of Psychiatry, Section of Child and Adolescent Psychiatry, Indiana University School of Medicine, James Whitcomb Riley Hospital for Children, Indianapolis, Indiana

Marc Lerner, M.D., University of California, Irvine, Irvine, California

Joan L. Luby, M.D., Department of Psychiatry, Washington University School of Medicine, St. Louis, Missouri

Carlene MacMillan, B.A., Psychopharmacology Program, Department of Psychiatry, Children's Hospital Boston and Harvard Medical School, Boston, Massachusetts

John S. March, M.D., M.P.H., Duke University Medical Center, Durham, North Carolina

Jonathan Martinez, M.A., University of California, Irvine, Irvine, California[6]

Donald R. Mattison, M.D., U.S. Public Health Service, Obstetric and Pediatric Pharmacology Branch, National Institutes of Health, Bethesda, Maryland

Michelle L. Mayfield-Jorgensen, M.D., University of Nebraska Medical Center, Omaha, Nebraska[7]

James T. McCracken, M.D., UCLA Semel Institute for Neuroscience and Human Behavior, Los Angeles, California

James J. McGough, M.D., UCLA Semel Institute for Neuroscience and Human Behavior, Los Angeles, California

---

[4]Current affiliation: Impax Pharmaceuticals, Hayward, California
[5]Current affiliation: New York University Child Study Center, Hackensack, New Jersey
[6]Current affiliation: Department of Psychology, UCLA, Los Angeles, California
[7]Current affiliation: Child Psychiatry Services and Eating Disorder Unit, Meritcare Hospital, Fargo, North Dakota; and University of North Dakota Medical School, Grand Forks, North Dakota

Karen G. Meighen, M.D., Department of Psychiatry, Section of Child and Adolescent Psychiatry, Indiana University School of Medicine, James Whitcomb Riley Hospital for Children, Indianapolis, Indiana

Glenn A. Melvin, Ph.D., New York State Psychiatric Institute/ Columbia University, New York, New York

Nishit B. Modi, Ph.D., ALZA Corporation, Mountainview, California[8]

Robert K. Moyzis, Ph.D., Department of Biological Chemistry, University of California, Irvine, Irvine, California

Christine Mrakotsky, Ph.D., Department of Psychiatry, Children's Hospital/ Harvard Medical School, Boston, Massachusetts

Desiree W. Murray, Ph.D., Duke University Medical Center, Durham, North Carolina

Eitan Nahshoni, M.D., M.Sc., Geha Mental Health Center, Liaison Service, Rabin Medical Center, Petach Tikva, Israel; and Sackler Faculty of Medicine, Tel Aviv University, Tel Aviv, Israel

Ginger Nicol, M.D., Department of Psychiatry, Washington University School of Medicine, St. Louis, Missouri

Natalya Paykina, M.A., New York State Psychiatric Institute/ Columbia University, New York, New York

Kelly Posner, Ph.D., New York State Psychiatric Institute/ Columbia University, New York, New York

Iva Pravdova, M.D., Formerly at Psychopharmacology Program, Department of Psychiatry, Children's Hospital Boston and Harvard Medical School, Boston, Massachusetts

Darcy Raches, M.A., Psychopharmacology Program, Department of Psychiatry, Children's Hospital Boston and Harvard Medical School, Boston, Massachusetts[9]

Hima Ravi, M.D., Duke University Medical Center, Durham, North Carolina

Mark A. Riddle, M.D., Division of Child and Adolescent Psychiatry, Johns Hopkins University School of Medicine, Baltimore, Maryland

Daniel J. Safer, M.D., Departments of Psychiatry and Pediatrics, Johns Hopkins Medical Institutions, Baltimore, Maryland

Alexander M. Scharko M.D., Department of Psychiatry and Behavioral Medicine, Division of Child and Adolescent Psychiatry, Medical College of Wisconsin, Milwaukee, Wisconsin; and Attending Child and Adolescent Psychiatrist, Mendota Mental Health Institute, Madison, Wisconsin

Gal Shoval, M.D., Child Cardiology Department, Schneider Children's Hospital, Petach Tikva, Israel and Sackler Faculty of Medicine, Tel Aviv University, Tel Aviv, Israel

Anne M. Skrobala, M.A., New York State Psychiatric Institute/ Columbia University, New York, New York

Susan L. Smalley, Ph.D., UCLA Semel Institute for Neuroscience and Human Behavior, Los Angeles, California

Sara Spitzer, M.D., Child Psychiatry Day Hospital, Geha Mental Health Center, Petach Tikva, Israel; and Sackler Faculty of Medicine, Tel Aviv University, Tel Aviv, Israel

Edward Spitznagel, Ph.D., Department of Mathematics, Washington University, St. Louis, Missouri

Melissa Meade Stalets, M.A., Department of Psychiatry, Washington University School of Medicine, St. Louis, Missouri

Annamarie Stehli, M.P.H., University of California, Irvine, Irvine, California

---

[8]Current affiliation: Impax Pharmaceuticals, Maywood, California
[9]Current affiliation: Texas Children's Hospital, Houston, Texas

Kenneth Steinhoff, M.D., University of California, Irvine, Irvine, California

Julie Stoner, Ph.D., University of Nebraska Medical Center, Omaha, Nebraska[10]

James M. Swanson, Ph.D., University of California, Irvine, Irvine, California

Aysegul Yolga Tahiroglu, M.D., Department of Child and Adolescent Psychiatry, Cukurova University, Adana, Turkey

Mini Tandon, D.O., Department of Psychiatry, Washington University School of Medicine, St. Louis, Missouri

Rebecca Tillman, M.S., Department of Psychiatry, Washington University School of Medicine, St. Louis, Missouri

Satish Valluri, M.S., M.P.H., Department of Pharmaceutical Health Services Research, School of Pharmacy, University of Maryland, Baltimore, Maryland

Brigette S. Vaughan, M.S.N., A.P.R.N., University of Nebraska Medical Center, Omaha, Nebraska

Brigid L. Vaughan, M.D., Psychopharmacology Program, Department of Psychiatry, Children's Hospital Boston and Harvard Medical School, Boston, Massachusetts

Benedetto Vitiello, M.D., Child and Adolescent Treatment and Preventive Intervention Research Branch, National Institute of Mental Health, Bethesda, Maryland

Abraham Weizman, M.D., Geha Mental Health Center, Liaison Service, Rabin Medical Center, Petach Tikva, Israel; Felsenstein Medical Research Center, Rabin Medical Center, Petach Tikva, Israel; and Sackler Faculty of Medicine, Tel Aviv University, Tel Aviv, Israel

Jane Whitney, B.A., Psychopharmacology Program, Department of Psychiatry, Children's Hospital Boston and Harvard Medical School, Boston, Massachusetts

Sharon B. Wigal, Ph.D., University of California, Irvine, Irvine, California

Tim Wigal, Ph.D., University of California, Irvine, Irvine, California

Meghan Williams, B.A., Department of Psychiatry, Washington University School of Medicine, St. Louis, Missouri

Aleksandra Yakhkind, B.A., Psychopharmacology Program, Department of Psychiatry, Children's Hospital Boston and Harvard Medical School, Boston, Massachusetts

Gil Zalsman, M.D., Child Cardiology Department, Schneider Children's Hospital, Petach Tikva, Israel; and Sackler Faculty of Medicine, Tel Aviv University, Tel Aviv, Israel

Julie M. Zito, Ph.D., Department of Pharmaceutical Health Services Research, School of Pharmacy and Department of Psychiatry, School of Medicine, University of Maryland, Baltimore, Maryland

Marcia L. Zuckerman, M.D., Psychopharmacology Program, Department of Psychiatry, Children's Hospital Boston and Harvard Medical School, Boston, Massachusetts[11]

---

[10]Current affiliation: Department of Biostatistics and Epidemiology, University of Oklahoma Health Sciences Center, College of Public Health, Oklahoma City, Oklahoma
[11]Current affiliation: Vinfen/DMH PACT Team, Lawrence, Massachusetts

Advances in
Preschool
Psychopharmacology

PART 1

Psychopharmacology of Preschool Mood, Anxiety, and Autistic Spectrum Disorders

ADVANCES IN PRESCHOOL PSYCHOPHARMACOLOGY
© 2009 Mary Ann Liebert, Inc.
140 Huguenot Street, 3rd Floor
New Rochelle, NY 10801-5215

Introduction

Psychopharmacology of Psychiatric Disorders in the Preschool Period

Joan L. Luby, M.D.

THE USE OF PSYCHOPHARMACOLOGY in preschool aged children has become the focus of significant attention over the last decade. Of primary interest to the general mental health community has been the high, and rising, rate of psychotropic prescribing to very young children. Although many details of the sources of this public health trend remain unclear, such as the forces, circumstances and practitioners primarily responsible for necessary as well as inappropriate prescribing, it is of significant concern. At the same time, progress has been made in the validation and characterization of several psychiatric disorders in the preschool period (for review see Task Force 2003). Yet, despite these significant advances, data on treatment (both psychotherapeutic and pharmacologic) have been slow to follow. The articles in Part One of this book aim to begin to address this problem but more clearly stand as a testament to the tremendous amount of research that remains to be done in this area.

One diagnostic area in which the most significant amount of psychopharmacologic progress has been made to date has been in the treatment of attention-deficit/hyperactivity disorder (ADHD) in the preschool period and this is the focus of Part Two of this book. An area that has also been the focus of relatively more empirical investigation has been autistic spectrum disorders. While these data are not comprehensively reviewed here, the paper by Luby et al., elucidates the promising findings in the use of second generation anti-psychotics for the control of some core symptoms of autism in young children.

More generally, there is a smaller body of literature already available demonstrating that there are clinically important developmental differences in the way psychopharmacologic agents are metabolized and exert their effect. The retrospective chart reviews by Zuckerman et al. and Nahshoni et al., demonstrate that developmental differences in both behavioral and cardiac side effects can be observed with selective serotonin re-uptake inhibitors (SSRIs). In this class of agents, behavioral adverse effects appear more prevalent in younger children. In the case of atypical anti-psychotics, cardiac adverse effects known in older populations were not observed in preschoolers. Zuckerman et al.'s finding of higher rates of activation in young children prescribed SSRIs has tangible implications for clinical practice and surely decreases the feasibility of this treatment option in young children. These findings taken together emphasize the need for specific study of the safety and efficacy of psychotropic medications in preschool populations and the correlate limitations of extrapolating from available data in older children.

Kratochvil et al. provide promising findings from an open label study of atomoxetine in young children suggesting that further more controlled study of this agent would be worthwhile in preschool populations. Meighan et al.

Department of Psychiatry, Washington University School of Medicine, St. Louis, Missouri.

describe several compelling cases of "acute stress disorder" among preschool-aged burn victims. Although this diagnosis itself remains somewhat controversial, low-dose risperidone appears to have benefited these emotionally and physically ill children beyond what was possible using psychosocial and developmental interventions, helping them to tolerate the invasive medical care that was necessary for their treatment. This paper illuminates the severity of mood and behavioral disturbances that can arise in young children and the circumstances in which the risk benefit ratio appears to clearly support the decision to treat despite the absence of a sufficient body of controlled data upon which to rely.

Celik and colleagues describe a case report of Turkish twins with a posttraumatic eating disorder. These toddlers, who presented with an iatrogenic form of feeding disorder, had failed numerous other treatment trials until they finally responded well to low-dose fluoxetine. Of note was the severity of impairment displayed and the marked improvement that was associated with the addition of fluoxetine. While the drug was well tolerated in these two cases, controlled trials are needed to investigate the tolerability, safety, and efficacy of this medication for this condition as well as related anxiety disorders.

Geller et al. provide an important position paper on the need for a clear definition of episodes and cycles in pediatric bipolar disorder, an area in which much nosologic controversy prevails. Clarity and uniformity in the definitions of symptoms and duration terms are essential to establish the appropriate inclusion criteria necessary for investigations of treatment. Further, the definition of these features using terms that can be applied in developmentally appropriate variations across the age span is also critical. As Geller et al. point out and as the Luby et al. preschool case paper illustrates, greater fluctuation in mood states known in early childhood provides a compelling example of the need to clearly delineate normative variation in mood "cycling" from clinically significant deviations in this phenomenon.

More globally, these papers underscore the remarkable dearth of controlled psychopharmacologic treatment data for preschoolers available as of 2007. This is noteworthy for two reasons. One is highlighted by the Zito et al. paper providing further details on the ongoing high rates of use of these medications in clinical settings and further detailing the link to diagnosis. Further, the paper by Luby et al. points to the finding that the majority of these prescriptions in a sample of mood and disruptive disordered preschoolers were written for those with Axis I disorders and high levels of impairment.

The other important issue is how sharply this paucity of treatment data stands out given the advances that have been made in the characterization of preschool disorders and the concurrent recognition of the need for early intervention in so many other areas of development. Investigators who have conducted multi-site trials in older children and/or who have participated in the only multi-site psychopharmacological trial conducted to date for preschoolers, the Preschool Attention-Deficit/Hyperactivity Disorder Treatment Study (PATS) have described the dangers and scientific complexities that must be addressed in such endeavors (Greenhill 1998; Vitiello 2005).

Perhaps equally foreboding, and less openly described however, have been the political and social forces that serve to impede progress in this area. While caution is well founded and surely in order, attempts to relieve the psychic suffering of young children and to intervene early and potentially more effectively continue to be thwarted by underlying fundamental resistance to the acceptance of mental disorders in young children. These trends are further abetted by oversimplified media sounds bytes reporting on tragic cases that serve only to enhance public fear and oversimplify the issues (Carey, 2007).

It is my hope that the papers in Part One of this book, the few ongoing controlled investigations that have been launched, combined with the increasing body of literature defining the clinical characteristics of preschoolers with mental disorders, will begin to shed light and diminish heat on this controversial area. The findings from these case studies, retrospective chart reviews, open label and controlled studies should in some cases help practitioners on the front lines navigate the difficult balance between reason and caution in pharmacologic treatment decisions. Most importantly, the articles illustrate that the scientific study of preschool psychopharmacology is an area truly in its infancy. This dearth of necessary scientific data in the midst of high rates of prescribing to this population underscores the urgent need for controlled studies in preschool populations.

REFERENCES

Carey B: Charges in the death of a girl, 4: Raise issue of giving psychiatric drugs to children. The New York Times, 2007, January 15.

Greenhill LL: The use of psychotropic medication in preschoolers: Indications, safety, and efficacy. Can J Psychiatry 43:576–581, 1998.

Task force on research diagnostic criteria: Infancy and preschool: Research diagnostic criteria for infants and preschool children: The process and empirical support.

Special communication. J Am Acad Child Adolesc Psychiatry 42:1504–1512, 2003.

Vitiello B: Pharmacoepidemiology and pediatric psychopharmacology research. J Child Adolesc Psychopharmacol 15:10–11, 2005.

ADVANCES IN PRESCHOOL PSYCHOPHARMACOLOGY
© 2009 Mary Ann Liebert, Inc.
140 Huguenot Street, 3rd Floor
New Rochelle, NY 10801-5215

Tolerability of Selective Serotonin Reuptake Inhibitors in Thirty-Nine Children Under Age Seven: A Retrospective Chart Review

Marcia L. Zuckerman, M.D., Brigid L. Vaughan, M.D., Jane Whitney, B.A., Alice Dodds, B.A., Aleksandra Yakhkind, B.A., Carlene MacMillan, B.A., Darcy Raches, M.A., Iva Pravdova, M.D., David Ray DeMaso, M.D., William R. Beardslee, M.D., and Joseph Gonzalez-Heydrich, M.D.

ABSTRACT

Objective: **To characterize the adverse effects of treatment with selective serotonin reuptake inhibitors (SSRIs) started in children under age 7 yr.**

Methods: **We conducted a retrospective review of medical records for all children who had begun treatment with an SSRI under age 7 at an academic psychiatry department in Boston.**

Results: **Thirty-nine children (26 males, 13 females) met the inclusion criteria. Mean age at start of treatment was 5.9 ± 0.8 yr, and median treatment duration was 5.0 months. The target diagnoses for SSRI treatment were anxiety disorders in 54%, depressive disorders in 23%, and both anxiety and depressive disorders in 20% of patients. There were no reports of suicidal ideation or attempt. No children were medically or psychiatrically hospitalized for adverse effects (AEs). Eleven patients (28%) reported an AE of at least moderate severity; 7 (18%) discontinued the SSRI due to the AE. Six patients discontinued due to behavioral activation and 1 due to gastrointestinal upset. The median time to onset of an AE was 23 days, and median resolution was 19 days from onset.**

Conclusions: **The high rate of adverse effects, especially activation, in this sample argues for continued caution in using SSRIs in young children. Controlled trials are warranted.**

INTRODUCTION

DESPITE THE INCREASING interest in and study of psychiatric disorders in children under the age of 7, there is still limited research to guide clinicians in treating these young children. Research by Eggar and Angold (2006) on psychiatric disorders in preschool children suggests that psychiatric disorders in this population share many of the same characteristics, including rate and pattern of comorbidities, with psychiatric disorders diagnosed in older children. In contrast to the idea that preschool children are too developmentally immature to experience depression, research by Luby et al. (2003) highlights that depressed preschool children display many of the typical symptoms and vegetative signs of depression. Similarly,

From the Psychopharmacology Program, Department of Psychiatry, Children's Hospital Boston and Harvard Medical School.

Statistical consultant: Joseph Gonzalez-Heydrich, M.D., Psychopharmacology Program, Children's Hospital Boston.

research by Spence et al. (2001) has suggested that the anxiety symptoms endorsed by preschoolers are consistent with past research on anxiety symptoms endorsed by primary schoolchildren. The estimated prevalence rates of psychiatric disorders in preschool children are as follows: any anxiety disorder (0.3% to 11.5%), major depressive disorder (0.9% to 1.1%), posttraumatic stress disorder (0.1% to 0.4%), attention-deficit/hyperactivity disorder (0.5% to 6.5%), oppositional defiant disorder (0.7% to 26.5%), and conduct disorder (0.8% to 4.6%) (McDonnell and Glod, 2003).

Although there is limited evidence of efficacy, selective serotonin reuptake inhibitors (SSRIs) are being used in the treatment of psychiatric conditions experienced by preschool and early primary grade children. The U.S. Food and Drug Administration has not given approval for their usage in younger children, although it has approved fluoxetine for depression and obsessive compulsive disorder (OCD) in children as young as age 7, sertraline for OCD in children as young as age 6, and fluvoxamine for OCD in children as young as age 8.

The rate of SSRI use under the age of 7 is difficult to determine precisely because many childhood medication utilization studies do not include children of less than 7 yr, do not break the data down by age, and/or do not separate SSRIs from other antidepressants. Nevertheless, an estimate of the prevalence of SSRIs in these younger children can be gleaned from published data on overlapping age groups. Hunkeler et al. (2005) found the rate of SSRI use in children 5 to 9 yr was 2.62 per 1000 for girls and 4.75 per 1000 for boys. Data from 1998 and 2003 have suggested a prevalence rate of SSRIs prescribed to children to be ≤1 in 1000 for children under the age of 6 and between 11 in 1000 for children 6 to 12 yr (Vitello et al., 2006), and 15 in 1000 for children 6 to 14 (Rushton and Whitmire, 2001). Taken together, these studies show that SSRIs are used in children under age 7, and that there is a sharp utilization increase between the ages of 6 and 12 years of age.

Wagner et al. (2003) suggests that younger children have different reactions to SSRIs than adolescents or adults. Many neurotransmitter systems do not fully develop until late adolescence, a fact that is likely to influence the effects of these medications. Additionally, there are age-related differences in SSRI pharmacokinetics (Vitiello and Jansen, 1995). When Safer and Zito (2006) compared published data on adverse effects (AEs) of SSRIs in preadolescents, adolescents, and adults, AEs were found to be more prevalent in preadolescents than in either adolescents or adults. The higher prevalence of AEs in preadolescents suggests that children under 7 may also be more prone to experience AEs and highlights the importance of careful side-effect screening in these younger children.

Unfortunately, like the prevalence research cited earlier, prior studies evaluating AEs have not included very young children and/or have not analyzed the data by age group. Research by Gualtieri and Johnson (2006) with 128 patients less than 18 yr old found that 28% experienced "behavioral side effects." Wilens et al. (2003) found that psychiatric AEs occurred in 22% of those between age 3 and 18 yr who were taking SSRIs. However, neither study stratified data by age. The average ages of participants in these studies were 13 yr (Gualtieri and Johnson, 2006) and 12.2 yr (Wilens et al., 2003), making it difficult to determine the rates of behavioral side effects experienced by the younger children.

Therefore, we set out to retrospectively characterize AEs experienced by children under 7 yr treated with SSRIs in our outpatient psychopharmacology clinic. To be helpful to clinicians, we wanted to identify the most common AEs in this population, the time it took for them to appear (onset), and the time it took for them to resolve (resolution), whether by discontinuation of the drug or by adaptation. In addition, we looked at how many patients discontinued their medication because of AEs. Finally, we explored whether children with a family history of bipolar disorder or those with a diagnosis of attention-deficit hyperactivity disorder (ADHD) were more likely to experience behavioral AEs.

METHODS

This was an investigator-initiated study. With institutional review board approval, we reviewed outpatient medical records of children who were first prescribed SSRIs while under the age of 7 yr. Target symptoms for initiating treatment included: anxiety, disabling depression, posttraumatic stress disorder (PTSD), affective/behavioral problems not otherwise specified (NOS), and obsessions or compulsions. Diagnoses were made by the clinician prescribing SSRIs according to DSM-IV criteria (American Psychiatric Association, 1994). In all cases, this clinician was a child and adolescent psychiatrist, a child psychiatry resident, or a nurse practitioner. For patients treated by a resident or nurse practitioner, the diagnosis was reviewed by a board-certified child and adolescent psychiatrist.

The children were treated in an outpatient pediatric psychopharmacology clinic at an academic medical center between January 1998 and September 2004. In accordance with clinic policy and professional practice guidelines (American Academy of Child & Adolescent Psychiatry, 1998a,b,c), all children in this study were receiving psychological treatment that included individual or family counseling, and this alone had not proved helpful in controlling the child's target symptoms. Informed consent for the use of SSRIs for all children had been obtained from legal guardians.

Appropriate patients were identified by querying the psychopharmacology program's electronic medical record system (Gonzalez-Heydrich et al., 2000), a relational database that includes historical, demographic, and diagnostic information for each patient, as well as a separate record for each patient visit that includes fields for medications, diagnoses, progress note text, and adverse effects.

From the total database (6408 patients), our initial search identified 66 children who were first prescribed an SSRI before their seventh birthday. Of those, 12 were excluded from the study because they had diagnoses of mental retardation, autism, and/or pervasive developmental disorder, all of which could complicate their response to antidepressant treatment (Safer and Zito, 2006). Of the 54 patients for whom records were reviewed, another 15 were eliminated either because they never started the prescribed medication (reasons included insurance problems, parental reconsideration, or other unspecified reasons) or because they

had been started on the medication elsewhere, meaning that any adverse effects on initiation would not be noted. For patients who had successive trials of 2 different SSRIs before turning 7, we used the first trial for our analysis.

For the 39 patients that met our inclusion criteria, each electronic record was reviewed by a trained and supervised research assistant and a psychiatrist (MLZ). Neither was involved in the care of these patients. Psychiatric diagnoses, medication dosages, duration of treatment, prior and concurrent medications, and co-occurring physical conditions were abstracted from the records. Individual results were also reviewed by a senior pediatric psychopharmacologist (either JG or BLV). No formal checklist of AEs was used when these patients visited the clinic. Thus AEs recorded in the electronic medical record by the treating clinician were based on spontaneous reports by the patient or his caretakers. Information on AEs also came from clinically directed inquiry about AEs by the treating clinician. AEs were abstracted using the following procedure.

A list of potential adverse events developed by Wilens et al. (2003) was reviewed. To improve the reliability of assigning a single term to an AE from its description in the medical record, the psychiatrist directly reviewing the records consolidated Wilen's AE descriptions into a smaller set of standard terms for AEs. The two senior psychopharmacologists supervising the study reviewed and amended the terminology, resulting in a total of 10 terms that effectively conveyed all the adverse effects described in the electronic medical records. The study psychiatrists then met to review notations found in the records that indicated that a particular type of AE had occurred in order to reach consensus on how to assign a term to an AE from the description in the medical record. For example, it was agreed that, if an emergent AE was described in the record with adjectives such as "anxious," "nervous," or "worried," this AE should be categorized as "anxiety." The AE terms were then grouped into three categories for analysis: behavioral, somatic, and anxiety or mood.

The research assistant and psychiatrist reviewing each medical record used all available documentation to determine if an AE occurred and to which standard term for AE it should be assigned. Additionally, they rated the severity of the AE using the descriptors "mild" if it did not interfere with functioning, "moderate" if it interfered with functioning, but not to an excessive or extreme degree, and "severe" if it interfered with functioning to the point that the child was completely or almost completely prevented from doing age-appropriate daily activities because of the AE. Moderate and severe AEs were further investigated to determine when they first occurred and when they resolved relative to the start of the SSRI treatment. These dates were based on an interval mentioned in the progress note, the date of the visit when the AE was first reported, and/or the visit when it was last noted.

For the statistical treatment of our data, we report mean and standard deviation for continuous data (e.g., treatment duration) and include the median for skewed data so as to better describe the distribution of the sample. We used the Breslow–Day test for homogeneity of odds ratios to evaluate whether the rates of AEs on each SSRI used could be combined. Fisher's Exact Test and logistic regression were used to explore associations between the presence of ADHD or a family history of bipolar disorder and the occurrence of agitation as an AE of SSRI treatment. Fisher's Exact Test was also used to explore a possible relationship between experiencing an AE and being younger than 6 versus older than 6 yr. Logistic regression was used to explore the possible relationship between age, as calculated by days before (−) or after (+) a patient's sixth birthday, and any of the following: experiencing an AE, discontinuing the present SSRI trial, or taking a concomitant medication. Logistic regression was also used to explore any relationship between experiencing an AE, discontinuing the index SSRI due to an AE, and the following: number of psychiatric diagnoses, number concurrent medications, number of past psychotropic trials, and whether there was a past trial of a SSRI.

RESULTS

Patient treatment characteristics

The 39 children (26 males and 13 females) were prescribed 1 of 5 SSRIs: citalopram ($n =$ 8), fluvoxamine ($n = 4$), paroxetine ($n = 6$), fluoxetine ($n = 3$), and sertraline ($n = 18$). Children in different medication groups did not differ with respect to age, duration of treatment, number of previous and concurrent medications, and number of comorbid psychiatric and medical diagnoses. The mean age at treatment start was 5.9 ± 0.8 yr, and 16 of the children were under 6. The mean duration of treatment was 10.1 ± 10.4 months (median 5.0 months).

The mean daily dose for each medication was as follows: citalopram, 14.6 mg $\pm$ 9.7; fluvoxamine, 37.5 mg $\pm$ 14.4; paroxetine, 11.7 mg $\pm$ 4.1; fluoxetine, 15.0 mg $\pm$ 7.8; sertraline, 22.5 mg $\pm$ 3.5.

The target diagnoses for SSRI treatment were anxiety disorders in 54%, depressive disorders in 23%, and both anxiety and depressive disorders in 20% of patients. Table 1 describes in more detail the diagnoses for which the medications were prescribed and the mean age of patients.

There was a high prevalence of psychiatric comorbidity, with patients having an average of 2.2 ± 1.0 DSM-IV Axis I diagnoses. In addition to the above target diagnosis, a diagnosis of attention-deficit hyperactivity disorder (ADHD) was found in 51% of the sample, and 10% were diagnosed with bipolar disorder I, II, or NOS. Other comorbid psychiatric disorders included learning ($n = 5$), adjustment ($n = 4$), oppositional defiant ($n = 4$), conduct ($n = 1$), and psychotic NOS ($n = 1$) disorders.

TABLE 1. TARGET DIAGNOSIS FOR SSRI TREATMENT AND MEAN AGE OF PATIENTS

Diagnosis	Number (%) of patients	Mean age
Anxiety disorders[a]	18 (46%)	6.06
MDD	9 (23%)	6.04
MDD and anxiety disorders	4 (10%)	6.58
MDD and PTSD	4 (10%)	5.43
OCD	2 (5%)	5.1
PTSD	1 (2.6%)	6.5
Affective/Behavioral problems NOS	1 (2.6%)	4.3

[a]Anxiety disorders do not account for OCD and PTSD diagnoses, which are captured in separate rows designated for these disorders.

MDD, major depressive disorder; OCD, obsessive compulsive disorder; PTSD, posttraumatic stress disorder; affective/behavioral NOS, Not otherwise specified.

The prevalence of medical comorbidity was also high, with 7 patients (18%) diagnosed with a significant medical condition. The medical conditions noted in these patients and the number and percent of patients affected were asthma (3, 8%), epilepsy (2, 5%), liver disease (1, 3%), history of neonatal apnea (1, 3%), and end-stage renal disease (1, 3%).

A prior trial of a psychotropic medication was found in 28% of the patients starting treatment with the index SSRI. Five patients (13%) with ADHD had been treated with psychostimulants. Four patients (10%) had been treated with an antidepressant, 6 (15%) with an α-adrenergic agonist, and 1 (3%) with an anticonvulsant mood stabilizer. During the index SSRI treatment, 54% were concurrently taking another psychotropic medication. These included 14 patients (36%) taking concurrent psychostimulants, 9 patients (23%) taking concurrent α-adrenergic agonists, 5 patients (13%) taking concurrent atomoxetine, 5 patients (13%) taking second-generation antipsychotics (2 of whom were also taking an anticonvulsant mood stabilizer), and 2 patients (5%) taking anxiolytics. An additional 4 patients (10%) took mood stabilizers, but not antipsychotics. While these findings are limited due to the small sample size and low power, an exploratory analysis was run and showed no relationship between taking a concurrent medication and experiencing an AE (Fisher's Exact Test, $p =$ ns). In recognition of the limited power of this study to detect a relationship, we cannot rule out a Type II error.

Tolerability

There were no reports of suicidal ideation and/or suicide attempts at any point in the study period in any of the children whose charts were reviewed. No children were medically or psychiatrically hospitalized for adverse effects. Although the power to detect a difference among the rate of AEs for each of the SSRIs is very low due to the small sample size, we performed the Breslow–Day test on the odds of having an AE of at least moderate severity on each SSRI studied. No statistically significant difference in the odds was found, so we report both an overall rate of these AEs and

the observed rates for individual SSRIs. It should be noted that our limited sample size could prevent us from detecting a true difference among the rate of AEs for different SSRIs.

A total of 11 patients (28%) reported an AE of at least moderate severity. The median time to the onset of an adverse effect of this severity was 23 days (range: 2 to 144). The median time to resolution of the AE was 19 days from its onset (range: 2 to 79). Some patients reported more than 1 AE, so 27 occurrences of adverse effects were reported and these occurred in 13 patients. Nine (23%) patients had a behavioral AE, 6 (15%) had somatic AEs, and 3 (8%) had an anxiety or mood-related AE. The most commonly reported AE in this population was behavioral activation, with 8 patients (21%) reporting this AE. Eight patients (21%) experienced more than 1 type of AE. Thirteen (33%) patients experienced any type of AE. Seven patients (18% of the total sample and 54% of those who experienced AEs) found the AE sufficiently severe to cause them to discontinue the medication (Table 2). For over 40% of the patients who experienced an AE, the difficulty resolved while they remained on the SSRI.

Of the 7 patients in the entire sample who discontinued their SSRI due to AEs, 1 did so due to gastrointestinal upset that resolved after stopping the medication. The other 6 patients discontinued their SSRI due to behavioral activation. One patient who discontinued due to behavioral activation also discontinued due to aggression and the development of hives. An exploratory analysis was run to see if the prevalence of a family history of bipolar disorder as noted in the medical record or the presence of ADHD increased the odds of experiencing agitation, because an AE of SSRI treatment failed to show a significant relationship between these variables. While these results are limited by a small sample size and low power to detect differences, and the chance of a Type II error cannot be ruled out, no relationships were found. It is noteworthy that 4 of the 7 patients who discontinued their SSRI did so following a dose increase; that is, the medication had been well tolerated at a lower dose.

The 3 patients who had severe AEs all discontinued treatment with the SSRI due to the

TABLE 2. PATIENTS WHO DISCONTINUED DUE TO ADVERSE EFFECTS

ID	Drug	Sex	Age at start (yr)	Adverse effect (AE) leading to discontinuation	Days to onset	Days to offset	Discontinuation following a dose increase?	Description of AE
1	Citalopram	Male	6.2	Activation	101	30	Yes	"Parents report significant increase of aggression, irritability, increased energy. Physically aggressive toward parents. Today at school punched school psychologist in the eye and was suspended for two days. Seemed irritable today in the waiting room, but once he came into the office he was playful and interactive. Psychomotor agitation was noticeable. Possible SSRI-induced hypomania. No difficulty sleeping."
2	Fluoxetine	Male	6.4	Activation	2	9	No	"Significant worsening in behavior in recent weeks. Increased motor activity, not listening, more oppositional behaviors and some aggression both at home and in day care."
3	Sertraline	Male	6.8	Activation	14	75	Yes	Following an increase in sertraline, "he's been more distractible and more risk taking [and doing], a lot of swearing. He seems to be speaking and moving faster. His temper tantrums seem to be a bit better still however. He is also impulsively affectionate."
4	Sertraline	Female	4.5	Activation, agression, hives	3	4	No	After 3 doses, patient "was very jumpy, loud, and generally horrible."
5	Sertraline	Male	6.1	Activation	42	20	Yes	"The teacher had sent home a note that he did not have a good afternoon yesterday at school. She reports that he is jumping on the couch and somewhat more active . . ."
6	Sertraline	Male	6.6	Activation	41	22	Yes	"The teachers and mom felt he was more anxious and agitated with the increase of Zoloft . . ." to 37.5 mg.
7	Sertraline	Male	6.8	Gastrointestinal upset	59	18	No	"Decreased appetite for 3 weeks. Said stomach bothering him."

AE. One patient on fluoxetine had a severe AE of activation, which had an onset of 2 days and an offset of 9 days. The other 2 patients with severe AEs were taking sertraline: 1 had activation and aggression with an onset of 3 days and an offset of 4 days; the other had gastrointestinal upset with an onset of 59 days and an offset of 18 days.

Influence of age: Comparing patients under six with those at least six years old

Sixteen patients (41%) began SSRI treatment before the age of 6. When tolerability of the SSRI treatment was broken down by age, 2 (13%) patients under the age of 6 and 9 (39%) patients who were at least 6 yr old experienced an adverse event of at least moderate severity. The AEs reported by children under 6 were as follows: 1 patient experienced activation and compulsions, and 1 patient experienced activation, aggression, and hives. For the patient who reported activation, aggression, and hives, the AEs were severe enough to cause discontinuation of the SSRI trial.

Fisher's Exact Tests were conducted to explore the baseline characteristics and SSRI trial outcomes of patients under the age of 6 and patients at least 6 yr old. No significant relationships were found between age (being younger than 6 or at least 6 yr old) and the following variables: experiencing an AE, taking concomitant medications, having more than 1 psychiatric disorder, or having a previous antidepressant medication trial (Fisher's Exact Test, p = ns). There was, however, a nonsignificant trend for children under 6 to be antidepressant-naïve, with all 4 patients who had had a previous antidepressant trial being at least 6 yr old (Fisher's Exact Test, p = 0.130). To better discern this relationship, a logistic regression was conducted to see if having a previous antidepressant trial was related to discontinuation. No significant relationship was found between these two variables. The influence age might have on baseline characteristics and outcome was further explored using a logistic regressions. To enhance our power to detect a difference, age at beginning of trial was calculated based on days before (−) or after (+) a patient's sixth birthday. A logistic regression was used to explore the relationship between this recalculated age (days before or after sixth birthday) and the following variables: experiencing an AE, discontinuing the SSRI trial, or taking concomitant medications. No significant relationships were found.

Although these results are intriguing, they are limited by the small sample size and low power to detect differences. Since the limited power of this study opens the possibility of a Type II error, these results should be seen as hypothesis generating and an area for future research.

DISCUSSION

In this retrospective case series of 39 children who began SSRI treatment while less than 7 yr of age, 28% had an AE of at least moderate severity, with behavioral activation being the most prevalent side effect (21%). This finding is similar to other studies of SSRI use in children. For example, Gualtieri and Johnson (2006) reported that 28% of 128 children and adolescents on various "modern" antidepressants, including SSRIs, experienced behavioral adverse effects.

Interestingly, the relative frequency of types of AEs noted in studies involving older children treated with SSRIs differs significantly from our findings in young children. Nixon et al. (2001) found that in 23 children 12 to 18 yr old treated with sertraline, the most prevalent AEs were nausea, headache, and behavioral activation/agitation. Safer and Zito (2006) noted that the adverse effects of activation or restlessness associated with taking an SSRI are less likely in older children compared to younger children; they speculate that this may be because young children are in general more likely to become activated than adolescents or adults.

Eighteen percent of patients in this study discontinued their medications because of adverse effects. This rate of discontinuation is twice as high as rates reported in studies of older children and adolescents. In a trial of 275 adolescents with major depression treated with paroxetine, imipramine, or placebo, Keller et al. (2001) found a 9.7% rate of discontinuation due to AE in those adolescents treated with paroxetine. Research by Wagner et al. (2003) on sertraline for child and adolescent depression showed an overall discontinuation rate due to AEs of 9% on active versus 3% on placebo, with a higher rate of discontinuation on sertraline due to AEs among children aged 6 to 11 yr (13 out of 86 children, 15%) compared to adolescents aged 12 to 17 yr (4 out of 103 adolescents, 4%). The higher rates of discontinuation due to AE found in children by Wagner et al. (2003) and by the present study support the suggestion by Brent et al. (2004) that younger children are in general more vulnerable to AEs.

In our study the median time to onset of AE was 23 days. In contrast, Masi et al. (2001) noted that most AEs in their pediatric study of paroxetine took place in the first days of treatment or when the dose was increased. The discrepancy with the findings of the present study could be partially explained by the way we measured the length of time to onset of AEs. We measured this time from the first dose of the drug to the reporting of an AE. However, in many cases the AE took place after a dose increase later in the course of treatment. This phenomenon would tend to lengthen the apparent time to onset of an AE. Also, clinic visits in our program are scheduled at intervals of between 2 and 6 weeks. Although some parents called the clinic as soon as they noted the emergence of an AE, as they were instructed to do, most reports of AE were at subsequent visits; this may have caused the observed onset time to be artificially long.

Our median time to onset of AE was shorter than the 91 days found by Wilens et al. (2003). These authors note, however, that of the patients, who developed an AE in the first 3 months, the majority emerged within the first 21 days, suggesting that patients whose onset of AE was later than that may actually be experiencing new illness symptoms. Our findings are closer to those of Safer and Zito (2006) who note that in the studies they reviewed activation was more prominent in the first 2 to 3 weeks of treatment. The average time to resolution of AEs in our study was 19 days, which is close to the mean duration of 18 days for agitation found by Riddle et al. (2001). Our finding that 55% of children were taking 1 or more medications concurrently with SSRI treatment is comparable to the 52% found by Duffy et al. (2005).

The absence of suicidal ideation and attempted suicide in the present study is in accordance with past research that has suggested lower rates of suicidal ideation and attempt in children (10.5 ± 1.8 yr) diagnosed with major depressive disorder compared to adolescents (15.7 ± 1.3 yr) with the same diagnosis (Yorbik et al., 2004). Yorbik et al. (2004) also found a significant correlation between older age and suicidal ideation, seriousness of suicidal acts, and medical lethality of suicidal acts.

Given the limitations of the present study's findings due to small sample size and limited power, the exploratory analyses of potential relationships between being younger than 6 and having a comorbid psychiatric diagnosis, a previous medication trial, a concurrent medication trial, or an AE while taking an SSRI, or between a family history of bipolar disorder and having an AE, need to be repeated in larger studies.

Limitations

There are several limitations in interpreting this study. This is a retrospective chart review. There is no comparison group or control group. Treatment assignment was not randomized. The relatively small sample size makes it difficult to generalize from its findings. This small sample size limits the study's power to detect relationships between specific variables and leaves area for a Type II error to be made. In addition, comparison to other studies is imprecise because there is no standard vocabulary for AEs and no standard grouping of them. The time to onset of AEs may be overestimated because AEs were most often reported at the next visit rather than at the time of initiation, leaving the investigators to estimate when the AE began. Another source of overestimation is the fact that some AEs occurred in the setting of a dose increase after the medication was initiated.

Despite these limitations, this study's focus on the effect of a commonly used treatment in an actual clinic population is important. The multiple comorbidities and concomitant medications that characterize this sample make it more representative of the children who actually present for treatment in clinics.

CONCLUSION

The present study highlights the relatively high rate of adverse effects in this sample and the importance of continued caution in treating young children with SSRIs. Specifically, clinicians and parents should be aware that younger children may be at higher risk for behavioral activation on SSRIs than older children or adults and should be monitored appropriately. Randomized controlled studies of adverse effects in this younger age group should be conducted in the future.

ACKNOWLEDGMENTS

Statistical data were analyzed by Joseph Gonzalez-Heydrich, Brigid Vaughan, Jane Whitney, Alice Dodds, and Carlene MacMillan. The statistical analysis was supervised by Joseph Gonzalez-Heydrich.

DISCLOSURES

Marcia L. Zuckerman, M.D., Brigid L. Vaughan, M.D., Jane Whitney, B.A., Alice Dodds, B.A., Aleksandra Yakhkind, B.A., Carlene MacMillan, B.A., Darcy Raches, B.A., Iva Pravdova, M.D., David Ray DeMaso, M.D., and William R. Beardslee, M.D., have no conflicts of interest or disclosures.

Joseph Gonzalez-Heydrich, M.D. has received research support from the following sources: Abbott Laboratories, Cyberonics, and Janssen Pharmaceutica Research Foundation. He is currently supported by NIMH grant K23 MH066835-02. He has been a consultant to McNeil Consumer and Specialty Pharmaceuticals, Novartis, Glaxo-SmithKline, and Eli Lilly. He has been on the speaker's bureau for Novartis, Pfizer, and Abbott Laboratories. He has been on the advisory board for McNeil Consumer and Specialty Pharmaceuticals and Cyberonics.

REFERENCES

American Academy of Child & Adolescent Psychiatry: Practice parameters for the assessment and treatment of children and adolescents with depressive disorders. AACAP. J Am Acad Child Adolesc Psychiatry 37:63S–83S, 1998a.

American Academy of Child & Adolescent Psychiatry: Practice parameters for the assessment and treatment of children and adolescents with obsessive–compulsive disorder. AACAP. J Am Acad Child Adolesc Psychiatry 37:27S–45S, 1998b.

American Academy of Child & Adolescent Psychiatry: Practice parameters for the assessment and treatment of children and adolescents with posttraumatic stress disorder. J Am Acad Child Adolesc Psychiatry 37:4S–26S, 1998c.

American Psychiatric Association: Diagnostic and Statistical Manual of Mental Disorders, 4th ed. (DSM-IV). Washington, DC: American Psychiatric Association, 1994.

Brent RL, Tanski S, Weitzman M: A pediatric perspective on the unique vulnerability and resilience of the embryo and the child to environmental toxicants: The importance of rigorous research concerning age and agent. Pediatrics 113:935–944, 2004.

Duffy FF, Narrow WE, Rae DS, West JC, Zarin DA, Rubio-Stipec M, Pincus HA, Regier DA: Concomitant pharmacotherapy among youths treated in routine psychiatric practice. J Child Adolesc Psychopharmacol 15:12–25, 2005.

Egger HL, Angold A: Common emotional and behavioral disorders in preschool children: Presentation, nosology, and epidemiology. J Child Psychol Psychiatry 47:313–337, 2006.

Gonzalez-Heydrich J, DeMaso DR, Irwin C, Steingard RJ, Kohane IS, Beardslee WR: Implementation of an electronic medical record system in a pediatric psychopharmacology program. Int J Med Information 57:109–116, 2000.

Gualtieri CT, Johnson LG: Antidepressant side effects in children and adolescents. J Child Adolesc Psychopharmacol 16:147–157, 2006.

Hunkeler EM, Fireman B, Lee J, Diamond R, Hamilton J, He CX, Dea R, Nwell WB, Hargreaves WA: Trends in use of antidepressants, lithium, and anticonvulsants in Kaiser Permanente-insured youths, 1994–2003. J Child Adolesc Psychopharmacol 15:26–37, 2005.

Keller MB, Ryan ND, Strober M, Klein RG, Kutcher SP, Birmaher B, Hagino OR, Koplewicz H, Carlson GA, Clarke GN, Emslie GJ, Feinberg D, Geller B, Kusumakar V, Papatheodorou G, Sack WH, Sweeney M, Wagner KD, Weller EB, Winters NC, Oake, R, McCafferty JP: Efficacy of paroxetine in the treatment of adolescent major depression: A randomized, controlled trial. J Am Acad Child Adolesc Psychiatry 40:762–772, 2001.

Luby JL, Heffelfinger AK, Mrakotsky C, Brown KM, Hessler MJ, Wallis JM, Spitznagel EL: The clinical picture of depression in preschool children. J Am Acad Child Adolesc Psychiatry 42:340–348, 2003.

Masi G, Toni C, Mucci M, Millepiedi S, Mata B, Perugi G: Paroxetine in child and adolescent outpatients with panic disorder. J Child Adolesc Psychopharmacol 11:151–157, 2001.

McDonnell MA, Glod C: Prevalence of psychopathology in preschool-age children. J Child Adolesc Psychiatr Nursing 16:141–152, 2003.

Nixon MK, Milin R, Simeon JG, Cloutier P, Spenst W: Sertraline effects in adolescent major depression and dysthymia: A six-month open trial. J Child Adolesc Psychopharmacol 11:131–142, 2001.

Riddle MA, Reeve EA, Yaryura-Tobias JA, Yang HM, Claghorn JL, Gaffney G, Greist JH, Holland D, McConville BJ, Pigott T, Walkup JT: Fluvoxamine for children and adolescents with obsessive–compulsive disorder: A randomized, controlled, multicenter trial. J Am Acad Child Adolesc Psychiatry 40:222–229, 2001.

Rushton JL, Whitmire JT: Pediatric stimulant and selective serotonin reuptake inhibitor prescription trends: 1992 to 1998. Arch Pediatr Adolesc Med 155:560–565, 2001.

Safer DJ, Zito JM: Treatment-emergent adverse events from selective serotonin reuptake inhibitors by age group: Children versus adolescents. J Child Adolesc Psychopharmacol 16:159–169, 2006.

Spence SH, Rapee R, McDonald C, Ingram M: The structure of anxiety symptoms among preschoolers. Behav Res Ther 39:1293–1316, 2001.

Vitiello B, Jensen PS: Developmental perspectives in pediatric psychopharmacology. Psychopharmacol Bull 31:75–81, 1995.

Vitiello B, Zuvekas SH, Norquist GS: National estimates of antidepressant medication use among U S children, 1997–2002. J Am Acad Child Adolesc Psychiatry 45:271–279, 2006.

Wagner KD, Ambrosini P, Rynn M, Wohlberg C, Yang R, Greenbaum MS, Childress A, Donnelly C, Deas D: Efficacy of sertraline in the treatment of children and adolescents with major depressive disorder: Two randomized controlled trials. JAMA 290:1033–1041, 2003.

Wilens TE, Biederman J, Kwon A, Chase R, Greenberg L, Mick E, Spencer TJ: A systematic chart review of the nature of psychiatric adverse events in children and adolescents treated with selective serotonin reuptake inhibitors. J Child Adolesc Psychopharmacol 13:143–152, 2003.

Yorbik O, Birmaher B, Axelson D, Williamson DE, Ryan ND: Clinical characteristics of depressive symptoms in children and adolescents with major depressive disorder. J Clin Psychiatry 65:1654–1659, 2004.

ADVANCES IN PRESCHOOL PSYCHOPHARMACOLOGY
© 2009 Mary Ann Liebert, Inc.
140 Huguenot Street, 3rd Floor
New Rochelle, NY 10801-5215

A Pilot Study of Atomoxetine in Young Children With Attention-Deficit/Hyperactivity Disorder

Christopher J. Kratochvil, M.D.,[1] Brigette S. Vaughan, M.S.N., A.P.R.N.,[1]
Michelle L. Mayfield-Jorgensen, M.D.,[1] John S. March, M.D., M.P.H.,[2]
Scott H. Kollins, Ph.D.,[2] Desiree W. Murray, Ph.D.,[2] Hima Ravi, M.D.,[2]
Laurence L. Greenhill, M.D.,[3] Lisa A. Kotler, M.D.,[3] Natalya Paykina, M.A.,[3]
Patricia Biggins, B.A.,[3] and Julie Stoner, Ph.D.[1]

ABSTRACT

Objective: The purpose of this study was to assess the effectiveness and tolerability of atomoxetine during acute treatment of attention-deficit/hyperactivity disorder (ADHD) in 5 and 6 year olds.

Method: Twenty two children (male $n = 19$, 86%) with ADHD were treated with atomoxetine for 8 weeks in a three-site, open-label pilot study. Dosing was flexible, with titration to a maximum of 1.8 mg/kg per day. Parent education on behavior management was provided as part of each pharmacotherapy visit.

Results: Subjects demonstrated a mean decrease of 20.68 points (SD = 12.80, $p < 0.001$)) on the ADHD Rating Scale-IV (ADHD-IV-RS) total score, 10.18 (SD = 7.48, $p < 0.001$) on the inattentive subscale and 10.50 (SD = 7.04, $p < 0.001$) on the hyperactive/impulsive subscale. Clinical Global Impression–Severity (CGI-S) was improved in 82% of the children (95% CI, 66–98%) and Children's Global Assessment (CGAS) scores improved 18.91 points on average (SD = 12.20, $p < 0.001$). The mean final dose of atomoxetine was 1.25 mg/kg per day (SD = 0.35 mg/kg per day). Mood lability was the most commonly reported adverse event ($n = 12$, 54.5%). Eleven subjects (50%) reported decreased appetite and a mean weight loss of 1.04 kg (SD = 0.80 kg) ($p < 0.001$) was observed for the group. Vital sign changes were mild and not clinically significant. There were no discontinuations due to adverse events or lack of efficacy.

Conclusion: Atomoxetine was generally effective for reducing core ADHD symptoms in the 5 and 6 year olds in this open-label study.

INTRODUCTION

APPROXIMATELY 3–7% of school-aged children are affected by attention-deficit/hy-peractivity disorder (ADHD), yet limited data are available regarding treatment of youngsters early in its course (American Psychiatric Association 2000). Symptoms of this neurodevelop-

[1]University of Nebraska Medical Center, Omaha, Nebraska.
[2]Duke University Medical Center, Durham, North Carolina.
[3]Columbia University/New York State Psychiatric Institute, New York, New York.
This work was supported by NIMH Grant 5K23MH06612701A1, as well as grants from Eli Lilly & Company to Duke University Medical Center and Columbia University/New York State Psychiatric Institute. The study drug was provided by Eli Lilly & Company.

mental disorder are often identifiable at an early age, with epidemiological data indicating that approximately 2% of children ages 3–5 years meet diagnostic criteria for ADHD (Lavigne et al. 1996). When compared to their unaffected counterparts, preschool children with ADHD are at significant risk for behavioral, social, familial, and school difficulties (DuPaul et al. 2001). In a study of 94 3- to 5-year-old children, DuPaul and colleagues showed that not only were children with ADHD demonstrating more behavioral problems than children without ADHD, but the difference in behavioral ratings between the groups was significant, greater than 2 SD. Additionally, skill deficits in basic math concepts, prereading, and fine motor abilities are more likely seen in children entering school with ADHD than in those without the disorder (Lahey et al. 1998; Mariani and Barkley 1997; Shelton et al. 1998). When these deficits are combined with the potential for significant social and behavioral difficulties, impairment may result and ultimately persist if appropriate interventions are not initiated. In addition, ADHD symptoms can tax parent and caregiver resources, resulting in a strained home environment for these young children. A study by Escobar and colleagues demonstrated that parents of children with ADHD perceived the level of interference in daily life to be greater than that reported by parents of normal controls, as well as parents of asthmatic children (Escobar et al. 2005).

Despite evidence suggesting that the initial symptoms of ADHD often present by 3 years of age, systematic study of the use of medications in 3- to 6-year-old children with ADHD has been quite limited (Food and Drug Administration 1997; Food and Drug Administration 1997; National Institutes of Health 1998). The need for additional research on the safety and efficacy of psychotropic medication use in preschoolers has been emphasized, especially in light of the rates of prescriptions for this age group (Greenhill 1998). Zito and colleagues found a three-fold increase in the use of psychotropic agents in 2- to 5-year-old children from 1991 to 1995 (Zito et al. 2000). Zuvekas et al. analyzed data from the Medical Expenditure Panel Survey (MEPS) and found that an estimated 0.3% of children under age 6 were

treated with psychostimulants from 1997 to 2002 (Zuvekas et al. 2006). While stimulant use in children under age 18 increased from 2.7% to 2.9% during those 5 years, the rate of use in the preschool age group remained stable, indicating that prescription of ADHD medications in young children may be leveling off in this group. Another database, however, indicated that use of stimulants in this population may be increasing, as a 2004 report by Medco Health Solutions showed a 49% increase in the number of stimulant prescriptions written for preschoolers from 2000 to 2003 (Greenhill et al. 2006).

Unfortunately, until recently, only 10 of over 160 controlled trials of psychostimulants for school-aged children included preschoolers ages 4–6, and all 10 assessed the use of methylphenidate (MPH) (Conners 1975; Schleifer et al. 1975; Cohen et al. 1981; Barkley et al. 1984; Barkley 1988; Mayes et al. 1994; Musten et al. 1997; Firestone et al. 1998; Handen et al. 1999; Chacko et al. 2005). Even in these few trials, not all of the samples were made up entirely of young children. By merging samples of younger and older children, limitations present, in that the studies are not necessarily specifically designed to evaluate and monitor symptoms in younger children. Scales may not be normed for both groups, appropriateness of diagnostic assessments may vary, and the studies may be underpowered solely to examine the younger children in the sample. The recently completed Preschool ADHD Treatment Study (PATS), a multisite trial of 303 preschoolers with ADHD added significantly to this literature base in that it was designed solely for young children and adequately powered, but again this study examined MPH (Greenhill et al. 2006).

Although stimulants have been shown to be safe and effective in the treatment of ADHD in children, adolescents, and adults, a range of factors have led parents and clinicians to seek alternative medication treatments, especially for younger children. As such, there has been considerable interest in developing additional treatments, including nonstimulant options, for ADHD.

Although information on the use of stimulants in preschoolers is limited, data on the use of nonstimulants in young children with ADHD is virtually nonexistent. A review of the PharMetrics database shows that a significant number of prescriptions of atomoxetine are written for children under 5 years of age, despite the lack of data on its use in children younger than 6 years old (Van Brunt et al. 2005). Thus, the management of preschool ADHD with nonstimulant pharmacotherapy currently requires clinicians to extrapolate from the data available on use of these medications in older children and adolescents to guide their clinical practice.

Atomoxetine is a nonstimulant medication that received Food and Drug Administration (FDA) approval for the treatment of ADHD in children 6 years and older, adolescents, and adults in November, 2002. Atomoxetine acts by selectively blocking the presynaptic norepinephrine transporter, increasing noradrenergic tone. It is highly specific, with minimal affinity for other receptors or other neuronal transporters (Spencer et al. 1998). To date, approximately 5,500 children and adolescents have been treated with atomoxetine in clinical trials.

As the only nonstimulant medication FDA approved for the treatment of ADHD, and one clinically used off-label in the treatment of ADHD in young children, atomoxetine was selected as the medication to be examined in this clinical trial. The goal of this pilot study was to evaluate systematically the effectiveness and tolerability of atomoxetine for the treatment of ADHD in children 5 and 6 years of age, and to collect pilot data for a larger double-blind, placebo-controlled trial.

METHODS

This study was a 22-subject feasibility trial that included children aged 5 and 6 years old who met Diagnostic and Statistical Manual of Mental Disorders, 4th edition, Text Revision (DSM-IV-TR) (American Psychiatric Association 2000) criteria for ADHD, any subtype, as confirmed by the Diagnostic Interview Schedule for Children-IV (DISC-IV) (Shaffer et al. 2000) and clinical interview. Symptom severity as measured by the ADHD Rating Scale-IV, by parent interview (ADHD-IV-RS) (DuPaul et al.

1998) at entry was required to be at least 1.5 SD above age and gender norms. Impairment as measured by the Clinical Global Impression–ADHD–Severity scale (CGI-S) (Guy 1976) had to be at least 4 (moderate severity), with a Children's Global Assessment Scale (CGAS) ≤55. Subjects were required to have estimated IQ's of ≥70. Patients who previously failed a trial of atomoxetine or who were already being effectively treated with atomoxetine were not included in the study. Diagnoses of an adjustment disorder, autism, psychosis, bipolar disorder, significant suicidality, or any other psychiatric disorder requiring treatment with additional medications were exclusionary, as was the presence of current or previous clinically significant hepatic disease, or any significant medical condition that would interfere with the study medication. Each case was discussed on a conference call, which included study personnel from each of the three sites, and a consensus decision regarding appropriateness for enrollment was required prior to initiation of study treatment. Several of these inclusion criteria were chosen to be consistent with the PATS, and also to provide a relatively conservative approach to inclusion.

The study was conducted at three sites in the United States: University of Nebraska Medical Center in Omaha, NE; Duke University Medical Center in Durham, NC; and Columbia University/New York State Psychiatric Institute in New York, NY. Prior to entering the study, there was a review of the consent document, oral description and discussion of the study, and written informed consent was obtained from a parent or guardian for each patient. The study was reviewed and approved by each site's ethical review board and was conducted in accordance with the ethical standards of the 1975 Declarations of Helsinki as revised in 2000 (World Medical Association 2000).

Measures

An initial assessment using the DISC-IV was completed interview style with the parent/guardian, followed by a clinical diagnostic assessment with a psychiatrist, psychologist or advanced practice registered nurse (APRN) trained and experienced in the assessment and treatment of pediatric mental health disorders. The clinical diagnostic assessment confirmed or refuted any co-morbid psychiatric diagnoses reported on the DISC-IV, and also evaluated the child for co-morbid diagnoses potentially missed by the computerized interview. The DISC-IV was used in PATS in a similar manner, despite lacking norms for children under the age of 6. The primary efficacy measure for the study was the ADHD-IV-RS, completed by investigator interview with the parent at study entry and at all subsequent visits, along with the CGI-S and CGAS. The Clinical Global Impression–Improvement (CGI-I) was completed at each visit following baseline. All of these measures were completed by the pharmacotherapist, a physician, or APRN with extensive experience using pharmacotherapy to treat young children with ADHD. An effort was made to have the same pharmacotherapist follow each child throughout his or her study participation.

Additional measures completed at the study screening visit included the Multidimensional Anxiety Scale for Children (MASC) (March et al. 1997), Children's Depression Inventory (CDI) (Kovacs 2001), and Childhood Autism Rating Scale (CARS) (Garfin et al. 1988). The Peabody Picture Vocabulary Test (PPVT-IIIA) (Dunn and Dunn 1997), an assessment of receptive language abilities, was completed at the initial evaluation visit as a proxy for intelligence quotient (IQ), given the correlation of receptive language with general cognitive ability. Scales completed by the parent included the Conners' Parent Rating Scale-Revised (L) (CPRS) (Conners et al. 1998a) and Parent Stress Index (PSI) (Abidin 1995). The child's teacher, or structured day-care provider in the case of those children not yet enrolled in school, completed the Conners' Teacher Rating Scale–Revised (L) (CTRS) (Conners et al. 1998b) and the teacher version of the ADHD-IV rating scale. The teacher scales, as well as MASC, CDI, CPRS, and PSI, were repeated at visit 5 and again at study completion (visit 8 or early discontinuation).

Safety analyses

Baseline height, weight, and vital signs, including heart rate and blood pressure, were ob-tained at study entry. Weight and vital signs were assessed at each subsequent visit, and height was measured again at the final study visit. Laboratory tests [complete blood count (CBC), liver function tests (LFT's), electrolytes, blood urea nitrogen (BUN), creatinine, and lead level], an electrocardiogram (EKG), and physical examination were performed at the screening visit. Hematology, chemistry, EKG, and physical examination were repeated at the final study visit. Preexisting conditions were reviewed at the screening visit and monitored for changes during study participation. Adverse events and concomitant medications were assessed by the physician or APRN prescribing and monitoring the study medication at each visit via open-ended discussion with the parent/guardian. The prescribing clinician evaluated the relatedness to the study drug for each event. Clinically significant laboratory and EKG results were documented as adverse events.

Study design

Once approved to enter the trial, study treatment with open-label atomoxetine was initiated. Atomoxetine was dosed by weight and increased at the discretion of the investigator on the basis of tolerability and response. The initial dose of atomoxetine was 0.5 mg/kg per day, with titration to a maximum of 0.8 mg/kg per day at week 1, 1.2 mg/kg per day at week 2, 1.4 mg/kg per day at week 3, and 1.8 mg/kg per day at week 5. Patients could be dosed once or twice daily. The parent/guardian also participated in an 8-week parent education protocol administered by the pharmacotherapist during the course of each pharmacotherapy visit to be consistent with practice guidelines recommending nonpharmacological interventions for this age group. Approximately 10–15 minutes of each pharmacotherapy visit were spent in parent education using an eight-session protocol adapted in part from McMahon and Forehand's "Helping the Noncompliant Child: Family-Based Treatment for Oppositional Behavior" (McMahon and Forehand 2003). Education on ADHD and identification of target behaviors for improvement comprised the first session, with two subsequent sessions on rewarding positive and ignoring negative behavior, and giving clear instructions. Optional sessions at visits 5–7 included effective utilization of time out, challenges to time out, standing rules, and implementation of a token-reinforcement program or daily report card for home and school use. The optional modules were selected at the discretion of the pharmacotherapist to tailor the parent education to the needs of the child.

Data analysis

Descriptive statistics were used to describe the baseline patient characteristics and outcome variables. The Wilcoxon signed-rank test was used to determine whether the median change in the outcome variables was statistically significant (tested the null hypothesis that the median change over the treatment period was 0). Data analyses were conducted on the 22 patients who took study drug.

RESULTS

A total of 30 subjects completed the screening visit, with 22 of these meeting all entry criteria and initiating study treatment at visit two. Six of the 8 subjects who did not proceed to the treatment phase of the study were excluded due to a failure to meet criteria for a diagnosis of ADHD. One subject withdrew consent prior to beginning atomoxetine and 1 subject refused the required blood draw. Two subjects (6.7%) withdrew from the study after completion of visit 3 due to inability to consistently swallow the capsules containing study medication. Twenty of the 22 patients who began treatment (90.9%) completed the study.

Nineteen males and 3 females met all inclusion and no exclusion criteria and were eligible to begin study treatment (Table 1). These subjects had a mean age at baseline 6.06 years (SD 0.58 years). The majority of subjects met criteria for the combined subtype of ADHD ($n = 18$, 82%), with the remaining 4 subjects meeting criteria for the hyperactive/impulsive subtype. The mean baseline ADHD-IV-RS total score was 38.23 (SD 8.05), with a mean inattentive subscale of 18.23 (SD 4.21) and mean hyperactive impulsive subscale of 20.0 (SD =

5.43). Nearly three fourths of subjects ($n = 16$, 73%) had a baseline CGI-S of 5 (markedly ill), with a mean baseline CGAS for the group of 53.23 (SD 3.85). There were no significant differences in ADHD severity between the 5 year olds and the 6 year olds at baseline, as measured by the ADHD-IV-RS total score, subscales, CGI-S, or CGAS. Twelve subjects (55%) were identified as having co-morbid oppositional defiant disorder, 5 (23%) had enuresis, and 2 (9%) met criteria for simple phobia. The mean CARS score for the group was 17.07 (SD = 1.83), with a range of 15–21, which is in the nonautistic range. The mean standard score for the PPVT-IIIA was 106.50 (SD = 13.07). All subjects who participated in the treatment portion of the study were treatment naïve.

The final total daily dose of atomoxetine ranged from 10 to 45 mg/day, with a mean total daily dose of 30.23 mg/day (SD = 9.70). By weight, the final mean total daily dose was 1.25 mg/kg per day, SD = 0.35, with a range of 0.47–1.88 mg/kg per day. The atomoxetine was given in either a single morning dose ($n = 20$) or in divided doses given morning and afternoon ($n = 2$). Though slightly higher than the final mean doses of older children in prior atomoxetine studies, it was below the FDA-approved maximum dose of 1.4 mg/kg per day.

TABLE 1. DEMOGRAPHICS[a]

Characteristic	Count
Age at visit 1 (years)	
Mean (SD)	6.06 (0.58)
5 year old	10 (45%)
6 year old	12 (55%)
Gender	
Male	19 (86%)
Female	3 (14%)
Race	
Black or African American	4 (18%)
White	18 (82%)
ADHD Subtype	
Hyperactive/Impulsive	4 (18%)
Combined	18 (82%)
Co-morbidities	
ODD	12 (55%)
Enuresis	5 (23%)
Simple phobia	2 (9%)
Phonological disorder	1 (5%)

ADHD = Attention-deficit/hyperactivity disorder; ODD = oppositional defiant disorder; SD = standard deviation
[a]$N = 22$.

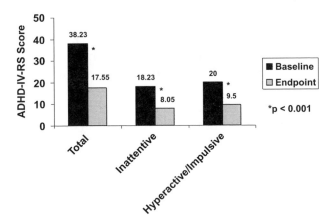

FIG. 1. ADHD-IV-RS. ADHD-IV-RS-Attention-Deficit/Hyperactivity–Rating Scale-IV.

The subjects demonstrated a mean decrease in the ADHD-IV-RS total score of 20.68 points (SD = 12.80, $p < 0.001$), with mean improvements in the inattentive subscale of 10.18 points (SD = 7.48, $p < 0.001$) and 10.50 points in the hyperactive/impulsive subscale (SD = 7.04, $p < 0.001$) (Fig. 1). At the end point, CGI-S was improved in 82% (95% CI, 66–98%) (Table 2) and mean improvement in CGAS score was 18.91 points (SD = 12.20, $p < 0.001$). Clinical improvement was reflected by the final CGI-I ratings, where 86% showed at least some improvement (95% CI, 72–100%). Sixteen of the 22 subjects who started study drug (72.7%) achieved the generally accepted criteria for response, a CGI-I score of 1 (very much improved) or 2 (much improved) by study end point (Fig. 2). The mean final total daily dose of atomoxetine (1.25 mg/kg per day, SD = 0.35) was below the FDA-approved maximum dose of 1.4 mg/kg per day, but near the approved target dose of 1.2 mg/kg per day.

Table 3 compares changes in outcome measures based upon age. Descriptively, the 5-year-old group appears to demonstrate greater improvement over time compared with the 6-year-old group, although with limited power, only the ADHD-IV inattentive subscale was statistically significant.

The most frequent spontaneously reported adverse event was mood lability, experienced by 12 of the 22 children (54.5%) at some point during the study, ranging from 13.6% to 31.8% at individual visits over 8 weeks (Fig. 3). Spontaneous mood-related adverse events classified as "mood lability" included: Angry/hostile, brittle mood, emotionally labile, fussy, mopey, rapid mood swings, tearful, and irritability. Half of the children (11 of 22) experienced decreased appetite (ranging from 9% to 45% at individual visits over 8 weeks). Additionally, a statistically significant mean decrease in weight of 1.04 kg (SD = 0.80, $p < 0.001$) was observed for the group. Parents/guardians were encouraged to use caloric supplementation to limit the effect of diminished appetite, and to give the medication after the child had eaten to minimize stomach upset. Five year olds did not differ significantly from 6 year olds in frequency or severity of adverse events reported.

Changes in vital signs were limited; with a mean change of systolic blood pressure of 2.98 mmHg (SD = 5.68) the only statistically significant change ($p = 0.03$) (Table 4). There were no clinically significant changes in heart rate, blood pressure, or on EKGs. No subjects discontinued due to adverse events or lack of efficacy.

DISCUSSION

The purpose of this open-label pilot study was to evaluate the general efficacy and tolerability of atomoxetine in 5 and 6 year olds with ADHD, prior to the initiation of a planned double-blind, placebo-controlled trial in this same population. Statistically and clinically significant improvement in symptoms of inattention and hyperactivity/impulsivity were observed in this open-label study, as evidenced by

TABLE 2. CLINICAL GLOBAL IMPRESSION–SEVERITY SCORES WERE DECREASED FROM BASELINE TO ENDPOINT ($p < 0.001$)

CGI-Severity	Baseline n (%)	End point n (%)
(1) Normal, not mentally ill	0 (0)	0 (0)
(2) Borderline mentally ill	0 (0)	8 (36)
(3) Mildly mentally ill	0 (0)	8 (36)
(4) Moderately mentally ill	3 (14)	3 (14)
(5) Markedly mentally ill	16 (73)	3 (14)
(6) Severely mentally ill	3 (14)	0 (0)
(7) Among the most extremely mentally ill	0 (0)	0 (0)

CGI-S = Clinical Global Impression–Severity.
Overall decrease in CGI-S was statistically significant ($p < 0.001$).

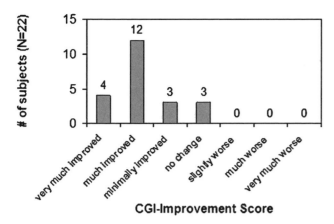

FIG. 2. CGI-I at end point. CGI-I = Clinical Global Impressions–Improvement.

decreases in the total and subscale scores of the investigator-scored ADHD-IV-RS. An improvement in functional status was also observed, evidenced by the changes in clinician-rated CGAS, CGI-S, and CGI-I scores. Because the MASC and CDI are not normed for use in this age group, they were not used to detect any significant changes in patient-reported anxiety or mood symptoms. Rather these scales were employed to support or rule out the presence of co-morbid disorders, particularly at the baseline visit as a part of the psychiatric assessment.

Atomoxetine is approved for use in children as young as 6 years old; however, it is being used in younger children in clinical practice. Because children are being identified and treated with pharmacotherapy at younger ages, it is worthwhile to examine the efficacy and safety of atomoxetine in a systematic fashion. This was the first study to assess atomoxetine use systematically in children younger than age 6 with ADHD. The authors' interest in identification and treatment of early-childhood ADHD, and well as their familiarity with atomoxetine from prior clinical trial experience, led to this study. Inclusion of children who were at least 5 years old allowed the investigators to collect data on younger children who were still likely to be in a structured setting such as a school or preschool. This provided investigators with an additional reporter of symptoms and impairment. Data obtained in this trial and its follow-up double-blind placebo-controlled study may lead to future studies that extend to younger children.

Despite the majority of children reporting at least one side effect, and at least half of the children reporting mood lability and half reporting diminished appetite, the medication was tolerated well enough so that no one discontinued the medication due to adverse effects. This is possibly due in part to the gradual and flexible titration schedule used over the course of treatment. There were no serious adverse events during the study, and the 2 chil-

TABLE 3.   OUTCOME MEASURES COMPARING 5 YEAR OLDS TO 6 YEAR OLDS

Outcome measure	5 year old		6 year old		Wilcoxon rank sum test p value comparing age groups
	n	Mean (SD)	n	Mean (SD)	
Parent ADHD-IV Total	10	−27.00 (9.19)	12	−15.42 (13.32)	0.06
Parent ADHD-IV Inattentive	10	−14.40 (4.22)	12	−6.67 (7.91)	0.04
Parent ADHD-IV Hyperactive	10	−12.60 (6.45)	12	−8.87 (7.30)	0.2
CGAS	10	22.40 (9.92)	12	16.00 (13.54)	0.2
	n	Count (%) improved	n	Count (%) improved	Fisher's exact test p value comparing age groups
CGI-S	10	10 (100%)	12	8 (67%)	0.1
CGI-I	10	10 (100%)	12	9 (75%)	0.2

ADHD = Attention-Deficit/Hyperactivity Disorder Rating Scale-IV; CGAS = Children's Global Assessment Scale; CGI-I = Clinical Global Impression–Improvement; CGI-S = Clinical Global Impression–Severity; SD = standard deviation.

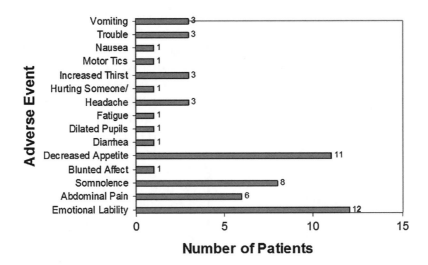

FIG. 3. Adverse events N = 22.

dren who discontinued the study after initiation of treatment were those who were unable to consistently swallow capsules. The most commonly reported adverse events, were mood lability ($n = 12$, 54.5%) and decreased appetite ($n = 11$, 50%), with a statistically significant decrease in weight of 1.04 kg (SD = 0.80, $p < 0.001$) observed for the group. The acute nature of the study, however, limits the ability to assess potential long-term effects on growth. Changes in vital signs were mild and not clinically significant. This is congruent with PATS, which demonstrated no significant changes in vital signs for subjects on MPH compared to those on placebo (Wigal et al. 2006). No clinically significant changes were observed in any of the laboratory tests or EKGs.

Mood lability was reported 1 week into treatment by 7 subjects, and was present for an average of 2½ weeks. This side effect persisted until the end of the 8-week treatment period for 2 of the 12 subjects. Many of the adverse effects categorized as "mood lability" have been demonstrated in other trials of psychotropic

medications in young children. In PATS, for example, 9 of the 14 children who discontinued due to adverse events did so because of emotionality or irritability (Greenhill et al. 2006). Also, Safer and Zito (2006) described a review of placebo-controlled clinical trials of serotonselective reuptake inhibitors (SSRIs) demonstrating that activation was consistently more prevalent in children than in adolescents (Safer and Zito 2006). All of these results indicate that younger children may be more prone to mood-related side effects than older children and adolescents. Decreased appetite appeared between the second and fourth weeks of treatment for the majority of the 11 subjects who reported it, and it was an ongoing adverse event at the end of the study for 8 subjects.

The frequency of adverse effects seen in this study, particularly the diminished appetite and mood lability, highlights the need for close monitoring of young children treated with pharmacotherapy for ADHD. Adjusting the rate of titration, total dose given, timing of doses, as well as caloric supplementation, can

TABLE 4. VITAL SIGNS

Measure	Baseline mean (SD)	End point mean (SD)	Change mean (SD)	
Weight (kg)	25.0 (38.1)	23.96 (3.45)	−1.04 (0.80)	$p < 0.001$
Systolic BP (mmHg)	94.25 (4.79)	100.10 (5.15)	2.89 (5.65)	$p = 0.03$
Diastolic BP (mmHg)	53.55 (5.25)	55.95 (6.58)	2.41 (6.80)	$p = 0.1$
Pulse (bpm)	93.36 (9.66)	92.05 (15.11)	−1.32 (14.37)	$p = 0.9$

BP = Blood pressure; bpm = beats per minute; kg = kilogram; mmHg = millimeters of mercury; SD = standard deviation.
Changes from baseline to end point were not statistically or clinically significant.

all potentially improve the tolerability when difficulties are identified.

Limitations

The results of this study are limited by its small sample size, predominantly Caucasian male population, and open-label design. Whereas boys constitute a higher proportion of preschoolers with ADHD, the ratio of males to females in this study was greater than that reported in clinical preschool samples. Additionally, it is difficult to identify the specific role of the atomoxetine, because the frequency of contact with the pharmacotherapist and the concomitant psychoeducational intervention may have also contributed to the overall robust response in this group. The parent education provided, while based on an evidence-based psychosocial treatment (McMahon and Forehand 2003), was very abbreviated and limited to eight 10- to 15-minute sessions (maximum of 2 hours). Parent training interventions demonstrating efficacy in this age group are much more intensive, averaging 8–12 hours duration, typically with significant behavioral rehearsal, modeling, and feedback components that the present intervention did not include (Pisterman et al. 1989; Strayhorn and Weidman 1989; Sonuga-Barke et al. 2001; Bor et al. 2002). Thus, although anecdotally many parents seemed to find the weekly discussions about behavior management strategies useful, it seems unlikely that this intervention alone provided significant direct benefits in reducing core ADHD symptoms. Nonetheless, it is certainly possible that the combination of psychoeducation with pharmacotherapy provided by the same physician contributed in some indirect ways to efficacy results. For example, psychoeducation may have enhanced the physician–patient relationship, which is believed to increase medication compliance.

Pharmacotherapists in this study had access to capsule strengths of atomoxetine that are not commercially available (2.5 mg, 5 mg, 20 mg), making smaller increases in study drug dose during titration possible. This allowed for dosing closer to the actual mg/kg dosing schedule, and a more gradual titration not possible or practical for clinicians in practice. Also, atomoxetine is only available in capsule form and

sprinkling of the capsule contents is discouraged. Therefore, participation in this study was limited to those children able to swallow the atomoxetine capsule whole. For young children, this may not always be possible, as evidenced by the two discontinuations in this study. This may be a limiting factor for clinicians in the use of atomoxetine in younger children.

Another limitation of this study is that it only provides data on the short-term treatment of a disorder that generally lasts years. Longer-term follow up with young children taking atomoxetine to determine safety and effectiveness over time will be important. The potential long-term effects on growth in this population would be of particular interest. An additional limitation was the monitoring of adverse events by spontaneous report from the parent/guardian. Despite the high rates of adverse events, this method of adverse event collection may have resulted in a lower reporting rate compared to use of a systematic collection measure.

CONCLUSIONS

This open-label study demonstrated atomoxetine to be effective in the treatment of 5 and 6 year olds with ADHD. Although a significant number of children experienced adverse events, they were often transient, and no subjects discontinued due to side effects. There were no unanticipated adverse events, although the rates of decreased appetite and mood lability were higher than expected. Close monitoring is clearly warranted when using atomoxetine in young children with ADHD.

The study demonstrated the feasibility of the diagnostic assessments and the atomoxetine dosing strategy used, and anecdotal comments from parents reinforced the utility of the parent education protocol. These data supported the initiation of a 120-subject randomized double-blind placebo-controlled clinical trial currently underway at the three clinical sites.

DISCLOSURES

Dr. Kratochvil received support from Eli Lilly and Company in the form of study drug supplies to conduct this study. No financial support was received from Eli Lilly and Company by Dr. Kratochvil. Dr. Kratochvil's research is supported by NIMH Grant 5K23MH06612701A1. He also receives grant support from Eli Lilly, McNeil and Cephalon, is a consultant for Eli Lilly, Shire, Cephalon, Organon, AstraZeneca, Boehringer-Ingelheim, and Pfizer, and a member of the Eli Lilly speaker's bureau.

Dr. March is a consultant or scientific advisor to Pfizer, Lilly, Wyeth, GSK, Jazz, and MedAvante and holds stock in MedAvante; he receives research support from Lilly and study drug for an NIMH-funded study from Lilly and Pfizer; he is the author of the MASC.

Dr. Kollins receives research support from Shire, Pfizer, Lilly, Psychogenics, Inc., New River Pharmaceuticals, NIDA, NIMH, NIEHS, EPA, and NINDS. He receives consultant support from Shire and Cephalon.

Dr. Murray receives research support from Eli Lilly and Company, Pfizer, NIMH, and the Department of Education.

Dr. Greenhill is a consultant for Pfizer, Janssen, Lilly, & Novartis. He is on the advisory Board for Lilly and the Data & Safety Monitoring Board for Pfizer and Janssen. He has research contracts with McNeil, New River Pharmaceuticals, and Novartis.

Ms. Vaughan, Dr. Jorgensen, Dr. Ravi, Dr. Kotler, Ms. Paykina, Ms. Biggins, and Dr. Stoner have no conflicts of interest to report.

REFERENCES

Abidin RA: Parenting Stress Index Third Edition Professional Manual. Odessa, Psychological Assessment Resources Inc., 1995.

American Psychiatric Association: Diagnostic and Statistical Manual of Mental Disorders, 4th ed. Text Revision. Washington, DC, American Psychiatric Association, 2000.

Barkley RA: The effects of methylphenidate on the interactions of preschool ADHD children with their mothers. J Am Acad Child Adolesc Psychiatry 27:336–341, 1988.

Barkley RA, Karlsson J, Strzelecki E, Murphy JV: Effects of age and Ritalin dosage on the mother-child interactions of hyperactive children. J Consult Clin Psychol 52:750–758, 1984.

Bor W, Sanders MR, Markie-Dadds C: The effects of the triple p-positive parenting program on preschool children with co-occurring disruptive behavior and attentional/hyperactive difficulties. J Abnorm Child Psychol 30:571–587, 2002.

Chacko A, Pelham WE, Gnagy EM, Greiner A, Vallano G, Bukstein O, Rancurello M: Stimulant medication effects in a summer treatment program among young children with attention-deficit/hyperactivity disorder. J Am Acad Child Adolesc Psychiatry 44:249–257, 2005.

Cohen NJ, Sullivan J, Minde K, Novak C, Helwig C: Evaluation of the relative effectiveness of methylphenidate and cognitive behavior modification in the treatment of kindergarten-aged hyperactive children. J Abnorm Child Psychol 9:43–54, 1981.

Conners CK: Controlled trial of methylphenidate in preschool children with minimal brain dysfunction. J Mental Heath 4:61–74, 1975.

Conners CK, Sitarenios G, Parker JD, Epstein JN: The revised Conners' Parent Rating Scale (CPRS-R): Factor structure, reliability, and criterion validity. J Abnorm Child Psychol 26:257–268, 1998a.

Conners CK, Sitarenios G, Parker JD, Epstein JN: Revision and restandardization of the Conners' Teacher Rating Scale (CTRS-R): Factor structure, reliability, and criterion validity. J Abnorm Child Psychol 26:279–291, 1998b.

Dunn LM, Dunn LM: Peabody Picture Vocabulary Test Third Edition Form IIIA and Form IIIB. Circle Pines, American Guidance Service, 1997.

DuPaul GJ, Power TJ, Anastopoulos AD, Reid R: ADHD Rating Scale-IV: Checklists, Norms, and Clinical Interpretations. New York, Guilford Press, 1998.

DuPaul GJ, McGoey KE, Eckert TL, VanBrakle J: Preschool children with attention-deficit/hyperactivity disorder: Impairments in behavioral, social, and school functioning. J Am Acad Child Adolesc Psychiatry 40:508–515, 2001.

Escobar R, Soutullo CA, Hervas A, Gastaminza X, Polavieja P, Gilaberte I: Worse quality of life for children with newly diagnosed attention-deficit/hyperactivity disorder, compared with asthmatic and healthy children. Pediatrics 116:e364–e369, 2005.

Firestone P, Musten LM, Pisterman S, Mercer J, Bennett S: Short-term side effects of stimulant medication are increased in preschool children with attention-deficit/hyperactivity disorder: A double-blind placebo-controlled study. J Child Adolesc Psychopharmacol 8:13–25, 1998.

Food and Drug Administration (1997). Modernization Act of 1997. 21 USC 321.

Food and Drug Administration (1997). Regulations requiring manufacturers to assess the safety and effectiveness of new drugs and biological products in pediatric patients. http://www.fda.gov/cder/guidance/pedrule.htm

Garfin DG, McCallon D, Cox R: Validity and reliability of the Childhood Autism Rating Scale with autistic adolescents. J Autism Dev Disord 18:367–378, 1988.

Greenhill LL: The use of psychotropic medication in preschoolers: Indications, safety, and efficacy. Can J Psychiatry 43:576–581, 1998.

Greenhill L, Kollins S, Abikoff H, McCracken J, Riddle M,

Swanson J, McGough J, Wigal S, Wigal T, Vitiello B, Skrobala A, Posner K, Ghuman J, Cunningham C, Davies M, Chuang S, Cooper T: Efficacy and safety of immediate-release methylphenidate treatment for preschoolers with ADHD. J Am Acad Child Adolesc Psychiatry 45:1284–1293, 2006.

Guy W: ECDEU Assessment Manual for Psychopharmacology, Revised. Bethesda, US Department of Health, Education, and Welfare, 1976.

Handen BL, Feldman HM, Lurier A, Murray PJ: Efficacy of methylphenidate among preschool children with developmental disabilities and ADHD. J Am Acad Child Adolesc Psychiatry 38:805–812, 1999.

Kovacs M: Children's Depression Inventory (CDI) Technical Manual. Toronto, Multi-Health Systems Inc., 2001.

Lahey BB, Pelham WE, Stein MA, Loney J, Trapani C, Nugent K, Kipp H, Schmidt E, Lee S, Cale M, Gold E, Hartung CM, Willcutt E, Baumann B: Validity of DSM-IV attention-deficit/hyperactivity disorder for younger children. J Am Acad Child Adolesc Psychiatry 37:695–702, 1998.

Lavigne JV, Gibbons RD, Christoffel KK, Arend R, Rosenbaum D, Binns H, Dawson N, Sobel H, Isaacs C: Prevalence rates and correlates of psychiatric disorders among preschool children. J Am Acad Child Adolesc Psychiatry 35:204–214, 1996.

March JS, Parker JD, Sullivan K, Stallings P, Conners CK: The Multidimensional Anxiety Scale for Children (MASC): Factor structure, reliability, and validity. J Am Acad Child Adolesc Psychiatry 36:554–565, 1997.

Mariani MA, Barkley RA: Neuropsychological and academic functioning in preschool boys with attention deficit hyperactivity disorder. Devel Neuropsychol 13:111–129, 1997.

Mayes SD, Crites DL, Bixler EO, Humphrey FJ, 2nd, Mattison RE: Methylphenidate and ADHD: Influence of age, IQ and neurodevelopmental status. Dev Med Child Neurol 36:1099–1107, 1994.

McMahon RJ, Forehand RL: Helping the Noncompliant Child. Family-Based Treatment for Oppositional Behavior. New York, The Guilford Press, 2003.

Musten LM, Firestone P, Pisterman S, Bennett S, Mercer J: Effects of methylphenidate on preschool children with ADHD: Cognitive and behavioral functions. J Am Acad Child Adolesc Psychiatry 36:1407–1415, 1997.

National Institutes of Health (1998). NIH policy and guidelines on the inclusion of children as participants in research involving human subjects. http://www.nih.gov/grants/guide/notice-files/not98-024.html

Pisterman S, McGrath P, Firestone P, Goodman JT, Webster I, Mallory R: Outcome of parent-mediated treatment of preschoolers with attention-deficit disorder with hyperactivity. J Consult Clin Psychol 57:628–635, 1989.

Safer DJ, Zito JM: Treatment-emergent adverse events from selective serotonin reuptake inhibitors by age group: children versus adolescents. J Child Adolesc Psychopharmacol 16:159–169, 2006.

Schleifer M, Weiss G, Cohen N, Elman M, Cvejic H, Kruger E: Hyperactivity in preschoolers and the effect of methylphenidate. Am J Orthopsychiatry 45:38–50, 1975.

Shaffer D, Fisher P, Lucas CP, Dulcan MK, Schwab-Stone ME: NIMH Diagnostic Interview Schedule for Children Version IV (NIMH DISC-IV): Description, differences from previous versions, and reliability of some common diagnoses. J Am Acad Child Adolesc Psychiatry 39:28–38, 2000.

Shelton TL, Barkley RA, Crosswait C, Moorehouse M, Fletcher K, Barrett S, Jenkins L, Metevia L: Psychiatric and psychological morbidity as a function of adaptive disability in preschool children with aggressive and hyperactive-impulsive-inattentive behavior. J Abnorm Child Psychol 26:475–494, 1998.

Sonuga-Barke EJS, Daley D, Thompson M, Laver-Bradbury C, Weeks A: Parent-based therapies for preschool attention-deficit/hyperactivity disorder: A randomized, controlled trial with a community sample. J Am Acad Child Adolesc Psychiatry 40:402–408, 2001.

Spencer T, Biederman J, Wilens T, Prince J, Hatch M, Jones J, Harding M, Faraone SV, Seidman L: Effectiveness and tolerability of tomoxetine in adults with attention deficit hyperactivity disorder. Am J Psychiatry 155:693–695, 1998.

Strayhorn JM, Weidman C: Reduction of attention deficit and internalizing symptoms in preschoolers through parent-child interaction training. J Am Acad Child Adolesc Psychiatry 28:888–896, 1989.

Van Brunt DL, Johnston JA, Ye W, Pohl GM, Sun PJ, Sterling KL, Davis ME: Predictors of selecting atomoxetine therapy for children with attention-deficit-hyperactivity disorder. Phamacotherapy 25:1541–1549, 2005.

Wigal T, Greenhill L, Chuang S, McGough J, Vitiello B, Skrobala A, Swanson J, Wigal S, Abikoff H, Kollins S, McCracken J, Riddle M, Posner K, Ghuman J, Davies M, Thorp B, Stehli A: Safety and tolerability of methylphenidate in preschool children with ADHD. J Am Acad Child Adolesc Psychiatry 45:1294–1303, 2006.

World Medical Association: Revising the Declaration of Helsinki. Bull Med Ethics 158:9–11, 2000.

Zito JM, Safer DJ, dosReis S, Gardner JF, Boles M, Lynch F: Trends in the prescribing of psychotropic medications to preschoolers. JAMA 283:1025–1030, 2000.

Zuvekas SH, Vitiello B, Norquist GS: Recent trends in stimulant medication use among U.S. children. Am J Psychiatry 163:579–585, 2006.

ADVANCES IN PRESCHOOL PSYCHOPHARMACOLOGY
© 2009 Mary Ann Liebert, Inc.
140 Huguenot Street, 3rd Floor
New Rochelle, NY 10801-5215

QT Interval and Dispersion in Very Young Children Treated with Antipsychotic Drugs: A Retrospective Chart Review

Eitan Nahshoni, M.D., M.Sc.,[1,5] Sara Spitzer, M.D.,[2,5] Michael Berant, M.D.,[3,5] Gal Shoval, M.D.,[3,5] Gil Zalsman, M.D.,[3,5] and Abraham Weizman, M.D.[1,4,5]

ABSTRACT

Objectives and background: QT dispersion (QTd) is a measure of interlead variations of the surface 12-lead electrocardiogram (ECG). Increased QTd, found in various cardiac diseases, reflects cardiac instability and risk for lethal cardiac arrhythmias. Research suggests a link between psychotropic treatment, ECG abnormalities (QT prolongation), and increased sudden cardiac mortality rates. Reports of sudden death in children treated with psychotropic drugs have raised concerns about cardiovascular monitoring and risk stratification. QTd analysis has not been investigated in very young children treated with antipsychotic drugs. In the present retrospective chart review study, we calculated QT interval, QTd, and their rate-corrected values in very young children treated with antipsychotics.

Methods: The charts of 12 children (ages 5.8 ± 0.98 yr; 4 girls, 8 boys) were examined before initiation of antipsychotic treatment [risperidone ($n = 7$), clotinapine ($n = 1$), and propericiazine ($n = 4$)] and during the maintenance period after achieving a positive clinical response. Three children were concomitantly maintained on methylphenidate. QT interval, QTd, and their rate-corrected values were calculated.

Results: QT interval, QTd, and their rate-corrected values were all within normal values both before and after successful drug treatment.

Conclusions: This preliminary, naturalistic, small-scale study suggests that antipsychotic treatment, with or without methylphenidate, in very young children is not commonly associated with significant alterations of QT interval and dispersion, suggesting the relative safety of these agents in this unique age group.

INTRODUCTION

PSYCHOTROPIC DRUGS, such as antipsychotics and antidepressants, have long been associated with risks for cardiac arrhythmias and sudden cardiac death (for a review, see Witchel et al., 2003). Furthermore, within the same class there might be a differential cardiac risk. For example, among the antidepressants, the tricyclic agents are associated with increased risk

[1] Geha Mental Health Center, Liaison Service, Rabin Medical Center, Petach Tikva, Israel.
[2] Child Psychiatry Day Hospital, Geha Mental Health Center, Petach Tikva, Israel.
[3] Child Cardiology Department, Schneider Children Hospital, Petach Tikva, Israel.
[4] Felsenstein Medical Research Center, Rabin Medical Center, Petach Tikva, Israel.
[5] Sackler Faculty of Medicine, Tel Aviv University, Tel Aviv, Israel.

for lethal cardiac arrhythmias through iatrogenic electrocardiographic (ECG) abnormalities, such as QT interval prolongation (Vieweg and Wood, 2004). A series of case reports has also associated antipsychotic treatment with the risk for serious ventricular arrhythmias and sudden cardiac death (Glassman and Bigger, 2001). Cohort studies of schizophrenia patients maintained on various antipsychotic agents have reported excess cardiovascular disease-related mortality (Ray et al. 2001; Curkendall et al. 2004). Moreover, clinical and animal studies of antipsychotic drugs point toward ECG abnormalities, including QTc prolongation, which is thought to increase the risk for serious ventricular arrhythmias (Zarate and Patel, 2001). In addition, an increase in cardiac death was reported with combined antipsychotic treatment (Waddington et al., 1998; Joukamaa et al., 2006).

Day et al. (1990) suggested that the maximal interlead difference in QT intervals in the surface 12-lead electrocardiogram (ECG), that is, the QT dispersion (QTd), may serve as a measure of myocardial repolarization inhomogeneity. Data from recent studies suggest that QTd usually measures 20 to 50 msec in normal subjects and 60 to 80 msec in patients with cardiac disease (Barr et al., 1994; Higham and Campbell, 1994; Statters et al., 1994; van de Loo et al., 1994; Roukema et al., 1998). Several researchers have therefore postulated that it may be a predisposing factor for arrhythmic events and sudden death (Manttari et al., 1997). According to experimental and clinical studies, the autonomic nervous system (ANS) modulates both the duration of cardiac ventricular repolarization, by conditioning ventricular repolarization to alterations in heart rate, and the spatial heterogeneity of repolarization. Ishida et al. (1997) correlated the circadian variation of QTd with heart rate variability (HRV) in normal subjects, using 24-h ECG recordings. Recently, Nakagawa et al. (1999) used the head-up tilt test to evaluate the influence of the ANS on HRV and QTd. QTd was positively correlated with HRV measures, indicating increased sympathetic tone and/or decreased vagal tone. Furthermore, plasma norepinephrine concentrations correlated positively with QTd. QTc interval and QTd values of >500 msec and >100

msec, respectively, are considered abnormal in adults (Haddad and Anderson, 2002). It is not clear whether these values should be adjusted for the pediatric population. However, children treated with psychotropic agents with QTc values >450 msec for boys and >460 msec for girls should be referred to a pediatric cardiologist (McNally et al., 2006).

The use of QTd in psychiatry was first reported in the context of electroconvulsive therapy, in order to depict patient vulnerability to arrhythmic events immediately after treatment (Guler et al., 1998). Indeed, the results paralleled the sequence of change in autonomic modulation: a vagal discharge followed by a sympathetic surge (Gaines and Rees, 1992). Recently, Nahshoni et al. (2000a) found that physically healthy patients with major depression have significantly higher values of QTd than normal controls. This observation supports the hypothesis of reduced vagal modulation in major depression, an alteration that may be a risk factor for sudden death in depressed patients (Agelink et al., 2002; Nahshoni et al., 2004b). Increased QTd was also reported for social anxiety disorder, pointing toward cardiac ANS imbalance (Nahshoni et al., 2004c). Recently, QTd analysis has been used in eating disorders and might show promise as a noninvasive measure for cardiac risk in anorectic patients (Takimoto et al., 2004). QTd analysis has also been recently used in an effort to evaluate the cardiotoxic effects of neuroleptics. Two reports have detected QT interval prolongation without a significant effect on QTd (Hartigan-Go et al., 1996; Warner et al., 1996), and a later report detected both increased QTc and QTc dispersion (Kitayama et al., 1999) in schizophrenia patients maintained on a long-term antipsychotic drug regimen. Recently, Nahshoni et al. (2004d) reported that, in psychotic schizophrenia inpatients maintained on antipsychotics and undergoing electroconvulsive therapy, QTd and the rate-corrected QTd showed a significant decrease after electroconvulsive therapy, concomitant with improvement in psychosis.

Early reports on sudden cardiac death of children and adolescents treated with psychotropic agents have raised concern regarding the suitability of psychotropic drug therapy, as well as monitoring and risk stratification schedules in this unique group of patients (Werry et al., 1995; Gutgesell et al., 1999). Today, the use of psychotropic agents, including psychostimulants, for children, is becoming more and more frequent (Nissen, 2006). This might be due to the greater availability of new agents with better side-effect profiles than the first-generation agents, concomitant with the remarkable progress and insight into the diagnosis of mental and emotional disorders among children. However, to date, to our best knowledge, there are no reports on the influence of antipsychotic agents on the QTd in children. It is of note that most studies in this area focused on QTc, but QTd is an important additional risk indicator for subsequent cardiovascular events, particularly arrhythmias and especially in vulnerable individuals (Tutar et al., 1998).

Since neuroleptic treatment might be associated with possible cardiac arrhythmias and autonomic imbalance, the present study was designed to assess QTd as a measure of cardiac ANS activity and repolarization heterogeneity, in relation to short-term clinical response of young children, before initiating treatment with antipsychotic drugs and during the maintenance period.

METHODS

This retrospective chart review study included 12 consecutive children (ages 5.8 ± 0.98 yr; 4 girls, 8 boys) admitted to the Psychiatry Day Department for very young children (age range from 4 to 7 yr) at Geha Mental Health Center, Petach Tikva, Israel. The diagnoses were established according to DSM-IV-TR criteria, following an interview according to the guidelines of the Schedule for Affective Disorders and Schizophrenia for School-Aged Children Lifetime Version (K-SADS-PL) (Shanee et al., 1997), as a part of a large follow-up study of the effectiveness of treatment in this day department. These diagnoses included pervasive developmental disorder (PDD) ($n = 5$), oppositional defiant disorder (ODD) ($n = 3$), attention deficit and hyperactivity disorder (ADHD) ($n = 3$), brief psychotic disorder ($n = 1$), psychotic disorder, NOS ($n = 1$), disruptive behavior disorder, NOS ($n = 1$), and mental re-

tardation ($n = 1$). Some patients had more than one diagnosis.

None of the included patients had a history, signs, or symptoms of cardiovascular, pulmonary, neurological, or endocrine disorders. As a standard practice of this day department, all patients underwent a comprehensive clinical examination, including a standard 12-lead surface ECG and routine blood biochemistry, which were within normal limits. An ECG tracing was performed before commencing with psychotropic drug treatment and again after a stabilization period on a clinically effective drug regimen. The average follow-up period was 181 ± 99 days. These ECG tracings were first evaluated by an experienced child cardiologist (MB), a routine policy of the department. All tracings were within normal limits consistent with the children's ages, except one child with P wave abnormal morphology, who then underwent an echocardiogram examination, which was found to be normal.

All the included patients were psychotropic treatment naïve before the initiation of drug treatment. The patients started and were maintained on the following drug therapy: atypical antipsychotics: risperidone (0.125 to 0.5 mg/d, $n = 7$); conventional antipsychotics: propericiazine (2 to 3 mg/d, $n = 4$) or clotiapine (20 mg/d, $n = 1$); stimulants: methylphenidate (Ritalin, 5 mg/d, $n = 2$) or Concerta (18 mg/d, $n = 1$). Three children were treated with a combination of antipsychotic and a stimulant (Table 1). Over the entire course of the study, the drug regimen was not changed. The study was approved by the Helsinki committee of Geha Mental Health Center and, due to the retrospective chart review nature of the study, no informed consent was required.

ECG recordings and QT analysis

As a standard of this center, the ECG recordings were done in the same quiet room after 10 min of rest in a supine position, between 10:00 AM and 12:00 noon (to avoid circadian bias). The ECG recordings were performed at least 2 h after a light breakfast. None of the subjects consumed caffeine beverages. The second ECG tracings of these in-patients (in the day department) were recorded in the same condi-

TABLE 1. DEMOGRAPHIC AND CLINICAL DATA OF THE STUDY POPULATION

Age (years)	Gender	Diagnosis	CGI-S	Treatment (mg/day)	Follow-up duration (days)
6	M	ADHD	4	Risperidone, 0.5 Ritalin, 5	126
7	F	ODD, ADHD	4	Concerta, 18 Propericiazine, 3	225
4.5	M	ADHD	4	Propericiazine 2	264
6	F	PDD (unspecified)	3	Propericiazine, 2, Ritalin, 5	165
4.5	M	ODD	2	Risperidone, 0.25	188
6	M	ODD, disruptive behavior disorder (NOS)	3	Clotiapine, 20	200
7	F	Psychotic disorder (NOS)	5	Risperidone, 0.5	70
6.5	F	PDD, mental retardation	5	Propericiazine, 3	133
5	M	PDD (NOS)	4	Risperidone, 0.5	52
7	M	PDD (NOS)	3	Risperidone, 0.5	425
4.5	M	PDD (NOS)	3	Risperidone, 0.5	113
6	M	Brief psychotic disorder	4	Risperidone, 0.25	213

ADHD = attention-deficit/hyperactivity disorder; CGI-S = Clinical Global Impression-Severity, ODD = oppositional defiant disorder; PDD = pervasive developmental disorder; NOS = not otherwise specified.

tions after 1 to 9 months of stabilization on the maximal effective dose, as a precautious, routine, clinical follow-up practice to monitor possible drug-induced cardiac adverse effects.

All subjects were in normal sinus rhythm and none had bundle branch block or signs of cardiomyopathy. All QT interval measurements were performed manually with a caliber with an accuracy of 20 msec (20 msec = 0.5 mm with a paper speed of 25 mm/sec). The QT interval was measured from the onset of the QRS complex to the end of the T wave, defined as the return to the T-P isoelectric line. If a U wave was present, the QT interval was measured to the nadir between the T and the U waves. If the T wave could not be clearly determined, that lead was excluded. Only recordings with more than eight analyzable leads were included. QTd was defined as the difference between the longest and shortest QT intervals; rate correction was performed with Bazett's formula: QTc = QT/square root of the RR interval in milliseconds (Bazett, 1920). RR interval is the interbeat interval between normal heartbeats. This traditional corrections procedure is intended to obviate the dependence of the QT interval on the heart rate.

The QT interval assessors were blind to the clinical diagnosis and status of the patients. Intra- and interrater reliability values were evaluated in 10 randomly selected ECG tracings. Pearson's correlation analysis was used for the evaluation of these reliability values.

Clinical rating

The Clinical Global Impressions Scale-Severity (CGI-S) was scored concomitantly with the ECG recordings (Guy, 1976).

Statistical analysis

All data are presented as mean ± SD. Statistical comparisons of the clinical and electrocardiographic measures were performed by two-tailed Student's t-test. Intra- and interobserver reproducibilities were tested by means of Pearson's correlation analysis, using GraphPad InStat software (GraphPad Software, Inc., San Diego, CA). Statistical significance was accepted at a p level <0.05

RESULTS

The epidemiological and clinical data of our cohort is presented in Table 1. Within an average follow-up period of 181 ± 99 days, a significant decrease in scores on the CGIS was noted (from 3.67 ± 0.89 to 3.17 ± 0.83; $t = 2.2$, df = 11, $p = 0.026$). The cohort's mean electrocardiographic measures are summarized in Table 2. RR intervals, QT intervals, QTc, QTd, and the rate-corrected QTd were all within normal limits. No significant changes were noted after initiating drug treatment. Intra- and interobserver variabilities were highly reproducible ($r = 0.71$, $p = 0.02$; and $r = 0.65$, $p = 0.04$, respectively). No cardiovascular events were reported.

Although the results were calculated for the whole group, we also attempted to discern the possible separate influences of risperidone, as an antipsychotic drug, on the ECG indexes. Thus, the ECG measures of a subgroup of 7 children who were administered risperidone (one of them was concomitantly maintained on methylphenidate; Table 1) were calculated. The results of this subgroup were also within normal limits, both before and after drug treatment and did not alter significantly following the risperidone administration (Table 3).

DISCUSSION

The aim of this follow-up naturalistic report was to evaluate possible alterations in QTd and their rate-corrected values in very young children before and after drug treatment with risperidone, clotiapine, and propericiazine, alone or in combination with methylphenidate. The major finding of our study was that all electrocardiographic measures were within normal limits, both before and along the medication–maintenance phase, that is, after achieving clinical response. Our results were also highly reproducible. It is of note that the mean QTc and QTd values in our cohort of very young patients (4.5 to 7 yr) are in the range of a previous large-scale ($n = 372$) study in normal schoolchildren, aged 7 to 18 yr: QTc, 423 ± 22 msec; QTd, 30 ± 10 msec (Tutar et al., 1998).

Although, to the best of our knowledge, our study is the first attempt to calculate QT dispersion in very young medicated children, several limitations are worth mentioning. First, the small sample size is a significant limitation of the present study. Thus, larger cohorts are mandatory. Second, there is a lack of duplicate ECG measurement, because both QTc and QTd have intra-individual variability (Malik, 2000). Third, some of the children were maintained on more than one medication. In general, it would be preferable to control for ECG abnormalities under a single medication. In other words, theoretically, more than one medication might have an additive negative effect on QT interval and its dispersion. However, 58% ($n = 7$) of the children in our study were maintained on risperidone, as a single antipsychotic drug, and this subgroup did not show any abnormal

TABLE 2. ELECTROCARDIOGRAPHIC AND CLINICAL DATA [MEAN ± SD (RANGE)] IN TOTAL CHILDREN COHORT ($n = 12$) BEFORE AND ALONG THE MAINTENANCE PHASE

Parameter	Pretreatment	Maintenance	p Value
RRI (msec)	662 ± 96 (560–872)	732 ± 158 (560–872)	0.054
QT interval (msec)	355 ± 22 (333–387)	367 ± 16 (333–393)	0.13
QTc	435 ± 31 (388–465)	432 ± 33 (372–465)	0.75
QTd (msec)	39 ± 11 (27–60)	38 ± 15 (13–67)	0.95
Rate-corrected QTd (msec)	48 ± 15 (30–80)	47 ± 19 (14–89)	0.84
CGI-S	3.7 ± 0.9 (2–5)	3.2 ± 0.8 (2–5)	0.026 ($t = 2.2$)

CGIS = Clinical Global Impressions Scale-Severity; QTc = QT corrected; QTd = QT dispersion; RRI = RR interval.

TABLE 3. ELECTROCARDIOGRAPHIC AND CLINICAL DATA [MEAN ± SD (RANGE)] IN THE
RISPERIDONE SUBGROUP ($n = 7$) BEFORE AND ALONG THE MAINTENANCE PHASE

Parameter	Pretreatment	Maintenance	p Value
RRI (msec)	650 ± 78 (560–800)	705 ± 176 (560–1080)	0.28
QT interval (msec)	355 ± 16 (333–380)	366 ± 11 (353–387)	0.17
QTc	442 ± 31 (403–490)	442 ± 37 (372–490)	0.97
QTd (msec)	41 ± 9 (33–60)	43 ± 15 (27–66)	0.64
Rate-corrected QTd (msec)	51 ± 13 (41–80)	53 ± 20 (35–89)	0.82
CGI-S	3.6 ± 1.0 (2–5)	3.1 ± 0.9 (2–5)	0.078

CGI-S = Clinical Global Impressions Scale-Severity; QTc = QT corrected; QTd = QT dispersion; RRI = RR interval.

ECG measures, both before and along the maintenance period. Thus, it is suggested that risperidone, given in the doses in our study, did not confer a cardiac risk for the children along the study period. It is of note that antipsychotic monotherapy was employed in only about half our cohort due to the naturalistic nature of the present study.

Although our study design was retrospective, it did not have the limitations of a cross-sectional study, and each subject served as his or her own control. Fortunately, the drug regimen was not altered throughout the study. Thus, the impact of drug treatment on the ECG tracings was minimized by keeping the drug regimen fixed throughout the whole study course. We also attempted to control for organic causes that might influence the ECG measures by selecting physically healthy children. Issues such as smoking and alcohol or drug abuse were not relevant in the context of the present study. Diurnal variations in QTd were minimized by performing the ECG recordings during the morning hours. We could not account for the effect of symptom severity and improvement on QTd. For this purpose, another design should be implemented, such as a long-term follow-up study with concomitant monitoring of several QTd assessments, with corresponding appropriate detailed clinical ratings. However, since most

of the patients improved significantly during the study, while the QTd values remained unaltered, it seems that the severity of the symptoms does not affect the cardiac measures.

Measurement of the QT interval and its dispersion is not standardized. In this study we used the method suggested by Day et al. (1990) and Barr et al. (1994). Correction of the QT interval using Bazett's formula is controversial because of the hypercorrection with high heart rate and hypocorrection with low heart rate (Schweitzer, 1992). Of note, our cohort did not display a significant change in heart rate as measured from the ECG traces; hence, this limitation was minimized.

The mean values of QTd and the rate-corrected QTd in our study are found to be comparable to those reported previously for normal control groups of children (Tutar et al., 1998; Vialle et al., 1999).

In adult patients who receive antipsychotic drugs (e.g., schizophrenia patients), there are reports of increased cardiac death rates, which might be caused from both abnormal cardiac autonomic nervous system activity and pro-arrhythmic drug effects. It was hypothesized that part of the pathophysiology might stem from the presence of acute psychotic exacerbations in adult schizophrenia patients. Fortunately, such a phenomenon was not detected in our very young cohort. Furthermore, along the study period, no clinically relevant cardiovascular events were noticed.

In conclusion, calculation of QTc interval and QTd from the standard surface ECG seems to serve as a simple and reliable noninvasive tool for the assessment of repolarization heterogeneity of the ventricular myocardium. Increased QTd has been found to indicate an increased risk for arrhythmia and sudden death in various diseases. The present small-scale retrospective study did not show any abnormal changes in QT interval, QTd, and their rate-corrected values in a unique cohort of very young children maintained on antipsychotic treatment, suggesting the relative safety of these agents in this age group. It is of note that our findings apply to antipsychotic treatment that consisted mostly of risperidone. Obviously, other antipsychotic treatments need to be investigated, particularly ziprasidone and sertindole.

DISCLOSURES

There are no conflicts of interest for Drs. Nahshoni, Shpitzer, Berant, Shoval, Zalsman, or Weizman.

REFERENCES

Agelink MW, Boz C, Ullrich H, Andrich J: Relationship between major depression and heart rate variability. Clinical consequences and implications for antidepressive treatment. Psychiatry Res 113:139–149, 2002.

Barr CS, Naas A, Freeman M, Struthers AD: QT dispersion and sudden unexpected death in chronic heart failure. Lancet 343:327–329, 1994.

Bazett HC: The time relations of the blood-pressure changes after excision of the adrenal glands, with some observations on blood volume changes. J Physiology 53:320–339, 1920.

Curkendall SM, Mo J, Glasser DB, Rose Stang M, Jones JK: Cardiovascular disease in patients with schizophrenia in Saskatchewan. Can J Clin Psychiatry. 65:715–720, 2004.

Day CP, McComb JM, Campbell RWF: QT dispersion: An indication of arrhythmia risk in patients with long QT intervals. Br Heart J 63:342–344, 1990.

Gaines G.Y., III, Rees DI: Anesthetic considerations for electroconvulsive therapy. South Med J 85:469–482, 1992.

Glassman AH, Bigger JT: Antipsychotic drugs: Prolonged QTc interval, torsade de pointes, and sudden death. Am J Psychiatry 158:1774–1782, 2001.

Guler N, Bilge M, Eryonucu B, Kutanis R, Erkoc R: The effect of electroconvulsive therapy on QT dispersion. Acta Cardiologia 53:355–358, 1998.

Gutgesell H, Atkins D, Barst R, Buck M, Franklin W, Humes R, Ringel R, Shaddy R, Taubert KA: AHA Scientific Statement: Cardiovascular monitoring of children and adolescents receiving psychotropic drugs. J Am Acad Child Adolesc Psychiatry 38:1047–1050, 1999.

Guy W: Clinical global impressions. In: ECDEU Assessment Manual for Psychopharmacology. Revised DHEW Pub. (ADM). Rockville, MD: National Institute for Mental Health, 1976, pp 218–222.

Haddad PM, Anderson IM: Antipsychotic-related QTc prolongation, torsade de pointes and sudden death. Drugs 62:1649–1671, 2002.

Hartigan-Go K, Batemen N, Nyberg G, Martensson E, Thomas SHL: Concentration-related pharmacodynamic effect of thioridazine and its metabolites in humans. Clin Pharmacol Ther 60:543–553, 1996.

Higham PD, Campbell RW: QT dispersion. Br Heart J 71:508–510, 1994.

Ishida S, Nakagawa M, Fujino T, Yonemochi H, Saikawa T, Ito M: Circadian variation of QT interval dispersion: Correlation with heart rate variability. J Electrocardiol 30:205–210, 1997.

Joukamaa M, Heliovaara M, Knekt P, Aromaa A, Raitasalo R, Lehtinen V: Schizophrenia, neuroleptic medication and mortality. Br J Psychiatry 188:122–127, 2006.

Kitayama H, Kiuchi K, Nejima J, Katoh T, Takano T, Hayakawa H: Long-term treatment with antipsychotic drugs in conventional doses prolonged QTc dispersion, but did not increase ventricular tachyarrhythmias in patients with schizophrenia in the absence of cardiac disease. Eur J Clin Pharmacol 55:259–262, 1999.

Malik M: QT dispersion: Time for an obituary? Eur Heart J 21:955–957, 2000.

Manttari M, Oikarinen L, Manninen V, Viitasalo M: QT dispersion as a risk factor for sudden cardiac death and fatal myocardial infarction in a coronary risk population. Heart 78:268–272, 1997.

McNally P, McNicholas F, Oslizlok P: The QT interval and psychotropic medications in children: Recommendations for clinicians. Eur Child Adolesc Psychiatry. [Epub ahead of printing], 2006.

Nahshoni E, Aizenberg D, Strasberg B, Dorfman P, Sigler M, Imbar S, Weizman A: QT dispersion in the surface electrocardiogram in elderly patients with major depression. J Affective Disord 60:197–200, 2000a.

Nahshoni E, Aravot D, Aizenberg D, Sigler M, Zalsman G, Strasberg B, Imbar S, Adler E, Weizman A: Heart rate variability in patients with major depression. Psychosomatics 45: 129–134, 2004b.

Nahshoni E, Gur S, Marom S, Levin JB, Weizman A, Hermesh H: QT dispersion in patients with social phobia. J Affective Disord 78:21–26, 2004c.

Nahshoni E, Manor N, Bar F, Stryjer R, Zalsman G, Weizman A. Alterations in QT dispersion in medicated schizophrenia patients following electroconvulsive therapy. Eur Neuropsychopharmacol 14:121–125, 2004d.

Nakagawa M, Takahashi N, Iwao T, Yonemochi H, Ooie T, Hara M, Saikawa T, Ito M: Evaluation of autonomic influence on QT dispersion using head-up tilt test in healthy subjects. Pacing Clin Electrophysiol 22: 1158–1163, 1999.

Nissen SE: ADHD drugs and cardiovascular risk. N Engl J Med 354:1445–1448, 2006.

Ray WA, Meredith S, Thapa PB, Meador KG, Hall K, Murray KT: Antipsychotics and the risk of sudden cardiac death. Arch Gen Psychiatry 58:1161–1167, 2001.

Roukema G, Singh JP, Meijs M, Carvalho C, Hart G: Effects of exercise-induced ischemia on QT interval dispersion. Am Heart J 135:88–92, 1998.

Schweitzer P: The values and limitations of the QT interval in clinical practice. Am Heart J 124:1121–1124, 1992.

Shanee N, Apter A, Weizman A: Psychometric properties of the K-SADS-PL in an Israeli adolescent clinical population. Isr J Psychiatry Related Sci 34:179–186, 1997.

Statters DJ, Malik M, Ward DE, Camm AJ: QT dispersion: Problems of methodology and clinical significance. J Cardiovasc Electrophysiol 5:672–685, 1994.

Takimoto Y, Yoshiuchi K, Kumano H, Yamanaka G, Sasaki T, Suematsu H, Nagakawa Y, Kuboki T: QT interval and QT dispersion in eating disorders. Psychother Psychosom 73:324–328, 2004.

Tutar HE, Ocal B, Imamoglu A, Atalay S: Dispersion of QT and QTc interval in healthy children, and effects of sinus arrhythmia on QT dispersion. Heart 80:77–79, 1998.

van de Loo A, Arendts W, Hohloser SH: Variability of QT dispersion measurements in the surface electrocardiogram in patients with acute myocardial infarction and in normal subjects. Am J Cardiol 74: 1113–1118, 1994.

Vialle E, Albalkhi R, Zimmerman M, Friedli B: Normal values of signal-averaged electrocardiographic parameters and QT dispersion in infants and children. Cardiol Young 9:556–561, 1999.

Vieweg WV, Wood MA: Tricyclic antidepressants, QT interval prolongation, and torsade de pointes. Psychosomatics 45:371–377, 2004.

Waddington JL, Youssef HA, Kinsella A: Mortality in schizophrenia. Antipsychotic polypharmacy and absence of adjunctive anticholinergics over the course of a 10-year prospective study. Br J Psychiatry 173: 325–329, 1998.

Warner JP, Barnes TRE, Henry JA: Electrocardiographic changes in patients receiving neuroleptic medication. Acta Psychiatr Scand 93:311–313, 1996.

Werry JS, Biederman J, Thisted R, Greenhill L, Ryan N. Resolved: Cardiac arrhythmias make desipramine an unacceptable choice in children. J Am Acad Child Adolesc Psychiatry 34:1239–1245, 1995.

Witchel HJ, Hancox JC, Nutt DJ: Psychotropic drugs, cardiac arrhythmia, and sudden death. J Clin Psychopharmacol 23:58–77, 2003.

Zarate CA, Patel J: Sudden cardiac death and antipsychotic drugs. Arch Gen Psychiatry 58:1168–1171, 2001.

ADVANCES IN PRESCHOOL PSYCHOPHARMACOLOGY
© 2009 Mary Ann Liebert, Inc.
140 Huguenot Street, 3rd Floor
New Rochelle, NY 10801-5215

Psychotherapeutic Medication Prevalence in Medicaid-Insured Preschoolers

Julie M. Zito, Ph.D.,[1] Daniel J. Safer, M.D.,[2] Satish Valluri, M.S., M.P.H.,[3]
James F. Gardner, Sc.M.,[3] James J. Korelitz, Ph.D.,[4] and Donald R. Mattison, M.D.[5]

ABSTRACT

Objective: To update knowledge of the prevalence of the use of psychotherapeutic medications in preschoolers with Medicaid insurance as requested by the Best Pharmaceuticals for Children Act of 2002 (BPCA).

Method: Prescription, enrollment, and outpatient visit data from 7 state Medicaid programs were used to identify 274,518 youths continuously enrolled in 2001 and aged 2 to 4 on January 1, 2001. Annual prevalence of use was defined as one or more dispensed prescriptions for a psychotherapeutic medication and adjusted for anticonvulsant and anxiolytic/sedative/hypnotic use according to ICD-9 diagnostic groupings. Prevalence ratios adjusted for age, race/ethnicity, and gender were estimated.

Results: 2.30% (CI = 2.24, 2.36) of preschoolers received one or more dispensings for a psychotherapeutic medication in 2001, approximately doubling the usage of comparable youth from 2 other state Medicaid programs studied in 1995. Boys were 2.4 times more likely than girls to receive psychotherapeutic medication. Whites were 4 times more likely than Hispanics and twice as likely as Blacks to receive medication for psychiatric or behavioral conditions. Since the mid-1990s, usage increased, especially for atypical antipsychotics and antidepressants. The prominent use of anticonvulsants (78.8%) and anxiolytic/sedative/hypnotic drugs (91.4%) in those with no psychiatric diagnosis, but with other medical diagnoses, shows that much use therein reflects treatment for seizures, rather than mood stabilization, and for minor medical conditions, rather than psychiatric disorders.

Conclusion: Preschool psychotherapeutic medication use increased across ages 2 to 4 for stimulants, antipsychotics, and antidepressants, reflecting use for psychiatric/behavioral disorders. However, the use of anxiolytic/sedative/hypnotics and anticonvulsants was more stable across these years, suggesting medical usage. Additional research to assess the benefits and risks of psychotherapeutic drugs is needed, particularly when such usage is off-label for both psychiatric and nonpsychiatric conditions.

---

[1]Department of Pharmaceutical Health Services Research, School of Pharmacy and Department of Psychiatry, School of Medicine, University of Maryland, Baltimore, Maryland.

[2]Johns Hopkins Medical Institutions, Departments of Psychiatry and Pediatrics, Baltimore, Maryland.

[3]Department of Pharmaceutical Health Services Research, School of Pharmacy, University of Maryland, Baltimore, Maryland.

[4]Westat, 1650 Research Blvd., Rockville, Maryland.

[5]U.S. Public Health Service, Obstetric and Pediatric Pharmacology Branch, National Institutes of Health, Bethesda, Maryland.

Funding for this study was provided by the National Institute of Child Health and Human Development.

INTRODUCTION

THE UTILIZATION OF psychotherapeutic medication for preschool children has prominently increased over the last decade (Zito et al., 2000, 2003; Cooper et al., 2004; Habel et al., 2005; Patel et al., 2005). By insurance coverage type, the use of these drugs has been higher in Medicaid than in managed care HMO populations (Zito et al., 2000, 2003; DeBar et al., 2003), and in those insured through parent employment policies (Patel et al., 2005). No national medication prevalence figures are available in the United States, but Medicaid preschoolers represent over 40% of all preschoolers (American Academy of Pediatrics, 2001), so updating usage in this insurance population is critical to understanding approved and off-label treatment patterns and trends. Such information is also requested by the Best Pharmaceuticals for Children Act of 2002 (BPCA) to assist in determining which drugs need additional study to improve appropriate use in children. In addition, it should be noted that medications typically characterized as psychotropic or psychotherapeutic may have different uses in Medicaid preschoolers, where there are more chronically ill youths than in the general population (Shatin et al., 1998).

Another source of prevalence variation is geographical region, which is sizable (Olfson et al., 2002; Shatin & Drinkard, 2002; Cox et al., 2003; MMWR, 2005; Patel et al., 2005). Prevalence also varies with race/ethnicity, with Whites showing a two- to three-fold greater use than non-Whites in several state population-based studies (Zito et al., 1998; Safer & Malever, 2000). Consequently, it is an advantage to have large multistate data from different regions within the United States with their different racial/ethnic populations.

Previous data on preschoolers are limited either by sample size (Olfson et al., 2002) or in generalizability to the larger Medicaid population (Zito et al., 2000) and are rapidly becoming outdated. To address this problem, a descriptive study was undertaken to assess annual prevalence of use of psychotherapeutic drugs among preschoolers and to assess age, gender, and race/ethnicity disparities.

METHOD

The data were extracted from a large data set of 7 state Medicaid programs covering 2.27 million youth 2 to 17 year olds that originated from CMS produced-MAX administrative claims files. These included eligibility files for demographic variables, medical encounter files for ICD-9 coded medical diagnoses, and pharmacy claims files for drug use information. The primary data set was created to assess the frequency of use of pediatric medications as mandated by the Best Pharmaceuticals for Children Act (2002) National Institute of Child Health and Human Development, 2006). For the present study, youth aged 2 to 4 years on January 1 2001 who were continuously enrolled 10 or more months were analyzed according to year of age, race/ethnicity, and gender. Annual psychotherapeutic prevalence was defined as having one or more prescriptions dispensed for a psychotherapeutic drug (i.e., drugs intended to treat emotional or behavioral disorders). Seven classes of psychotherapeutic drugs were included in the analysis and subclasses were made for 5 of them: stimulants (methylphenidate, amphetamine), antipsychotics (conventional vs. atypical), antidepressants (selective serotonin reuptake inhibitors, SSRI; tricyclic antidepressants (TCAs), and other), anxiolytic/sedative/hypnotics (ASH) (benzodiazepine; clonazepam/diazepam; other ASH and hydroxyzine); anticonvulsants (mood stabilizers and others), lithium, and α-agonists. Anticonvulsant mood stabilizers included carbamazepine, divalproex, oxcarbazepine, and gabapentin, as suggested by prior research (Zito et al., 2006).

To measure psychotherapeutic drug usage in preschoolers, conservative estimates of psychiatric usage were made for 2 classes with very high usage: anticonvulsants and anxiolytic/sedative/hypnotics. ICD-9 CM codes from outpatient visits at any time during the year were used to categorize psychiatric disorders ($290.\times$-$319.\times$) and seizure disorder ($345.\times$); the remaining diagnoses were grouped as other medical diagnoses. The diagnostic categories associated with anticonvulsant users were identified according to whether there was a psychiatric diagnosis, a seizure diagnosis, both, neither, or no diagnosis. Only anticonvulsant users with a psychiatric diagnosis were included in the estimate of psychotherapeutic medication prevalence. Likewise, youth with anxiolytic/sedative/hypnotic (ASH) use were included if they had a psychiatric diagnosis, but not if they had a nonpsychiatric medical diagnosis or no diagnosis. This analytic method was utilized to reassess the psychotropic prevalence among 2 to 4 year-olds in the 1995 two-state Medicaid analysis (Zito et al., 2000). To establish disparities according to gender, race/ethnicity (White, Black, Hispanic, and Other (Alaskan Natives, Hawaiian, Pacific Islanders and Asians) and age (2, 3, and 4 years of age on January 1, 2001), adjusted prevalence ratios and 95% confidence intervals were analyzed using a GENMOD linear regression model (SAS vs. 9.13). Descriptive statistics included annual percent of prevalence, prevalence ratios, and frequency of use of drug class and subclass by year of age. Cross-tabulations were used to assess the frequency of youth with psychiatric diagnoses, seizure diagnoses, other diagnoses, and no diagnosis among those with dispensed anticonvulsants, and the frequency of psychiatric and nonpsychiatric medical diagnoses and no diagnosis among users of anxiolytic/sedative/hypnotics.

RESULTS

The prevalence of any psychotherapeutic medication use by Medicaid-insured youth in 7 states of the United States in 2001 was 2.3% among 274,518 continuously enrolled preschoolers (who represented 58.3% of all enrolled preschoolers). Boys had a prevalence of 3.21%, while girls had a prevalence of 1.34%. Whites had the highest prevalence (3.13%), followed by Blacks 1.55% and Hispanics 0.77%. Other race/ethnicity was 0.42%, which is a very unstable estimate because of very low usage among various Asian groups and Native Americans. The prevalence by year of age was 0.96% for age 2, 2.08% for age 3, and 3.99% for age 4. Overall, the prevalence ratios show that boys were 2.4 time more likely than girls and Whites were 4 times more likely than Hispan-

ics and twice as likely as Blacks to have psychotherapeutic dispensings. Four-year-olds were 4.3 times more likely than 2-year-olds, with 3-year-olds being intermediate in their likelihood of being medicated (Table 1).

To compare these 2001 seven-state data with previously published estimates of psychotherapeutic drug prevalence for 2- to 4-year-olds, we adjusted the 1995 Medicaid data from a mid-west and a mid-Atlantic state (Zito et al., 2003), which averaged 1.03% after removing 78.8% of anticonvulsants and 91.4% of anxiolytic/sedative/hypnotics from the 1995 estimates of preschooler prevalence. The result is an estimated doubling of usage in the 6-year period from1995 through 2001.

Table 2 reveals that two-thirds of users of psychotherapeutic medication received stimulants. Stimulants were fairly evenly split between methylphenidate and amphetamine products. Antipsychotics represented 17% of the total psychotherapeutic users, with 96% of these users receiving atypical antipsychotics. The frequency of antidepressant use was 20.5% of the total, and the 3 antidepressant subclasses proportionally were not remarkably different. α-Agonists were the second most commonly dispensed class (26%). Among ASH-treated youth, 79.6% received hydroxyzine. Anticonvulsants represented 11.2% of psychotherapeutic users, with the mood-stabilizer type being predominant.

A cross-tabulation analysis of two ICD-9 diagnostic groups (psychiatric vs. nonpsychiatric disorders) by ASH users revealed that only 8.6% of these youth had a psychiatric diagnosis, suggesting a predominance of nonpsychiatric medical usage (Table 3). Likewise, for anticonvulsant use, a cross-tabulation analysis of psychiatric versus seizure disorder revealed that only 21.2% of these medication users had a psychiatric diagnosis (Table 4). Regardless of diagnostic grouping, certain proportions of anticonvulsant usage were unexpectedly high, that is, phenobarbital (17.4%) and topiramate (11.7%) (Table 4).

Several patterns according to age were distinct. As age increased, α-agonist use increased, but to a lesser extent than the increase in stimulant use. Also, as age increased, psychiatric drug usage increased [stimulants (6.6-fold), an-

TABLE 1. PSYCHOTHERAPEUTIC DRUG PREVALENCE OF USE (PER 100 MEDICAID-ENROLLED YOUTH)[a] FOR THE TOTAL POPULATION AND RACE/ETHNICITY-, GENDER- AND AGE-SPECIFIC GROUPS (CY 2001) AMONG 274,518 PRESCHOOLERS

	Population		Prevalence of any psychotherapeutic use				
Grouping	n	%	n	%	95% CI[b]	Adjusted prevalence[c] ratio, (n = 258,663)	95% CI
Total population	274,518	100	6319	2.30	(2.24, 2.36)	—	—
Gender							
Boys	140,698	48.8	4523	3.21	(3.12, 3.3)	2.40	(2.27, 2.54)
Girls	133,820	51.3	1796	1.34	(1.28, 1.4)	1.00	
Race/ethnicity							
White	119,454	43.5	3742	3.13	(3.03, 3.23)	4.03	(3.59, 4.54)
Black	88,389	32.2	1374	1.55	(0.99, 2.39)	2.03	(1.79, 2.3)
Others	12,147	4.4	51	0.42	(0.05, 9.42)	0.54	(0.4, 0.72)
Hispanic	38,673	14.1	297	0.77	(0.14, 2.82)	1.00	
Unknown	15,885	5.8	855	5.39	(4.02, 7.18)	—	
Age							
4	88,061	32.1	3511	3.99	(3.38, 4.7)	4.25	(3.93, 4.59)
3	90,791	33.1	1888	2.08	(1.5, 2.86)	2.17	(1.99, 2.36)
2	95,666	34.9	920	0.96	(0.47, 1.9)	1.00	

[a]The estimate of prevalence includes only anticonvulsant mood stabilizer and anxiolytic/sedative/hypnotic users with an ICD-9 diagnosis of a psychiatric disorder.
[b]CI = 95% confidence interval.
[c]Prevalence ratios were adjusted for age, race/ethnicity, and gender; for unknown race/ethnicity, the adjustment is for age and gender.

tidepressants (4.1-fold), antipsychotics (3.1-fold)], while drug classes with both psychiatric and medical use [anticonvulsants (1.5-fold) and anxiolytic/sedative/hypnotics (0.5-fold)] either changed slightly or decreased with year of age (data not shown).

DISCUSSION

Preschool psychotherapeutic medication prevalence, although sizably increasing in the past decade, is still far lower than that of older youth. Utilization patterns of medication classes also differ prominently by age. For example, preschoolers in contrast to older youth are given anxiolytic/sedative /hypnotic drugs such as hydroxyzine primarily for medical indications (e.g., allergy or atopic dermatitis). Likewise, anticonvulsants are primarily prescribed for preschoolers for seizure control, whereas over 80% of youth over age 5 are prescribed these drugs for psychiatric indications (Zito et al., 2006). Furthermore, (TCAs) are used almost as much as SSRIs in preschoolers, although published antidepressant trends reveal that SSRIs in preado-

lescent youths are now most prominent and the use of TCAs is rapidly declining (Hunkeler et al., 2005). Interestingly, only 14% of TCA users were associated with a diagnosis of enuresis, which raises questions about the usage in view of the lack of efficacy of TCAs for depression in children. It is also possible that some TCAs are being used to treat insomnia.

Psychotherapeutic drug use was largely explained by stimulants (67.3%) and α-agonists (26.0%). The combined use of these classes should be distinguished from α-agonist monotherapy to better understand the relatively greater use of these drugs in 2-year-olds compared with 3- and 4-year-olds. Compared with 1995 usage in 2 Medicaid states, antipsychotic use in this 7-state data set was 5-fold greater and antidepressant use was 2-fold greater (Zito et al., 2000).

Except for 3 first-generation antipsychotics and the amphetamine compounds, nearly all the other psychotherapeutic medications are prescribed off-label for psychiatric and behavioral treatment of preschool-aged children (Luby, 2006). This has understandably created concern, because adverse drug events (ADEs)

TABLE 2. FREQUENCY (n, %) OF DRUG USE BY AGE GROUP AND TOTAL AMONG 6319 PSYCHOTHERAPEUTIC DRUG MEDICATED PRESCHOOLERS (CLASS IN BOLD, %) AND SUBCLASS USERS (REGULAR TYPE, %)

Psychotherapeutic drugs	2-year-olds		3-year-olds		4-year-olds		Total	
	n	%	n	%	n	%	n	%
Any psychotherapeutic	**920**	**100**	**1888**	**100**	**3511**	**100**	**6319**	**100**
Stimulants	**387**	**42.1**[a]	**1205**	**63.8**	**2658**	**75.7**	**4250**	**67.3**
Methylphenidate	214	55.3[a]	664	55.1	1601	60.2	2479	58.3
Amphetamines	245	63.3	759	63.0	1574	59.2	2578	60.7
Other	2	0.5	11	0.9	17	0.6	30	0.7
Antipsychotics	**150**	**16.3**	**339**	**18.0**	**585**	**16.7**	**1074**	**17.0**
Conventional	17	11.3	24	7.1	31	5.3	72	6.7
Atypical	137	91.3	327	96.5	568	97.1	1032	96.1
Antidepressants	**162**	**17.6**	**372**	**19.7**	**759**	**21.6**	**1293**	**20.5**
SSRI	72	44.4	141	37.9	315	41.5	528	40.8
Other	59	36.4	146	39.3	283	37.3	488	37.7
TCA	38	23.5	117	31.5	241	31.8	396	30.6
Lithium	**5**	**0.5**	**13**	**0.7**	**17**	**0.5**	**35**	**0.6**
α-Agonists	**240**	**26.1**	**539**	**28.5**	**864**	**24.6**	**1643**	**26.0**
Anxiolytic/sedative/ hypnotics[b]	**217**	**23.6**	**256**	**13.6**	**296**	**8.4**	**769**	**12.2**
Benzo–clonazepam/ diazepam	14	6.5	10	3.9	14	4.7	38	4.9
Benzo-other	17	7.8	14	5.5	14	4.7	46	6.0
Hydroxine	169	77.9	205	80.1	238	80.4	612	79.6
Other	46	21.2	45	17.6	55	18.6	146	19.0
Anticonvulsants[a]	**150**	**16.3**	**226**	**12.0**	**330**	**9.4**	**706**	**11.2**
ATC-MS[c]	101	67.3	163	72.1	269	81.5	533	75.5
ATC-other	63	42.0	63	27.9	76	23.0	202	28.6

[a,b]Only the anticonvulsant users with an ICD-9 diagnosis of a psychiatric disorder during the study year were included (n = 706) and, similarly, only anxiolytic/sedative/hypnotic users with an ICD-9 diagnosis of a psychiatric disorder during the study year (n = 769) were included in the estimate of psychotherapeutic drug prevalence.

[c]Only mood stabilizer anticonvulsant users with an ICD-9 diagnosis of a psychiatric disorder (n = 533) were included in the estimate of psychotherapeutic prevalence.

SSRI, selective serotonin reuptake inhibitors; TCA, tricyclic antidepressants; ATC-MS, anticonvulsants-mood stabilizer.

are more common with off-label drugs (Turner et al., 1999; Horan et al., 2002). Preschool data in the present study suggest certain specific ADE concerns. For example, phenobarbital was still commonly prescribed for seizure control in this age group, although it is not recommended by neurologists as a first-line treatment because of cognitive (Farwell et al., 1990) and behavioral side effects (Glauser, 2004). Similarly, topiramate, another commonly used anticonvulsant, is known to impair cognitive function (Lee et al., 2003; de Araujo Filho et al., 2006).

Dispensings of antipsychotic medications for preschoolers have grown (Cooper et al., 2004; Patel et al., 2002) along with associated ADE reports of metabolic dysfunction and significant weight gain (Correll and Carlson, 2006; Biederman et al., 2005). In addition, studies of

treatment with antipsychotics, as well as with stimulants and SSRIs, have shown that preschoolers are more sensitive to adverse events than their adolescent counterparts (Safer, 2004; Safer and Zito, 2006; Wigal et al., 2006). To deal with this important issue, more *age-specific* short- and long-term outcome research clearly needs to be conducted (Vitiello and Hoagwood, 1997; Brent, 2004).

LIMITATIONS

The findings from this computerized Medicaid data set reveal the 2001 psychotherapeutic medication prevalence from 7 states in the United States, not all 50. However, the 7 states were selected from 4 major geographical regions with a composite 2- to 4-year-old enrolled pop-

TABLE 3. FREQUENCY OF PSYCHIATRIC, NONPSYCHIATRIC MEDICAL DIAGNOSES AND NO DIAGNOSIS AMONG PRESCHOOLERS WITH DISPENSED MEDICATIONS FOR ANXIOLYTIC/SEDATIVE/HYPNOTICS

Dx	Alprazolam	Buspirone	Cloral hydrate	Clorazepate	Hydroxyzine	Lorazepam	Midazolam	[a]Others	Total
Other medical DX	35	17	452	46	6301	79	35	19	6882
%	77.8	26.2	70.3	73.0	77.5	65.3	74.5	54.3	76.5
Psychiatric Dx	4	42	106	10	612	29	2	5	769
%	8.9	64.6	16.5	15.9	7.5	24.0	4.3	14.3	8.6
No Dx	6	6	85	7	1222	13	10	11	1342
%	13.3	9.2	13.2	11.1	15.0	10.7	21.3	31.4	14.9
Total	45	65	643	63	8135	121	47	35	8993

[a]Other anxiolytics/sedatives/hypnotics with less than 20 users were combined: chlordiazepoxide, droperidol, flurazepam, pentobarbital, temazepam, triazolam, zaleplon, and zolpidem.

TABLE 4. FREQUENCY OF PSYCHIATRIC, SEIZURE, OTHER MEDICAL DIAGNOSES AND NO DIAGNOSIS AMONG PRESCHOOLERS WITH DISPENSED MEDICATIONS FOR ANTICONVULSANTS (ATC)

Dx	CBZ	CZM	DZM	CVX/VA	EXM	GBA	LTG	LVM	OXP	PB	PHN	TOP	ZON	aOther ATC	Unique row totals
Other medical DX	148	82	422	170	2	33	36	19	15	154	47	65	6	7	904
%	16.1	31.1	40.3	16.7	9.1	35.9	15.7	15.7	10.4	26.6	21.8	16.6	7.3	21.9	27.2
Only psychiatric	84	21	55	184	1	24	8	1	28	17	5	27	2	1	376
%	9.2	8.0	5.3	18.0	4.5	26.1	3.5	0.8	19.4	2.9	2.3	6.9	2.4	3.1	11.3
Only seizure	490	104	320	431	14	16	116	59	62	301	113	194	46	14	1305
%	53.4	39.4	30.6	42.2	63.6	17.4	50.7	48.8	43.1	51.9	52.3	49.6	56.1	43.8	39.3
Psychiatric and seizure	114	29	76	137	2	8	40	20	21	51	30	59	14	4	330
%	12.4	11.0	7.3	13.4	9.1	8.7	17.5	16.5	14.6	8.8	13.9	15.1	17.1	12.5	9.9
No Dx	82	28	173	99	3	11	29	22	18	57	21	46	14	6	409
%	8.9	10.6	16.5	9.7	13.6	12.0	12.7	18.2	12.5	9.8	9.7	11.8	17.1	18.8	12.3
Total	918	264	1046	1021	22	92	229	121	144	580	216	391	82	32	3324

aOther anticonvulsants with less than 20 users were combined: ethotoin, felbamate, fosphenytoin, mephobarbital, primidone, and tiagabine.
CBZ = carbamazepine, CZM = clonazepam, DZM = diazepam, DVX/VA = divalproex/valproic acid, EXM = ethosuximide, GBA = bagapentin, LTG = lamotrigine, LVM = levetiracetam, OXP = oxcarbazepine, PB = phenobarbital, PHN = phenytoin, TOP = topiramate, ZON = zonisamide.

ulation of 274,518. Furthermore, in the only comparable analysis of 2001 data in the literature, the antipsychotic prevalence range for 2- to 4-year-olds derived from 3 states (Patel et al., 2005) was 0.08% to 0.55%, and the prevalence found in the present study (0.39%) was within that range. Second, the diagnostic information used to characterize anxiolytic/sedative/hypnotic use for psychotherapeutic purposes is based on clinician-reported diagnoses, and when both psychiatric and nonpsychiatric diagnoses were recorded, it was not always clear which applied to the treatment utilized. In the case of anticonvulsant use among children with psychiatric and seizure disorder diagnoses, it is very likely they were treated for seizure disorder.

Nevertheless, the adjusted prevalence is far more likely to reflect current medical practice in preschoolers than if all users in these two drug classes were counted as receiving psychotherapeutic treatment. In addition, clinician-reported diagnoses lack demonstrated reliability, although they provide a window to understand the perceived need for drug treatment and offer clues to distinguish medical usage from psychiatric therapy.

POLICY IMPLICATIONS

As early as 1968, Shirkey identified children as therapeutic orphans (Shirkey, 1968). Since that time there have been many attempts to create an evidence-based framework for the rational use of drugs in children. Recently, Congress enacted legislation, the Best Pharmaceuticals for Children Act of 2002 (BPCA), to begin to address this issue. The BPCA mandates the federal government, that is, the National Institutes of Health, to sponsor pediatric studies of drugs approved for use in the United States but lacking evaluation in the pediatric population (BPCA, 2002). The selection of drugs for study is based on the frequency of use in the pediatric population, the prevalence and severity of the condition being treated, and the potential for providing a health benefit in the pediatric population. The present study was undertaken to provide input into the prioritization process for federal pediatric drug studies by evaluating the frequency of use of psychotherapeutic medications among preschool-aged children.

CONCLUSION

Increasing psychotherapeutic medication prevalence for preschool-aged children parallels that for older youth (Zito et al., 2003), but there are important age differences in diagnostic relationships and in off-label prescribing. As a group, preschoolers are more vulnerable to ADEs than adolescents, and most long-term consequences from these treatments are unknown. As Vitiello and Hoagwood (1997) have suggested, "Given the dearth of pediatric data for so many drugs, a good epidemiologic follow-up is really the minimum we owe to our children."

DISCLOSURES

Drs. Zito, Safer, Korelitz and Mattison and Mr. Valluri and Mr. Gardner have no conflicts of interest to report.

REFERENCES

American Academy of Pediatrics: Medicaid State Report. http://www.aap.org/research/pdf01/fy2001.pdf. 2001.

Biederman J, Mick E, Hammerness P, Harpold T, Aleardi M, Dougherty M, Wozniak J: Open-label, 8-week trial of olanzapine and risperidone for the treatment of bipolar disorder in preschool-age children. Biol Psychiatr 58:589–594, 2005.

BPCA: Best Pharmaceuticals for Children Act. Pub. L. No. 107-109, Pub. L. No. 107-109, 115 Stat. 1408 (2002) (codified as amended at 42 U.S.C.A. § 284m (West 2003), 21 U.S.C.A. § 355b (West Supp. 2003), 21 U.S.C.A. § 393a (West Supp. 2003). 2002.

Brent RL, Tanski S, Weitzman M: A pediatric perspective on the unique vulnerability and resilience of the embryo and the child to environmental toxicants: The importance of rigorous research concerning age and agent. Pediatrics 113:935–944, 2004.

Cooper WO, Hickson GB, Fuchs C, Arbogast PG, Ray WA:. New users of antipsychotic medications among children enrolled in TennCare. Arch Pediatr Adolesc Med 158:753–759, 2004.

Correll C, Carlson HE: Endocrine and metabolic adverse effects of psychotropic medications in children and adolescents. Am Acad Child Adolesc Psychiatry 45(7):771–791, 2006.

Cox ER, Motheral BR, Henderson RR, Mager D: Geographic variation in the prevalence of stimulant medication use among children 5 to 14 years old: Results from a commercially insured US sample. Pediatrics 111:237–243, 2003.

de Araujo Filho GM, Pascalicchio TF, Lin K, Sousa PS, Yacubian EM: Neuropsychiatric profiles of patients with juvenile myoclonic epilepsy treated with valproate or topiramate. Epilepsy Behav May 8, 606–609, 2006.

DeBar LL, Lynch F, Powell J, Gale J: Use of psychotropic agents in preschool children: Associated symptoms, diagnoses, and health care services in a health maintenance organization. Arch Pediatr Adolesc Med 157:121–123, 2003.

Farwell JR, Lee YJ, Hirtz DG, Sulzbacher SI, Ellenberg JH, Nelson KB: Phenobarbital for febrile seizures—effects on intelligence and on seizure recurrence. New Engl J Med 322:364–369, 1990.

Glauser TA: Behavioral and psychiatric adverse events associated with antiepileptic drugs commonly used in pediatric patients. J Child Neurol Aug 19, Suppl 1:S25–S38, 2004.

Habel LA, Schaefer CA, Levine P, Bhat AK, Elliott G: Treatment with stimulants among youths in a large California health plan. J Child Adolesc Psychopharmacol 15:62–67, 2005.

Horen B, Montastruc JL, Lapeyre-Mestre M: Adverse drug reactions and off-label drug use in paediatric outpatients. Br J Clin Pharmacol 54(6):665–670, 2002.

Hunkeler EM, Fireman B, Lee J, Diamond R, Hamilton J, He CX, Dea R, Nowell WB, Hargreaves WA: Trends in use of antidepressants, lithium and anticonvulsants in youth: 1994–2003. J Child Adolesc Psychopharmacol 15:26–37, 2005.

Lee S, Sziklas V, Andermann F, Farnham S, Risse G, Gustafson M, Gates J, Penovich P, Al-Asmi A, Dubeau F, Jones-Gotman M: The effects of adjunctive topiramate on cognitive function in patients with epilepsy. Epilepsia 44:339–347, 2003.

Luby JL: Psychopharmacology. In: Luby JL, editor. Handbook of Preschool Mental Health: Development, Disorders and Treatment. Guilford Press (New York), 2006, pp 311–330.

MMWR: Mental health in the United States: Prevalence of diagnosis and medication treatment for attention-deficit/hyperactivity disorder—United States, 2003. Morbidity and Mortality Weekly Report (MMWR) 54:842-847, 2005.

National Institute of Child Health and Human Development: Frequency of medication usage in the pediatric population (Rep. No. Contract # GS-23F-8144H), 2006.

Olfson M, Marcus SC, Weissman MM, Jensen PS: National trends in the use of psychotropic medications by children. J Am Acad Child Adoles Psychiatry 41:514–521, 2002.

Patel NC, Crismon ML, Hoagwood K, Johnsrud MT, Rascati KL, Wilson JP, Jensen PS: Trends in the use of typical and atypical antipsychotics in children and adolescents. Am Acad Child Adolesc Psychiatry 44:548–556, 2005.

Patel NC, Sanchez RJ, Johnsrud MT, Crismon ML: Trends in antipsychotic use in a Texas Medicaid population of children and adolescents: 1996 to 2000. J Child Adolesc Psychopharmacol 12(3):221–229, 2002.

Safer DJ: A comparison of risperidone-induced weight gain across the age span. J Clin Psychopharmacol 24:429–436, 2004.

Safer DJ, Malever M: Stimulant treatment in Maryland public schools. Pediatrics 106:533–539, 2000.

Safer DJ, Zito JM: Treatment-emergent adverse events from selective serotonin reuptake inhibitors by age group: Children versus adolescents. J Child Adolesc Psychopharmacol 16(1):203–213, 2006.

Shatin D, Drinkard CR: Ambulatory use of psychotropics by employer-insured children and adolescents in a national managed care organization. Ambulatory Pediatr 2:111–119, 2002.

Shatin D, Levin R, Ireys HT, Haller V: Health care utilization by children with chronic illnesses: A comparison of Medicaid and employer-insured managed care. Pediatrics 102:e44, 1998.

Shirkey H: Therapeutic orphans. J Pediatr 72:119, 1968.

Turner S, Nunn AJ, Fielding K, Choonara I: Adverse drug reactions to unlicensed and off-label drugs on paediatric wards: A prospective study. Acta Paediatr 88:965–968, 1999.

Vitiello B, Hoagwood K: Pediatric pharmacoepidemiology: Clinical applications and research priorities in children's mental health. J Child Adolesc Psychopharmacol 7(4):287–290, 1997.

Wigal T, Greenhill LL, Chuang S, McGough J, Vitiello B, Skrobala A, Swanson J, Wigal S, Abikoff H, Kollins S, McCracken J, Riddle M, Posner K, Ghuman J, Davies M, Thorp B, Stehli A: Safety and tolerability of methylphenidate in preschool children with ADHD. J Acad Child Adolesc Psychiatry 45:1294–1303, 2006.

Zito JM, Safer DJ, dosReis S, Gardner JF, Boles M, Lynch F: Trends in the prescribing of psychotropic medications to preschoolers. J Am Med Assoc 283:1025–1030, 2000.

Zito JM, Safer DJ, dosReis S, Gardner JF, Magder L, Soeken K, Boles M, Lynch F, Riddle MA: Psychotropic practice patterns for youth: A 10-year perspective. Arch Pediatr Adolesc Med 157:17–25, 2003.

Zito JM, Safer DJ, dosReis S, Riddle MA: Racial disparity in psychotropic medications prescribed for youths with Medicaid insurance in Maryland. J Am Acad Child Adolesc Psychiatry 37:179–184, 1998.

Zito JM, Safer DJ, Gardner JF, Soeken K, Ryu J: Anticonvulsant treatment for psychiatric and seizure indication among youths. Psychiatr Serv 57:681–685, 2006.

ADVANCES IN PRESCHOOL PSYCHOPHARMACOLOGY
© 2009 Mary Ann Liebert, Inc.
140 Huguenot Street, 3rd Floor
New Rochelle, NY 10801-5215

Psychotropic Prescriptions in a Sample Including Both Healthy and Mood and Disruptive Disordered Preschoolers: Relationships to Diagnosis, Impairment, Prescriber Type, and Assessment Methods

Joan L. Luby, M.D., Melissa Meade Stalets, M.A., and Andy C. Belden, Ph.D.

ABSTRACT

Objective: Epidemiological data has shown that psychotropic medications are being prescribed to preschoolers at increasing rates. The diagnostic context and functional impairment of these preschoolers remains unknown. This investigation aimed to address these questions in a sample of preschoolers who were either without symptoms (healthy) or with mood and disruptive disorders by assessing them using a structured diagnostic interview and measure of impairment.

Method: Preschoolers aged 3.0 to 5.11 without symptoms and those with symptoms of mood and disruptive disorders were recruited from primary care and daycare sites in the St. Louis area to participate in a psychiatric evaluation that included information about psychotropic prescriptions from community practitioners.

Results: Seven percent of preschoolers ($n = 19$) out of a total sample of $n = 267$ were prescribed psychotropic medications. Fifty-two percent of preschoolers in the total sample met criteria for an Axis I psychiatric disorder. Presence of an Axis I disorder was significantly related to psychotropic prescription ($p < 0.01$). Among preschoolers who met criteria for an Axis I disorder 12% received psychotropics (Dx/Rx group). The Dx/Rx group was more impaired than those with a diagnosis who were not prescribed psychotropics ($p < 0.001$). Among preschoolers taking psychotropic medications, two failed to meet criteria for any Axis I disorder.

Conclusion: In this sample, most psychotropic medications were prescribed for impaired preschoolers with an Axis I diagnosis. These findings shed some light on the prescribing trends among mood and disruptive disordered preschoolers.

INTRODUCTION

EPIDEMIOLOGICAL INVESTIGATIONS have revealed that psychotropic medications have been prescribed to preschool aged children over the last decade at rates that raise concern when the fact that they have not been tested for efficacy or approved by the Food and Drug Administration (FDA) for use in this young age group is considered (Coyle 2000). Prior studies

---

Washington University School of Medicine, Department of Psychiatry, St. Louis, Missouri.
The study was funded by NIMH R01 #064769 to Dr. Luby

also indicate that these prescribing trends have been accelerating in the past five years (Pathak et al. 2004; Rappley et al. 1999; Zito and Safer 2005; Zito et al. 2000). However, several important issues have yet to be addressed by the investigations done to date, preventing a full understanding of the key contributors and underlying factors giving rise to the public health problem. One issue is that most of the available data describes patterns of psychotropic medication prescribing in preschoolers enrolled in Medicaid or other federal or state funded insurance programs (Rushton and Whitmire 2001; Zito et al. 2000). While these samples give us a picture of psychotropic prescribing in specific subpopulations, they are not representative of the general population.

Another critical and unexplored issue in the available pharmaco-epidemiological studies is that the diagnostic context of these prescriptions remains unknown. One exception to this is a study that addressed prescriptions in relation to symptoms in a preschool sample from a health maintenance organization (DeBar et al.,2003). Further, it is unclear whether appropriate diagnostic assessments were conducted and what DSM-IV diagnoses if any, or types and degree of functional impairment, were being targeted by these prescriptions. A related factor that remains unknown is the medical specialty and training (e.g., general practitioner versus child psychiatrist) of prescribing practitioners. Yet another key question that needs to be addressed is whether medications are prescribed before, after, or in conjunction with a trial of psychotherapy or other psychosocial interventions in these very young children. Obtaining information about these issues would further clarify the nature of the preschool prescribing trend and could be useful to direct public health education and intervention efforts necessary to minimize and prevent inappropriate prescribing.

During the same period that these prescribing trends have arisen, significant progress has been made in the area of clarifying age-appropriate assessment techniques and diagnostic nosologies of mental disorders in preschool children (Task force on research diagnostic criteria: Infancy and Preschool 2003). However, it remains unclear whether these age-appropriate methods and/or diagnostic criteria are being utilized in the psychopharmacologic treatment decisions for pre-

school populations. In addition, the efficacy of a few early psychotherapeutic and behavioral techniques for the treatment of specific preschool onset disorders has now been established (e.g., Hood and Eyberg 2003; Faja and Dawson 2006). The positive and in some cases enduring ameliorative effects of early interventions in these specific areas suggests a possible window of opportunity for early intervention during the preschool period. Based on these new findings and current prescribing trends of psychotropic medications to preschool-age children, there is a clear need for additional information regarding the use of psychotropic medications among this young and potentially vulnerable and/or potentially uniquely treatable age group.

The aim of this investigation was to explore the rates and types of psychotropic medications prescribed by community practitioners in a sample of healthy or mood and disruptive disordered preschool children who had undergone a comprehensive research diagnostic assessment. We also sought to investigate the methods of clinical assessment used by these community practitioners as well as the recommendation and use of psychotherapy in advance of psychotropic prescribing.

METHOD

Participants and procedure

Preschoolers between 3.0 and 5 years 11 months of age (5.11) were recruited from community pediatric or primary care practices and preschools/daycares in the St. Louis metropolitan area for participation in a study of early emotional development and mood disorders. Participants were ascertained using the Preschool Feelings Checklist (PFC; Luby et al. 2004) a validated screening checklist that identified children with symptoms of depression and disruptive disorders as well as those without behavioral problems. To achieve an ethnically and socio-economically diverse sample, a demographically broad range of primary care and daycare settings in the St. Louis metropolitan area was selected for participation in the study.

Approximately 6,000 checklists were distributed to the recruiting sites and from those $n = 1,474$ checklists were returned to the Washington University School of Medicine (WUSM) Early Emotional Development Program (EEDP). Using the PFC, and previously established thresholds, the study population was over-sampled for preschoolers with mood and disruptive symptoms. This was done by design so that a large group of preschoolers with these disorders could be obtained to facilitate the main study aims, which were to investigate the nosology of preschool mood disorders. Previous findings have illustrated that a score ≥ 3 on the PFC is highly sensitive and moderately specific for mood disorders as well as moderately sensitive for disruptive disorders (Luby et al., 2004). Caregivers of preschoolers between 3.0 and 5.11 years of age and with a PFC score ≥ 3 and < 1, as well as those with a PFC scores $=1$ based on the presence of the symptom of anhedonia, were contacted by phone for a screening interview. Those without anhedonia and a score of 1 and those with a score of 2 were excluded. Eight hundred and ninety-nine ($n = 899$) caregivers of preschoolers were contacted by phone to establish if any exclusion criteria (e.g., neurological disorders, autistic spectrum disorders, developmental delays) were present and that all inclusion criteria were met. Those who met all inclusion and exclusion criteria ($n = 416$) were invited for study participation and $n = 302$ agreed and participated in the full assessment.

Trained research assistants (separate parent and child interviewers) evaluated preschool study participants and their primary caregivers at WUSM EEDP. The study protocol was reviewed and approved by the Human Research Protection Office. Prior to the evaluation, parents gave informed consent, and the children assented to the study protocol. Preschoolers participated in a comprehensive evaluation of developmental capacities and mental health status in both dyadic and individual testing formats. The primary caregiver (94% were biological mothers) was interviewed about their child's behaviors, emotions and development. In addition, caregivers completed four self-report take-home questionnaires.

For the purpose of this investigation, the primary caregivers of all preschool participants reported to be taking psychotropic medications were subsequently contacted by telephone. Additional information about the specialty of the prescribing practitioner as well as the method of clinical diagnostic assessment was obtained. Assessment methods were categorized in the following way: a specialty preschool mental health assessment was defined by the use of a multi-session dyadic play format, a general child mental health assessment was defined as being seen by a child psychiatrist in a format typically used for older children (without observations of dyadic play) and no formal mental health assessment was defined as being seen by a non-mental health practitioner in a single office visit. In addition, information about whether any form of psychotherapy was recommended or initiated prior to, or concurrent with, medication prescription was also sought. For the purpose of the following analyses, psychotherapy was defined broadly as any treatment by a clinician that focused directly on children's behaviors and emotions. This could include psychodynamic, cognitive and/or behavioral therapies. It did not include therapies such as physical therapy, speech and language or occupational therapy. These treatments were categorized as "developmental therapies" and were considered separately. Out of $n = 20$ preschoolers who were reported as receiving medication, $n = 18$ participants were successfully contacted by phone and provided the requested information, $n = 2$ could not be contacted or failed to return calls.

Measures

Information about mental health, prescriptions taken by the child, and treatment (i.e., developmental as well as psychotherapeutic) was obtained using the Health and Behavior Questionnaire (HBQ; Armstrong et al. 2003) an age-appropriate measure with established validity (Essex et al. 2002). The HBQ assessed "regular" medication use defined as "taken daily for at least one month." This measure was completed by caregivers prior to coming to the EEDP. Trained interviewers who remained blind to children's diagnostic status administered all other study measures. Preschoolers' degree of impairment, ranging from no impairment to severe impairment was established using the Preschool Early Childhood Functional Assessment Scale (PECFAS; Hodges 1994) an age appropriate measure of impairment with established validity. The PECFAS is rated by trained interviewers who achieve reliability with an outside site using standardized testing materials (Murphy 1999). The PECFAS is rated on the basis of parental response to probes about their child's functioning. Items are designed to address impairment in functioning as a result of symptoms and address 3 contexts (home, school and community) and 4 domains (behavior towards others, moods/emotions, self-harm, thinking and communication). Parents were also interviewed extensively by a trained interviewer about their child's moods and behaviors using the Preschool Age Psychiatric Assessment (PAPA; Egger et al. 1999), The PAPA is a comprehensive age-appropriate semi-structured interview with established construct validity and test-re-test reliability (Egger et al. 2006). Diagnostic modules of the PAPA contain developmentally sensitive translations of relevant mental health symptoms. Diagnoses were based on standard computerized DSM-IV algorithms. For mood disorders, symptom criteria only were used (duration criteria were set aside). Preschoolers in the study sample fell into the following diagnostic categories based on the application of DSM-IV algorithms: Major Depressive Disorders (MDD), Bipolar-I (BP), ADHD, Oppositional Defiant Disorder (ODD), Conduct Disorder (CD) and Anxiety Disorders (alone and in varying co-morbid combinations). Preschoolers who did not meet criteria for any of these disorders were categorized as healthy.

Data analysis

Chi-square analyses were conducted to test for differences between psychotropic medication use and demographic characteristics such as, age, gender, and gross household income. An odds ratio was computed to examine the expected increase in likelihood that children who were taking psychotropic medication(s) would have been diagnosed with a DSM-IV Axis-I disorder in the current study. Next, descriptive statistics (i.e., percentages) were calculated to examine the proportion of children taking certain classes of psychotropic medication in relation to diagnostic classification, prescriber-type, and assessment method. To test the likelihood that preschoolers taking psychotropic medications had or were receiving psychotherapy and/or developmental therapy,

odds ratio tests were calculated. Last, Mann-Whitney and odds ratio tests were calculated to examine expected differences between preschoolers' psychotropic medication use and functional impairment. Functional impairment was measured and tested as a dimensional as well as dichotomous (i.e., severe versus not severe functional impairment) variable.

RESULTS

Psychotropic prescriptions and demographic factors

Out of the total sample of $n = 302$, $n = 35$ were missing the pertinent prescribing information due to failing to complete the HBQ Thus, relevant data about psychotropic medication use was available for $n = 267$ preschoolers. There were no demographic or diagnostic differences between preschoolers of caregivers who completed the HBQ and those who did not. The study sample had a diverse socioeconomic and ethnic composition consistent with the ethnic composition of the St. Louis metropolitan area (see Table 1). Among the sub-sample with data about medication use, 7% (i.e., $n = 19$ out of $n = 267$) were reported to be taking psychotropic medication. Alpha agonists (guanfacine and clonidine) were included as psychotropic medications (although originally designed for cardiac treatments) due to their use (and some available investigations) in clinical practice to control impulsivity in young children. Gender was related to medication use, $\chi^2 (df1, n = 267) = 6.09, p < 0.01$, with rates of psychotropic medication use approximately four times higher among boys than girls. Gender was also related to meeting criteria for any DSM-IV Axis I diagnosis (i.e., yes or no). Boys were almost twice as likely to be diagnosed with any Axis I disorder compared to girls. Age was related to medication status, $\chi^2 (df2, n = 267) = 8.40$ $p < 0.01$, with $n = 1$, 3-year-old child taking psychotropics (stimulant & alpha agonist) compared to $n = 8$, 4-year olds ($n = 1$ stimulant and antipsychotic, $n = 1$ alpha agonist and antipsychotic, $n = 1$ lithium and antipsychotic, $n = 3$ stimulants, $n = 1$ antipsychotic, $n = 1$ alpha agonist,) and $n = 10$, 5-year-old children ($n = 1$ alpha agonist and

TABLE 1. DEMOGRAPHIC CHARACTERISTICS OF THE STUDY SAMPLE

	DSM		No DSM	
	DX/RX n = 17	DX/No RX n = 123	DX/RX n = 2	DX/No RX n = 125
Gender % (n)				
Male	77% (13)	55% (68)	100% (2)	44% (54)
Female	23% (4)	45% (55)	X	56% (70)
Age in Years				
3	6% (1)	32% (39)	X	28% (35)
4	47% (8)	40% (49)	X	48% (60)
5	47% (8)	29% (35)	100% (2)	23% (29)
Ethnicity (child)				
White	59% (10)	47% (57)	50% (1)	65% (81)
Black	35% (6)	43% (53)	50% (1)	39% (36)
Hispanic	6% (1)	4% (5)	X	2% (3)
Asian or Pacific Indian	X	3% (3)	X	2% (2)
Mixed racial background	X	3% (3)	X	2% (2)
Caregivers' education				
No college	23% (4)	20% (24)	X	14% (17)
Some college	53% (9)	42% (52)	50% (1)	31% (38)
4-year degree	6% (1)	20% (24)	50% (1)	26% (32)
Beyond 4-year degree	X	4% (5)	X	7% (8)
Professional degree	18% (3)	15% (18)	X	22% (26)
Marital status				
Married	59% (10)	50% (61)	50% (1)	67% (83)
Separated	X	4% (5)	X	2% (2)
Divorced	12% (2)	12% (15)	X	4% (5)
Widowed	X	X	X	2% (2)
Never married	29% (5)	34% (41)	50% (1)	26% (32)
Income				
0–$20,000	31% (5)	29% (31)	X	21% (24)
$20,001–$40,000	19% (3)	21% (23)	X	11% (13)
$40,001–$60,000	31% (5)	16% (17)	50% (1)	17% (20)
$60,000+	19% (3)	34% (37)	50% (1)	51% (59)

DSM DX/RX = *Diagnostic and Statistical Manual* Diagnosis, diagnosis/prescription; DX/No RX = *Diagnostic and Statistical Manual* Diagnosis, diagnosis/no prescription; No DSM = No *Diagnostic and Statistical Manual* Diagnosis

antipsychotic, $n = 7$ stimulants, $n = 2$ antipsychotics). Preschoolers' age did not differ as a function of diagnostic status (i.e., BP, MDD, ADHD/ODD/CD, anxiety, and healthy) in the sub-sample ($n = 267$) included in these analyses. When examining the presence or absence of a DSM-IV Axis I disorder (but not taking into account specific disorders), results indicated the presence of any Axis I disorder was significantly related to psychotropic medication use, χ^2 (df1, $n = 267$) = 11.25, $p < .01$. Preschoolers with a DSM-IV Axis I diagnosis were almost 9 (CI = 1.954 to 38.182) times more likely to be taking a psychotropic medication than those with no DSM-IV Axis I disorder (see Table 2).

Psychotropic prescriptions and DSM-IV diagnosis

Of the children with a DSM-IV Axis I diagnosis according to parent report on the PAPA, 12% ($n = 17$) were taking psychotropic med-

TABLE 2. VARIABLES ASSOCIATED WITH PSYCHOTROPIC MEDICATION
PRESCRIPTION DURING PRESCHOOL PERIOD

	Odds ratio	Confidence interval
Male gender	3.84**	1.24–11.90
≥55 months vs. ≤54 months	4.90**	1.58–15.21
In psychotherapy	46.46***	13.95–154.70
Met criteria for BP-1	21.36***	7.47–61.02
Met criteria for disruptive disorder (ADHD, ODD, CD)	7.73***	2.49–24.04
Met criteria for any Axis I disorder	8.63**	1.95–38.18

**$p < .01$; ***$p < .001$
BP-1 = bipolar 1; ADHD = attention-deficit/hyperactivity disorder; ODD = oppositional defiant disorder; CD = conduct disorder
Note: Confidence intervals above and throughout this paper are large simply because the point estimates are large. If one were to examine the log odds ratios of the gender and psychotherapy findings above, it becomes clear that distances between the lower and upper ends of the interval in relation to the point estimate are very similar.

ication. Five children (29%) of those on medications were prescribed two psychotropic medications. Among those taking psychotropic medications in the sample as a whole ($n = 19$), 11% ($n = 2$) did not meet diagnostic criteria for any of the DSM-IV Axis I disorders assessed. Of note, Autistic Spectrum Disorders (ASDs) were not assessed and attempts were made to screen out participants with ASDs (which was an exclusion criterion for study participation). Within the sub-group on medication, specific psychotropic medications prescribed within different diagnostic groups, are outlined in Table 3. Of particular interest was that all preschool participants taking an atypical antipsychotic met DSM-IV symptom criteria for a diagnosis of BP-1 with co-morbid MDD (see Table 3). Conversely, 42% of preschoolers who met symptom criteria for BP-1 had been prescribed a psychotropic medication.

Psychotropic prescriptions and prescriber type and assessment method

Among the $n = 19$ preschoolers who were taking a psychotropic medication, information regarding type of prescriber was available for 18 children (prescriber type unknown for 1 combination prescription). Of these preschoolers, 33% ($n = 6$: $n = 3$ atypical antipsychotic, $n = 2$ stimulant, $n = 1$ atypical antipsychotic and alpha agonist combination) of the prescriptions were written by child psychiatrists, 33% ($n = 6$: $n = 5$ stimulant, $n = 1$ alpha ago-

TABLE 3. DSM-IV DIAGNOSIS AND MEDICATION PRESCRIBED

	Healthy (n = 2)	Anxiety (n = 1)	MDD (n = 1)	CD (n = 1)	ADHD /ODD (n = 1)	MD/ADHD/ ODD (n = 2)	MDD/BP/≥ 1 Disruptive* (n = 11)	Total RX
Stimulant	2	0	1	1	1	2	5	12
Antipsychotic	0	0	0	0	0	0	7	7
Alpha Agonist	0	1	0	0	0	0	2	3
Lithium	0	0	0	0	0	0	1	1
Total n	2	1	1	1	1	2	11	

*Within this group four children were taking two separate psychotropic medications concurrently
MDD = major depressive disorder; CD = conduct disorder; ADHD/ODD = attention-deficit/hyperactivity disorder/oppositional defiant disorder; MDD/ADHD/ODD = major depressive disorder/attention-deficit/hyperactivity disorder/oppositional defiant disorder; MDD/BP = major depressive disorder/bipolar disorder; RX = prescription

nist) were written by pediatricians, 22% ($n = 4$: $n = 2$ stimulants, $n = 1$ atypical antipsychotic and alpha agonist combination, $n = 1$ stimulant and alpha agonist combination) by pediatric neurologists and 11% ($n = 2$: $n = 1$ stimulant, $n = 1$ stimulant and atypical antipsychotic combination) were written by nurse practitioners working in a child psychiatry office. Information about the type of assessment received prior to psychotropic prescription was available for $n = 17$ preschoolers. Nine (53%) caregivers reported their child did not receive any formal mental health assessment prior to being prescribed medication. Six preschoolers (35%) received a general child mental health assessment and two preschoolers (12%) received a specialized preschool mental health assessment. All preschool subjects who received prescriptions from their pediatrician or neurologist did not receive a formal mental health evaluation (defined above). Among those who were prescribed by a child psychiatrist $n = 4$ received a general mental health assessment and $n = 2$ received a specialized infant/preschool assessment. Both subjects ($n = 2$) prescribed by a nurse practitioner working under the supervision of a child psychiatrist received a general mental health evaluation. Of note was that both participants who received medications but who did not meet criteria for an Axis I DSM-IV diagnosis based on the PAPA received their prescriptions from a pediatrician. Regarding the type of assessment conducted for this subgroup, this data was missing from one and the mother of the second preschooler reported receiving no formal psychiatric assessment. Both medicated preschoolers without a DSM-IV diagnosis were boys (see Table 1).

Psychotropic prescriptions and psychotherapy and developmental therapies

Fifteen out of $n = 19$ or 79% of preschoolers taking psychotropic medications had previous or current psychotherapy of some form. Within the entire study sample (i.e., $n = 267$) $n = 30$ preschoolers had previously or were currently participating in some form of psychotherapy (broadly defined as described above). Preschoolers in psychotherapy were 46.45 (CI = 13.952 to 154.704) times more likely to be pre-

scribed a psychotropic medication than preschoolers who were not in psychotherapy. Among the 2 preschoolers who were on medication and did not meet criteria for a DSM-IV diagnosis, 1 received no psychotherapy either prior to or concurrent with the medication treatment. Of the $n = 19$ preschoolers prescribed psychotropic medications, 16% ($n = 3$) had received some form of developmental therapy (i.e., school resource room, speech/language therapy, physical and/or occupational therapy) in the last year.

Psychotropic prescriptions and functional impairment

Mann-Whitney U tests were conducted to evaluate potential differences in preschoolers' impairment scores in relation to psychotropic medication use and the presence or absence of a DSM-IV Axis I diagnosis. The first analysis examined whether there was a significant difference in impairment between children prescribed psychotropic medication versus not taking medication among preschoolers with an Axis I diagnosis. Results indicated that preschoolers who were prescribed psychotropic medication and who had an Axis I diagnosis had significantly higher impairment scores on all seven subscales of the PECFAS as well as on the PECFAS total impairment score, $z = -4.66$, $p < 0.0001$, compared to preschoolers with an Axis I diagnosis who were not prescribed psychotropic medications.

To examine the likelihood that preschoolers taking psychotropic medications would be rated as severely impaired on the PECFAS overall as well as within its seven subscales, odd ratios were computed. Analyses indicated that preschoolers who had been prescribed a psychotropic medication were 11 (CI = 3.48 to 32.25) times more likely to have been given the most severe rating on one or more of the PECFAS subscales compared to those not on medication. Odds ratios (and confidence intervals) for specific subscales are provided in Table 4. Of particular interest was the finding that preschoolers taking psychotropic medication were 20 (CI = 5.63 to 76.85) times more likely to have been rated "severely impaired" on the social subscale and 16 (CI = 1.38 to 188.78)

TABLE 4. ODDS OF RATING OF "SEVERE" IMPAIRMENT BY DOMAIN MEDICATED VERSUS NOT MEDICATED

	Odds ratios	Confidence interval
School	11.78***	3.09–44.96
Home	7.84***	2.45–25.07
Community	Did not occur	Did not occur
Social	20.80***	5.63–76.85
Mood	16.13**	1.38–188.77
Self-harm	3.69 (ns)	0.32–43.05
Thinking/communication	1.06 (ns)	0.943–1.20

$**p < .01$; $***p < .001$

Note: Large confidence interval explanation as in Table 2.

times more likely to have rated as severely impaired on the mood subscale.

Mann-Whitney U tests were conducted to test whether preschoolers who were prescribed an antipsychotic (in this study all were atypical antipsychotics) were more impaired than preschoolers who were prescribed any psychotropic medication outside of this class (e.g., stimulant, alpha agonist, other mood stabilizer). Results indicated that preschoolers who were prescribed antipsychotics were significantly more impaired on the PECFAS home behavior ($z = -3.11$, $p < 0.005$), social behavior ($z = -2.40$, $p < 0.01$), moods/emotions ($z = -2.19$, $p < 0.02$), self-harm ($z = -2.88$, $p < 0.01$), thinking/communication ($z = -2.85$, $p < 0.01$) subscales, as well as on the total PECFAS impairment scale ($z = -2.78$, $p < 0.01$) compared to preschoolers prescribed psychotropic medication outside of this class.

DISCUSSION

Study findings report on psychotropic medication use in a sample of preschoolers for whom structured research diagnostic assessments and measures of impairment have also been obtained. These data provide new information about the association between diagnosis from a validated age-appropriate semistructured diagnostic interview and level of functional impairment and their relationship to psychotropic medication use in specific diagnostic areas in preschool aged children. While the available literature has consistently reported high rates of psychotropic prescribing to preschoolers, the available data to date have not yet informed the issue of whether the children receiving these prescriptions met criteria for DSM-IV Axis I psychiatric disorders and if so which disorders were the primary target of treatment. Of note was the finding that 90% (17 out of 19) of preschoolers between the ages of 3.0 and 5.11 who were prescribed a psychotropic medication met criteria for a DSM-IV Axis 1 disorder based on an age appropriate structured research diagnostic interview. In keeping with these findings, preschoolers on psychotropic medications had a much higher likelihood of being rated as "severely impaired" on a structured measure. The highest odds ratios for impairment were found in the social and mood domains suggesting that difficulty in these areas may trigger pharmacologic interventions.

Another clear and notable finding was the higher rate of psychopharmacological treatment of externalizing/disruptive behavioral problems compared to those with internalizing disorders only. In particular, psychopharmacologic treatment for preschoolers meeting symptom criteria for BP-I (42% of those prescribed a medication met symptom criteria for BP-I), in which disruptive features are prominent, was the highest of any disorder targeted. Further, every atypical antipsychotic prescription written was for a child who met symptom criteria for BP-I (in addition to other co-morbid disorders). In contrast, no antidepressants were prescribed in this preschool population that contained $n = 72$ (27%) preschoolers who met all DSM-IV symptom criteria for MDD. This difference in rates of prescribing antidepressants compared to antipsychotics is of interest because both classes of medications are similarly lacking in safety and efficacy data for preschool aged children. Several factors may have contributed to the difference in prescribing of these two classes of medications, including the under identification of depressive syndromes and the recent FDA "Black Box" warning for antidepressants. However, the socially disruptive nature of the externalizing disorders for which antipsychotics were prescribed may be the most important factor. The finding of one depressed preschooler who was prescribed a stimulant medication was notable along these lines. The disruptive disorders are often viewed by caregivers and clinicians as requiring greater urgency for behavioral control, given the potential for self-harm and aggression towards others.

Another notable finding was the unique characteristics of the two preschoolers who did not meet criteria for a DSM-IV diagnosis but who were prescribed stimulants. Both prescriptions were written by pediatricians and at least one was known to be administered without formal psychiatric evaluations. Further both participants were boys and one also received psychotherapy. Notably, these two children were significantly less impaired (according to the PECFAS) compared to the $n = 17$ preschoolers taking medications who also met criteria for a DSM-IV Axis 1 disorder. It is possible that these children received clinical diagnoses from their prescribing community practitioner even though they did not meet criteria for the DSM-IV diagnoses assessed as a part of our research assessment. The use of stimulants in both "undiagnosed" preschoolers suggests that disruptive behavior that included inattention and/or impulsivity was being targeted. Alternatively, it is also possible that medication was effective in minimizing symptoms to a point below diagnostic thresholds at the time of the research diagnostic assessment. Based on

the very small number of children in this interesting group, it is premature to draw conclusions. However larger scale studies that address the relationship between diagnosis and stimulant prescriptions among primary care physicians would be of interest to investigate this issue further.

Results suggest that the overall rate of psychopharmacological treatment in the study sample was comparable or lower than (when sampling differences are considered) those reported in population based samples. However, this comparison is not straightforward based on the fact that this study sample was oversampled for preschoolers with behavioral and emotional symptoms and therefore is not a representative community sample. Seven percent (7%) of preschoolers in the study sample were found to be on psychotropic medications. This rate in a sample with high rates of psychiatric disorders would seem to represent a lower rate than the 5.9-6.3% prevalence rate of psychotropics found in a recent population based study of youths less than 20 years of age (Zito et al. 2003). However, in a more targeted preschool-age Oregon HMO study of psychotropic usage, 16% of a sample of 743 preschoolers was taking psychotropics (DeBar et al. 2003). Based on differences in sampling characteristics, it is difficult to compare this rate to the prescription rate found in the study sample presented here.

Further, among preschoolers meeting diagnostic criteria for Axis I disorders (which included ADHD, ODD, CD, MDD, BP and anxiety disorders) rates of prescribing in the study sample were also lower than those reported in preschool pharmacoepidemiology studies. For example, among $n = 223$ Medicaid enrollees in Michigan younger than age 4 with a clinical diagnosis of ADHD, 57% took at least 1 medication (Rappley et al. 2002). This compares to only 22% of those with a diagnosis of ADHD based on a structured research interview in the study sample presented here.

The finding that boys are more likely to be treated with psychotropic medication than girls is consistent with previous findings in larger and older samples (Shireman et al. 2005; Rushton and Whitmire 2001) as well as in other larger and younger Health Maintenance Organization (HMO) samples (Zito et al. 2003). These findings may be explained by the fact that disruptive behaviors were the most common target of psychopharmacologic treatment, and higher rates of disruptive behavioral disorders have been found in preschool aged boys (Egger and Angold, 2006).

Notably, preschoolers meeting DSM-IV symptom criteria for BP-I (with other co-morbid disorders) had the highest rate of psychotropic medication use. While this diagnosis remains highly controversial in preschool children, preliminary evidence for the validity of the BP-I syndrome has been previously provided (Luby and Belden 2006). This finding is consistent with other findings from the same study sample showing that this group demonstrated the highest levels of impairment; levels significantly higher even than those groups with other Axis 1 disorders (Luby and Belden 2006). However, given the absence of prospective, double-blind, placebo-controlled studies of treatment for preschool onset BP, this finding suggests that prescriptions to preschoolers with symptoms of mania and/or severe mood instability may be an important source of the public health problem in preschool psychotropic prescribing. These findings suggest that studies of age-appropriate treatments, to include both psychotherapeutic and psychopharmacologic, as well as further studies of the nosology of early onset BP are now needed.

The prescription of more than 1 psychotropic medication to preschool children (found in 5 cases) is also of interest given the higher risks involved and the paucity of data, not only on use of single agents, but even further on the use of combinations. Of note was that none of these combination prescriptions was written by a pediatrician. Although the sub-sample of preschoolers on multiple psychotropic medications was too small for further analysis in this sample, further investigation of this prescribing practice would be of paramount importance.

Another issue apparent from the study findings was the high rates of impairment found among the group of children undergoing treatment with a psychotropic medication. While details of pre- and post-treatment impairment are not known, and it is also unclear for how long the study participants were treated beyond the 1 month period assessed by the HBQ, this finding is notable. This finding taken together with other study findings and the extant literature underscores the need for specific study of the efficacy of these medications.

Several features of the study design and sample characteristics limit these findings. The relatively small subgroup of preschoolers on psychotropic medication on which many of the analyses are based is a limitation. The reliance of this small group suggests the reader should interpret the findings with caution due to an increased likelihood of statistical error, such as a lack of power to identify potentially important but small effect sizes. The fact that the same rater conducted the psychiatric interview (although was not privy to formal diagnostic group classification) and the measure of impairment could have given rise to rater bias. The sole reliance on parent report to derive psychiatric diagnosis without accounting for observation of the child and child informant measures is a design limitation. Another limitation is the restricted focus on mood and disruptive disorders and the exclusion of preschoolers with ASDs. The latter group is of importance as preschoolers with ASDs are a frequent target of psychotropic medications and are worthy of independent study.

The nosology of many preschool disorders, and internalizing disorders in particular, remains understudied and substantial ambiguities remain in the application of several psychiatric diagnoses to preschool age children. Nevertheless, these findings from a diagnostically well-characterized sample are informative and add new details to the relatively small body of empirical data regarding psychotropic medication use in preschool age children. These findings underscore the need for continued investigation in this area. They also provide some reassurance that based on standardized research assessments, those children who meet criteria for Axis I diagnoses and who are impaired appear to be the primary targets of psychotropic treatment in the community. Also reassuring was the majority of preschoolers on psychotropic medications were also in some form of psychotherapy. While this does not confirm that these psychotropic treatments were the optimal or even appropriate treatments in each case, it does suggest that children who are symptomatic and impaired as a group were being targeted in this sample of mood and disruptive disordered preschoolers.

AUTHOR DISCLOSURE

The authors do not have any corporate, commercial, or financial relationships that pose conflicts of interest.

REFERENCES

Armstrong JG, Goldstein LH, The MacArthur Working Group on Outcome Assessment: Manual for the MacArthur Health and Behavior Questionnaire (HBQ 1.0). MacArthur Foundation Research Network on Psychopathology and Development (David J. Kupfer, Chair), University of Pittsburgh, 2003.

Biederman J: Does attention-deficit hyperactivity disorder impact the developmental course of drug and alcohol abuse and dependence? Bio Psychiatry 44: 269–273, 1998.

Coyle JT: Psychotropic drug use in very young children. JAMA 283:1059–1060, 2000.

DeBar LL, Lynch F, Powell J, Gale J: Use of psychotropic agents in preschool children: Associated symptoms, diagnoses, and health care services in a health maintenance organization. Arch Pediatr Adolesc Med 157: 150–157, 2003.

Egger HL, Ascher B, Angold A: Preschool Age Psychiatric Assessment (PAPA): Version1.1. Durham, NC: Center for Developmental Epidemiology, Department of Psychiatry and Behavioral Sciences, Duke University Medical Center, 1999.

Egger HL, Angold A: Common emotional and behavioral disorders in preschool children: Presentation, nosology, and epidemiology. J Child Psychol Psychiatry 47: 313–337, 2006.

Egger HL, Erkanli A, Keeler G, Potts E, Walter B, Angold A: The test-retest reliability of the preschool age psychiatric assessment. J Am Acad Child Adolesc Psychiatry 45:538–549, 2006.

Essex MJ, Boyce WT, Goldstein LH: The confluence of mental, physical, social, and academic difficulties in middle childhood II: Developing the MacArthur Health and Behavior Questionnaire. J Am Acad Child Adolesc Psychiatry 41:588–603, 2002.

Faja S, Dawson G: Early Intervention for Autism, In: Handbook of Preschool Mental Health, Luby J, ed. New York: Guilford Press, pp 388–416, 2006.

Hodges K: The Preschool and Early Childhood Functional Assessment Scale (PECFAS). Eastern Michigan University, Ypsilanti, MI, 1994.

Hood KK, Eyberg SM: Outcomes of parent child interaction therapy: Mothers' reports of maintenance three to six years after treatment. J Clin Child Adolesc Psychology 32: 419–429, 2003.

Luby J, Heffelfinger A, Koenig-McNaught A, Brown K, Spitznagel E: The preschool feelings checklist: A brief and sensitive screening measure for depression in young children. J Am Acad Child Adolesc Psychiatry 43:708–717, 2004.

Luby J, Belden A: Defining and validating bipolar disorder in the preschool period. Dev Psychopathol 18: 971–988, 2006.

Murphy MJ, Ramirez A, Anaya Y, Nowlin C, Jellinek MS: Validation of the preschool and early childhood functional assessment. J Child Fam Studies, 8:343–356, 1999.

Pathak S, Arszman SP, Danielyan A, Johns E, Smirnov A, Kowatch R: Psychotropic utilization and psychiatric presentation of hospitalized very young children. J Child Adolesc Psychopharmacol 14:433–442, 2004.

Rappley M, Mullan P, Alvarez F, Eneli F, Wang J, Gardiner J: Diagnosis of ADHD and the use of psychotropic medication in very young children. Arch Pediatr Adolesc Med 153:1039–1045, 1999.

Rappley M, Eneli I, Mullan P, Alvarez F, Wang J, Ino Z, Gardiner J: Patterns of psychotropic medication use in very young children with ADHD. J Dev Behav Pediatr 23:23–30, 2002.

Rushton J, Whitmire T: Pediatric stimulant and SSRI prescription trends. Arch Pediatr Adolesc Med 155:560–565, 2001.

Shireman TI, Reichard A, Rigler SK: Psychotropic medication use among Kansas medicaid youths with disabilities. J Child Adolesc Psychopharmacol 15:107–115, 2005.

Task force on research diagnostic criteria: Infancy and preschool: Research diagnostic criteria for infants and preschool children: The process and empirical support. Special communication. J Am Acad Child Adolesc Psychiatry 42:1504–1512, 2003.

Zito JM, Safer DJ: Recent child pharmacoepidemiological findings. J Child Adolesc Psychopharmacol 15:5–9, 2005.

Zito JM, Safer DJ, dosReis S, Gardner JF, Boles M, Lynch F: Trends in the prescribing of psychotropic medications to preschoolers. JAMA 283:1025–1030, 2000.

Zito JM, Safer DJ, dosReis S, Gardner J, Boles M, Lynch F: Psychotropic practice patterns for youth: A 10-year perspective. Arch Pediatr Adolesc Med 157:17–25, 2003.

ADVANCES IN PRESCHOOL PSYCHOPHARMACOLOGY
© 2009 Mary Ann Liebert, Inc.
140 Huguenot Street, 3rd Floor
New Rochelle, NY 10801-5215

Proposed Definitions of Bipolar I Disorder Episodes and Daily Rapid Cycling Phenomena in Preschoolers, School-Aged Children, Adolescents, and Adults

Barbara Geller, M.D., Rebecca Tillman, M.S., and Kristine Bolhofner, B.S.

ABSTRACT

Objective: Recent data from several large studies of pediatric bipolar I disorder reported baseline (current) episode duration ranging from less than a month to ≥1 year. These data may reflect actual sample differences, but the absence of uniformly applied definitions of episode duration, number of lifetime episodes and daily rapid cycling patterns during episodes may also account for these differences.

Method: Proposals for definitions of episode and cycling phenomena were based upon data from the Washington University in St. Louis Kiddie Schedule for Affective Disorders and Schizophrenia (WASH-U-KSADS).

Result: Episode would be used for the interval between onset and offset of full DSM-IV criteria for bipolar I disorder. Cycling would be used only to describe daily (ultradian) switching of mood states that occurs during an episode.

Conclusion: Historically, in the adult bipolar literature the words "episode" and "cycle" were used interchangeably. "Rapid cycling," in this earlier literature, actually referred to multiple episodes per year. To avoid confusing episodes with daily cycling, the proposal is to use "episode" for the duration of DSM-IV criteria, to use "cycling" for daily switching phenomena during an episode, and to replace the historical term "rapid cycling" with "multiple episodes per year." These clarifications will be especially important for phenomenological research on preschool populations.

OUR UNIT PREVIOUSLY communicated about the need for uniformly applied definitions of episode and cycling to provide comparability of data across studies (Tillman and Geller, 2003). But, recent data from several large studies (see Table 1) demonstrate the need for further clarification. Three studies reported baseline (current) episode duration (Geller et al., 2004; Birmaher et al., 2006; TEAM Study, unpublished data) of at least one year. By contrast, Wagner et al. (2006) reported 17.1 ± 18.9 episodes per year; implying that the mean episode duration was less than one month. Because the Wagner et al. (2006) study reported

Washington University School of Medicine, Department of Psychiatry, St. Louis, Missouri.
Supported by NIMH grants R01 MH-53063 and U01 MH-64846 to Dr. Geller.

TABLE 1. CURRENT (BASELINE) EPISODE DURATION, N LIFETIME EPISODES, AND % DAILY (ULTRADIAN) CYCLING IN CHILDREN WITH FULL DSM-IV CRITERIA FOR BIPOLAR I DISORDER

Author (year)	N	Age ± SD	Prospective	Recruitment	SADS Series tool	Blinded & controlled assessment	Current episode duration	% First episode	N lifetime episodes	% Subjects with daily cycling
Geller et al. (2004)	86	10.8 ± 2.7	yes	consecutive new case	WASH-U[b]	Yes	79.2 ± 66.7 weeks	81.4	1.2 ± 0.4	77.9
Biederman et al. (2005)	197	8.4 (SD N/A)	no	consecutive referrals	E[c]	No	N/A	N/A	N/A	N/A
Birmaher et al. (2006)	152	13.2 ± 3.0	partly	convenience	P/L[d]	No	median 52.0 weeks	N/A	N/A	N/A[f]
Wagner et al. (2006)	115	Range 7–18 yr	no	convenience	P/L	No	N/A	N/A	17.1 ± 18.9[e]	N/A
TEAM[a] study (still recruiting)	283	10.1 ± 2.7	no	convenience	WASH-U	No	4.8 ± 2.5 years	90.8	1.1 ± 0.3	98.9

[a]TEAM = Ongoing NIMH-funded multisite "Treatment of Early Age Mania (TEAM)" study.
[b]WASH-U-KSADS = Washington University in St. Louis Kiddie Schedule for Affective Disorders and Schizophrenia (Geller et al., 2001).
[c]KSADS-E = Kiddie Schedule for Affective Disorders and Schizophrenia—Epidemiologic Version (Orvaschel and Puig-Antich, 1987).
[d]KSADS-P/L = Kiddie Schedule for Affective Disorders and Schizophrenia—Present and Lifetime Version (Kaufman et al., 1997).
[e]Number of episodes within past year in active drug group.
[f]These investigators reported 82.3% with mood lability, which may be measuring the same concept as daily cycling (Axelson et al., 2006).
N/A = not applicable.

17.1 ± 18.9 episodes per year, the mean duration of the current episode must have been far less than the minimum of one year found in the three other studies in Table 1. Two studies reported a mean lifetime number of episodes of 1.1–1.2, and in these studies 81.4%–90.8% of subjects were in their first episode (Geller et al., 2004; TEAM Study, unpublished data). These striking differences in number of lifetime episodes and in current episode duration between studies strongly support the need for definitions of episode and daily cycling that will provide comparable data across studies. It is possible that the apparent differences between Wagner et al. (2006) and the other studies in Table 1 are definitional rather than phenomenological.

This issue of daily cycling, i.e., mood switching during a single day for every day of the episode, is especially cogent to the preschool population. One of the most challenging aspects of assessing preschool children for psychopathology is the oftentimes protean nature of the symptoms (Luby et al., 2007). Preschool manic symptoms noted in Luby et al. (2007) were typical of mania but occurred for multiple brief periods daily for years, similar to descriptions in older children.

Another problem extant for all ages, but more so for preschoolers, is what constitutes pathological, impairing mood states. For depressed moods, this is relatively more straightforward, because *any* sustained sadness or anhedonia is considered abnormal. For example, there would be little disagreement that the anhedonic preschoolers reported by Luby et al. (2004) are impaired, as all children are expected to play. By contrast, Geller et al. (2002) have published on the counterintuitive conception that children can be psychopathologically too happy or too grandiose. And this would be even more so for preschoolers who are not yet "burdened" with school regulations or homework (Luby and Belden, 2006).

These observations on the pattern of manic symptoms in preschool children are highly similar to those reported for children aged 7 and older. In subjects aged 7 and older (Geller et al., 2004) and in those aged 6 and older (TEAM Study, unpublished data), daily mood switching during an episode was the most common presentation in studies that used the WASH-U-KSADS tool, which documents onset and offset of each current and lifetime episode (see Table 1). This tool also asks about the presence and number of daily cycles, and mood state during the daily cycle (Geller et al., 2001).

A problem has been how to define and document these daily phenomena so that comparable data across studies can be obtained. Authors studying both pediatric and adult samples have used the phrase "rapid cycling" in diverse contexts. Historically in the adult bipolar literature, "rapid cycling" was defined as four or more episodes per year (see Table 2). Thus, rapid cycling was defined as equivalent to multiple episodes per year, i.e., one episode equaled one cycle, as depicted in Table 2.

Episode duration in the Geller et al. (2004) and Birmaher et al. (2006) studies in Table 2 was defined using the Frank et al. (1991) criteria, which were developed for adults. These criteria were that recovery was defined as 8 consecutive weeks without meeting DSM-IV criteria for mania or hypomania, remission was defined as 2–7 weeks without meeting DSM-IV criteria for mania or hypomania, and relapse after recovery was defined as 2 consecutive weeks of meeting DSM-IV criteria for mania or hypomania with clinically significant impairment. Thus, investigators across the age span have used similar definitions of remission, recovery, and relapse.

TABLE 2. PROBLEM WITH THE HISTORICAL DEFINITIONS OF RAPID
CYCLING IN THE ADULT BIPOLAR I DISORDER LITERATURE

Historically: The words "episodes" and "cycling" were used interchangeably so that ≥4 episodes/year = rapid cycling.
Problem: This definition did not account for daily cycling during episodes.
Proposal: "Rapid cycling" be used only for daily switching phenomena that occur during an episode.

TABLE 3. PROPOSED DEFINITIONS OF EPISODES AND CYCLING PHENOMENA

Phenomenon	Definition
episode	onset to offset of full DSM-IV criteria for bipolar I disorder[b]
ultra-rapid cycling[a]	mood switches every few days during an episode
ultradian cycling[a]	mood switches multiple times daily during an episode

[a]These terms are from Kramlinger and Post (1996).
[b]Episodes are defined using Frank et al. (1991) criteria.

One important question is whether these daily rapid cycling definitions would pertain to adults with bipolar I disorder (BP-I). To examine this issue, data on daily cycling were collected in a blindly rated, controlled study of psychopathology of parents of BP-I probands who had BP-I themselves (Geller et al., 2006). Among these parents, 40.3% had daily cycling (Geller et al., unpublished data).

Uniform definitions of episode and cycling would help to clarify developmental, age-specific manifestations of mania. Therefore (see

TABLE 4. EXAMPLES OF EPISODE DURATION AND DAILY (ULTRADIAN) CYCLING IN PRESCHOOLERS, SCHOOL-AGE CHILDREN, AND ADULTS

Note that most children are in their first episode at baseline. Therefore, there may be a history of onset of DSM-IV bipolar I disorder but not of offset.

Example 1: Preschooler

A 6-year-old had an onset of DSM-IV symptoms of bipolar I disorder one year ago. During this year, there was a mean of 4 cycles per day. Cycles were from mania to euthymia. Child would be said to be in a current episode (and first episode) of bipolar I disorder symptoms that has a duration of one year, and the episode is characterized by daily cycling.

Example 2: School-Aged Child

An 8-year-old had an onset of DSM-IV bipolar I disorder two years ago. During these two years, there was a mean of 3 cycles per day. Cycles were from mania to depression or mania to euthymia. Child would be said to be in a current episode (and first episode) of bipolar I disorder with a duration of two years, and the episode is characterized by daily cycling.

Example 3: Adult

A 25-year-old patient had a history of two prior episodes of DSM-IV bipolar I disorder. One of these episodes was mania with a duration of three months and was without daily cycling. The second of these prior episodes was MDD for four weeks without daily cycling, immediately followed by two weeks of mania, also without daily cycling. This second episode, therefore, had a duration of six weeks characterized by four weeks of MDD and two weeks of mania, and without daily cycling. The current DSM-IV manic episode began 1 week ago and is without daily cycling.

Example 4: Adult

A 35-year-old patient had a history of onset of DSM-IV bipolar I disorder at age 16 characterized by 2–3 daily cycles from mania to depression or mania to euthymia and without a DSM-IV bipolar I disorder free period of at least eight weeks.[a] Thus, this adult had a current (and first) episode of bipolar I disorder with a duration of 19 years (no intervening euthymic period of at least eight weeks), characterized by daily (ultradian) cycling.

[a]The definition of separate episodes defined by eight week intervals of not meeting full DSM-IV criteria is used by multiple authors (Findling et al., 2001; Frank et al., 1991; Geller et al., 2004).
MDD = major depressive disorder.

Table 3), the proposal is as follows. A definition of episode that best fits the data is that episode refer to the onset and offset of full DSM-IV bipolar I disorder. Cycling would be used only to describe daily (ultradian) switching of mood states that occurs during an episode. Examples of the use of these definitions of episode and of cycling appear in Table 4. These examples also include how depressive states are incorporated into episode and cycling definitions.

For these definitions to have clinical utility, clinicians will need to ask parents and, separately, children whether they have daily cycles. If they say yes, then the number of cycles per day and the character of the cycles (elated, depressed, etc.) needs to be documented.

In summary, historically the words "episode" and "cycle" were used interchangeably. "Rapid cycling," in this historical schema, actually referred to multiple episodes per year. To avoid confusing episodes with daily cycling, the proposal is to use "episode" only for the duration of DSM-IV criteria, to use "cycling" only for daily phenomena during an episode, and to replace the historical term "rapid cycling" with "multiple episodes per year."

TREATMENT OF EARLY AGE MANIA (TEAM)

The Treatment of Early Age Mania (TEAM) study (NCT00057681) is conducted with the participation of the following sites: Washington University in St. Louis, St. Louis (coordinating site): Barbara Geller, M.D., Rebecca Tillman, M.S., Kristine Bolhofner, B.S., Betsy Zimerman, M.A., Jeanne Frazier, B.S.N., Linda Beringer, R.N., Nancy Strauss, B.S.N., Patricia Kaufmann, M.S.N., Jan Lautenschlager, B.S.; Children's National Medical Center, Washington D.C.: Paramjit Joshi, M.D., Adelaide Robb, M.D., Jay A. Salpekar, M.D., Nasima Nusrat, M.D.; Johns Hopkins Medical Institutions, Baltimore: John Walkup, M.D., Mark Riddle, M.D., Elizabeth Kastelic, M.D., Shannon Barnett, M.D., Shauna Reinblatt, M.D., Maria Rodowski, M.D., Jessica Foster, B.A., Andrea Galatis, B.S., Maureen Masarik, M.S., Samuel Walford, M.A.; University of Pittsburgh, Pittsburgh: David Axelson, M.D., Boris Birmaher, M.D., Neal Ryan, M.D., Annette Baughman, B.S.N., Leah Giovengo, B.A., Susan Wassick, R.N., Jennifer Fretwell, B.A., Christine Hoover, M.S.N.; University of Texas, Southwestern, Dallas: Graham Emslie, M.D.; University of Texas Medical Branch, Galveston: Karen Dineen Wagner, M.D., Ph.D., Melissa Martinez, M.D., Aileen Oandasan, M.D.; Washington University in St. Louis, St. Louis: Joan Luby, M.D., Samantha Blankenship, M.S.W., Mary Nail, M.A., Molly McGrath, L.C.S.W.; National Institute of Mental Health, Bethesda, MD: Benedetto Vitiello, M.D. (scientific collaborator), Joanne B. Severe, M.S. (operations staff). Please note that there are two separate sites at Washington University in St. Louis.

ACKNOWLEDGEMENT

We would like to thank Joan Luby, M.D. and Karen Dineen Wagner M.D., Ph.D. for their helpful comments on the manuscript.

AUTHOR DISCLOSURE

The authors have no conflicts of interest to disclose.

REFERENCES

Axelson D, Birmaher B, Strober M, Gill MK, Valeri S, Chiappetta L, Ryan N, Leonard H, Hunt J, Iyengar S, Bridge J, Keller M: Phenomenology of children and adolescents with bipolar spectrum disorders. Arch Gen Psychiatry 63:1139–1148, 2006.

Biederman J, Faraone SV, Wozniak J, Mick E, Kwon A, Cayton GA, Clark SV: Clinical correlates of bipolar disorder in a large, referred sample of children and adolescents. J Psychiatr Res 39:611–622, 2005.

Birmaher B, Axelson D, Strober M, Gill MK, Valeri S, Chiappetta L, Ryan N, Leonard H, Hunt J, Iyengar S, Keller M: Clinical course of children and adolescents with bipolar spectrum disorders. Arch Gen Psychiatry 63:175–183, 2006.

Findling RL, Gracious BL, McNamara NK, Youngstrom EA, Demeter CA, Branicky LA, Calabrese JR: Rapid, continuous cycling and psychiatric co-morbidity in pediatric bipolar I disorder. Bipolar Disord 3:202–210, 2001.

Frank E, Prien RF, Jarrett RB, Keller MB, Kupfer DJ, Lavori PW, Rush AJ, Weissman MM: Conceptualization and rationale for consensus definitions of terms in major depressive disorder. Arch Gen Psychiatry 48:851–855, 1991.

Geller B, Zimerman B, Williams M, Bolhofner K, Craney JL, DelBello MP, Soutullo C: Reliability of the Washington University in St. Louis Kiddie Schedule for Affective Disorders and Schizophrenia (WASH-U-KSADS) mania and rapid cycling sections. J Am Acad Child Adolesc Psychiatry 40:450–455, 2001.

Geller B, Zimerman B, Williams M, Delbello MP, Frazier J, Beringer L: Phenomenology of prepubertal and early adolescent bipolar disorder: examples of elated mood, grandiose behaviors, decreased need for sleep, racing thoughts and hypersexuality. J Child Adolesc Psychopharmacol 12:3–9, 2002.

Geller B, Tillman R, Craney JL, Bolhofner K: Four-year prospective outcome and natural history of mania in children with a prepubertal and early adolescent bipolar disorder phenotype. Arch Gen Psychiatry 61:459–467, 2004.

Geller B, Tillman R, Bolhofner K, Zimerman B, Strauss NA, Kaufmann P: Controlled, blindly rated, direct-interview family study of a prepubertal and early-adolescent bipolar I disorder phenotype: morbid risk, age at onset, and comorbidity. Arch Gen Psychiatry 63:1130–1138, 2006.

Kaufman J, Birmaher B, Brent D, Rao U, Flynn C, Moreci P, Williamson D, Ryan N: Schedule for Affective Disorders and Schizophrenia for School-Age Children—Present and Lifetime Version (K-SADS-PL): Initial reliability and validity data. J Am Acad Child Adolesc Psychiatry 36:980–988, 1997.

Kramlinger KG, Post RM: Ultra-rapid and ultradian cycling in bipolar affective illness. Br J Psychiatry 168:314–323, 1996.

Luby J, Belden A: Defining and validating bipolar disorder in the preschool period. Dev Psychopathol 18:971–988, 2006.

Luby JL, Mrakotsky C, Heffelfinger A, Brown K, Spitznagel E: Characteristics of depressed preschoolers with and without anhedonia: Evidence for a melancholic depressive subtype in young children. Am J Psychiatry 161:1998–2004, 2004.

Luby JL, Tandon M, Nicol G: Three clinical cases of DSM-IV mania symptoms in preschoolers. J Child Adolesc Psychopharmacol 17:237–243, 2007.

Orvaschel H, Puig-Antich J. Schedule for affective disorders and schizophrenia for school-age children: Epidemiologic version. Fort Lauderdale (FL), Nova University, 1987.

Tillman R, Geller B: Definitions of rapid, ultrarapid, and ultradian cycling and of episode duration in pediatric and adult bipolar disorders: A proposal to distinguish episodes from cycles. J Child Adolesc Psychopharmacol 13:267–271, 2003.

Wagner KD, Kowatch RA, Emslie GJ, Findling RL, Wilens TE, McCague K, D'Souza J, Wamil A, Lehman RB, Berv D, Linden D: A double-blind, randomized, placebo-controlled trial of oxcarbazepine in the treatment of bipolar disorder in children and adolescents. Am J Psychiatry 163:1179–1186, 2006.

ADVANCES IN PRESCHOOL PSYCHOPHARMACOLOGY
© 2009 Mary Ann Liebert, Inc.
140 Huguenot Street, 3rd Floor
New Rochelle, NY 10801-5215

Risperidone Treatment of Preschool Children with Thermal Burns and Acute Stress Disorder

Karen G. Meighen, M.D., Lori A. Hines, R.N., and Ann M. Lagges, Ph.D.

ABSTRACT

Pharmacologic treatment of acute stress disorder (ASD) is a novel area of investigation across all age groups. Very few clinical drug trials have been reported in children and adolescents diagnosed with ASD. Most of the available, potentially relevant, data are from studies of adults with posttraumatic stress disorder (PTSD). The atypical antipsychotic agents have been reported to be effective as an adjunctive treatment for adults with PTSD. There have been a limited number of studies published regarding atypical antipsychotic treatment of PTSD in children and adolescents, and there is no current literature available on the use of these agents for children with ASD. This report describes the successful treatment of three preschool-aged children with serious thermal burns as a result of physical abuse or neglect. Each of these children was hospitalized in a tertiary-care children's hospital and was diagnosed with ASD. In all cases, risperidone provided rapid and sustained improvement across all symptom clusters of ASD at moderate dosages. Minimal to no adverse effects were reported. These cases present preliminary evidence for the potential use of risperidone in the treatment of ASD in childhood.

INTRODUCTION

THE PREVALENCE OF PSYCHOLOGICAL SEQUELAE in pediatric burn survivors is estimated to be between 25% and 30% (Meyer et al. 1995; Altier et al. 2002). Many of these children develop acute stress disorder (ASD) (Stoddard 1990), which was first defined as a separate entity from posttraumatic stress disorder (PTSD) in the *Diagnostic and Statistical Manual of Mental Disorders*, 4th edition (DSM-IV) (American Psychiatric Association 1994). ASD is diagnosed when symptoms are present within 1 month of a trauma, whereas PTSD may be diagnosed 30 days or more after the event. These two disorders share many symptoms, including reexperiencing, avoidance, and hyperarousal, but ASD requires that dissociative symptoms also be present.

ASD symptoms are grouped into distinctive clusters: (1) The person has been exposed to a traumatic event in which they experienced or witnessed actual or threatened death or serious injury, or threat to physical integrity of self or

Department of Psychiatry, Section of Child and Adolescent Psychiatry, Indiana University School of Medicine, James Whitcomb Riley Hospital for Children, Indianapolis, Indiana.

This work was supported in part by Clarian Health Partners, the Riley Children's Foundation, and the State of Indiana Division of Mental Health and Addictions.

others. The person responded with intense fear, helplessness or horror. (2) Dissociative symptoms include: Emotional numbing, detachment, absence of emotional responsiveness, reduced awareness of surroundings (dazed), derealization, depersonalization, and dissociative amnesia. (3) Reexperiencing of the event may occur through recurrent images, thoughts, dreams, illusions, flashbacks, a sense of reliving the experience, or distress on exposure to reminders of the event. (4) Avoidance of stimuli that arouse recollections of the trauma. (5) Anxiety/hyperarousal symptoms include: Difficulty sleeping, irritability, poor concentration, hypervigilance, exaggerated startle response, and motor restlessness. These symptoms often impact the care of seriously ill patients, whose compliance with wound care and immobilization for grafts, participation in physical therapy, need for sleep, and proper nourishment are vitally important to recovery.

The use of psychopharmacologic agents to treat ASD is an understudied area across the developmental spectrum. A limited number of drug studies of PTSD in children have been published and even fewer have been reported in youths with ASD. A significant amount of data have been generated from studies of adults with PTSD. It is unclear if data from studies of PTSD in children and adolescents or adults are applicable to pediatric ASD. On the basis of similarities in symptom presentation and etiology of PTSD and ASD, however, it is important to review the pertinent literature available regarding both diagnoses.

There are currently two drugs with a United States Food and Drug Administration (FDA) indication for the treatment of adults with PTSD, sertraline and paroxetine, which are both selective serotonin-reuptake inhibitors (SSRIs). Off-label psychopharmacologic interventions currently employed for the treatment of childhood PTSD include: SSRIs, tricyclic antidepressants, serotonin-norepinephrine reuptake inhibitors, alpha-2 receptor agonists, buspirone, cyproheptadine, atypical antipsychotics, and benzodiazepines (Donnelly et al. 1999; Donnelly 2003).

Neuroleptics were the mainstay of treatment for PTSD symptoms in adults in the 1970s, but these agents are currently reserved for patients with refractory PTSD who exhibit paranoid behavior, hallucinatory phenomena or intense flashbacks, self-destructive behavior, explosive or overwhelming anger, or thought disorder (Donnelly et al. 1999). There has been a shift in practice of both adult and child and adolescent psychiatry toward the use of newer, atypical antipsychotics such as riperidone, olanzapine, and quetiapine, owing to their apparent lower risk of adverse effects such as extrapyramidal symptoms and tardive dyskinesia (Stigler et al. 2001). As a result, there is an emerging literature on the use of atypical antipsychotics as primary or adjunctive therapy for PTSD in adults, as well as in children and adolescents. Risperidone was more effective than placebo for symptoms of reexperiencing, avoidance, and hyperarousal when used alone or as adjunctive therapy along with stable doses of antidepressants, anxiolytics or hypnotics in combat veterans with PTSD (Bartzokis et al. 2005). A 6-week open-label study of quetiapine (dosage range 50–200 mg/day) in 6 adolescents with PTSD found the drug effective for reducing symptoms of dissociation, anxiety, depression, and anger with no persisting side effects or adverse events (Stathis et al. 2005). Clozapine (mean dose, 102 mg/day) was found to be effective in 19 adolescents with treatment-refractory PTSD at two residential facilities. Associated side effects included orthostatic hypotension, sedation, excessive salivation, constipation, agranulocytosis, significant weight gain, and neutropenia (Kant et al. 2004). Fifteen of 18 children (83%) (mean age, 9.28 years) with PTSD and co-morbid bipolar disorder or attention-deficit/hyperactivity disorder (ADHD) experienced robust decreases in their PTSD symptoms when treated with risperidone (mean dose, 1.37 mg/day) with no acute or chronic side effects (Horrigan and Barnhill 1999).

There is evidence for the effectiveness of risperidone in treating ASD in adult patients. Risperidone reduced sleep disturbance, frequency of nightmares and flashbacks, and hyperarousal associated with ASD in 10 adult burn patients within 24–48 hours at a dosage of 0.5–2 mg nightly (Stanovic et al. 2001). Risperidone (mean dose, 1.6 mg/day) rapidly relieved symptoms of ASD in 4 adults who were hospitalized due to physical trauma (Eidelman et al. 2000). This report describes three preschool-aged children who were admitted to a tertiary care children's hospital due to severe thermal burns from scalding water and were subsequently diagnosed with ASD based on DSM-IV criteria. All 3 patients demonstrated a rapid and sustained response to risperidone at moderate dosages, defined as improved emotional responsiveness, reduced dissociative symptoms, less frequent and less intense episodes of reexperiencing, decreased avoidance of stimuli that arouse recollections of the event, and a decrease in hyperarousal.

Treatment-emergent side effects were assessed using clinical observation, nursing reports, physical examinations, and monitoring of changes in vital signs and laboratory measures. Blood pressure and heart rate were monitored daily and weight was checked twice weekly during hospitalization. Fasting glucose and lipid profiles were checked prior to initiation of risperidone and at discharge of each child.

CASE 1

N. was a 3-year 2-month-old Caucasian girl admitted to a tertiary care children's hospital with 9% total body surface area (TBSA) scald burns to both hands and her forearms. Her wounds were thought to have been caused by nonaccidental trauma and she was made a ward of the county court by child protective services (CPS) at the time of her admission. N.'s mother was suspected of perpetrating abuse on N., thus CPS did not allow her to visit with the child. The mother was able to provide informed consent for treatment at the time of N.'s admission and CPS gave written informed consent for treatment.

A child psychiatry consultation was sought 4 days after N. was admitted to the burn unit due to extensive complaints of her hands hurting, irritability, and minimal communication. At the time of psychiatric evaluation, N. demonstrated emotional detachment and she looked as if she was functioning in a daze. She did not appear to be responding to internal stimuli or to be having visual hallucinations.

She talked about her wounds frequently, even when not experiencing pain. She was having difficulty sleeping, and the nurses noted she would awaken with bad dreams. When allowed to speak with family members on the telephone, she would say, "Mommy burnt me, Mommy burnt me." N. tried to avoid water, especially hot water, but daily baths are a necessary part of the burn treatment protocol. She became extremely agitated and combative with the nurses during baths and dressing changes despite receiving multiple sedative medications prior to these procedures. N. demonstrated hypervigilance and an exaggerated startle response. She had not been eating, and her nutrition was not adequate for healing. The nursing staff limited the number of nurses assigned to N. to provide her with some consistency. N. had been responsive to these nurses, but her affect remained very restricted. She had been a quiet and easygoing child prior to this trauma per the CPS report from her mother. There were no reported premorbid developmental, behavioral, or emotional problems noted. There was a positive maternal family history for depression. The paternal family psychiatric history was unknown.

On physical examination, N. was found to have 9% TBSA burns of the upper extremities but was otherwise normal for age. Computerized tomography of the head and a skeletal survey were both normal, as were routine blood chemistries. Scheduled medications at the time of psychiatric consultation included: Acetaminophen with codeine, ascorbic acid, zinc supplement, multivitamin, metoclopramide, ducosate sodium, senna, and cefazolin. N. received adequate trials of midazolam, acetaminophen with codeine, fentanyl, diphenhydramine, and ibuprofen combinations prior to necessary procedures without significant benefit for her anxiety, agitation, or complaints of pain.

Initial mental status examination revealed an alert, disheveled 3-year-old Caucasian girl who was restless and roaming the open areas of the burn unit. She was very watchful of the interviewer and others on the unit. She made several complaints to the interviewer that her "boo-boo's hurt." She was difficult to redirect and often appeared to be in her own world. Her affect was constricted and irritable. She nodded her head "yes" to being scared, but responded negatively to feeling other emotions. She produced a limited amount of speech. Thought processes appeared concrete, fairly focused, and repetitive. Thought content primarily regarded her wounds.

N. was diagnosed with ASD with a rule-out diagnosis of child victim of physical abuse. Risperidone was started at 0.5 mg given 45 minutes prior to her once-daily bath and dressing change and 0.5 mg every night. N. continued to receive previously prescribed doses of fentanyl, diphenhydramine, and midazolam prior to each dressing change. On day 2 after starting risperidone, N. had tolerated baths without as much combativeness but was still anxious. She had been sleeping better and was communicating with the nurses more. She did not appear to be so detached or dazed. Her affect was less irritable. On day 2, no adverse effects were noted with risperidone use and the dosage was increased to 1 mg 45 minutes prior to each daily dressing change and 0.5 mg nightly. By day 5 of risperidone treatment, the dosage of scheduled fentanyl was being tapered and N. no longer required the larger amounts of midazolam and fentanyl previously needed during procedures. Her affect appeared brighter and N. was much more playful and interactive. She was more interested in coloring and playing games. She was sleeping 7–8 hours per night and denied having bad dreams. She had begun to help with her daily baths. When she spoke of her "boo-boo's," it was to speak proudly about how she had washed them and she raised the topic only in appropriate context. N. began to show an improved appetite, but she did require significant encouragement to ingest adequate calories. On day 14 of risperidone treatment, N. had continued to demonstrate improvement in the symptoms of ASD. Her fentanyl had been discontinued and her pain during procedures was well managed with oral opiates. She was significantly more interactive and playful. She was cooperative with nursing staff, as well as occupational and physical therapists who required her to use both of her hands. Her complaints of pain were minimal and consistent with what would be expected based upon the severity of her physical injuries. She continued to sleep well and had experienced only a single bad dream over the course of the previous 9 days. She only spoke about her wounds in an appropriate context. Telephone contacts with family continued to be a source of agitation for N. Baths, dressing changes, and other procedures became less extensive at this point in N.s care. In preparation for outpatient care, risperidone was changed to 1.5 mg nightly with no loss of clinical benefit. CPS substantiated physical abuse to N. by her mother. On day 19, N. was introduced to her potential foster family and she was discharged to foster care on day 22 of risperidone therapy.

CASE 2

Z. was a 3-year 6-month-old Caucasian male seen in psychiatric consultation 10 days after admission to a tertiary-care children's hospital for the treatment of 24% TBSA scald burns to his neck, back, and upper extremities. Z.'s case was being investigated by county CPS due to concerns for maternal neglect. The mother had been limited to 1 hour per day visits with Z. She and CPS provided written informed consent for treatment.

The burn unit staff noted that Z. had a labile mood since the day of admission. He would become spontaneously tearful. He had been screaming at night and had difficulty sleeping. He refused to be left alone and would climb out of bed day and night to sit in the hall and be near nursing staff. When he did fall asleep, he was notably restless. His appetite had been very poor and a nasogastric (NG) tube was being considered for nutrition if his oral intake did not rapidly improve. He refused to be around water, hot foods and beverages, as well as the heating vent in his room. Dressing changes with baths had been extremely traumatic for Z. despite receiving high doses of pain medications and sedatives in preparation for these procedures. He required physical restraint to accomplish these tasks. During visits with his mother, Z. was overheard repeatedly asking, "Are you my Mommy?" and he would appear to function in a trance for prolonged periods after her visits. He had one episode during which he grabbed a doll from the hands of a peer, looked as if in a trance, and screamed, "Baby burning!" Z. had refused to talk about his trauma with law enforcement specialists and CPS. He had not described to any of the staff what had happened to him.

Premorbidly, Z. had been living with his unemployed, 28-year-old mother and three older siblings. His biologic father had no contact with Z. His mother denied any developmental delays, health problems, or traumas in Z.'s past. She described Z. as sometimes having a difficult temperament and being demanding of her time but admitted that his older sister tended to have much worse behavior. She had not observed sleep problems or anxiety symptoms prior to his admission to the hospital.

Z. was found to be a healthy 3-year-old Caucasian male with 24% TBSA burns to the neck, upper back, and upper extremities on physical examination. Routine blood chemistries at the time of admission were normal. Scheduled medications at the time of psychiatric consultation included: Ducosate sodium, collagenase, and polysporin. His as-needed medicines were: Acetaminophen with codeine, fentanyl, midazolam, diphenhydramine, and ibuprofen. A one-time dose of ketamine had been tried during a dressing change, along with fentanyl, midazolam, and diphenhydramine, to try and achieve adequate sedation and anesthesia but without benefit.

On initial mental status examination, Z. was an alert 3-year-old male who had a frightened affect when seen in his hospital room. Psychomotor agitation was noted. He wanted to sit in the hallway and hugged a picture of his siblings throughout the interview. He was tearful for the remainder of the contact and frequently said, "I want my Nana," meaning his grandmother. His speech was very soft. Thought processes were concrete but logical and sequential. Thought content was focused on Z.'s fear for his safety and that of his brother and sisters. He was most afraid of water, especially hot water, but refused to expand upon that. He was also afraid of the dark and monsters. When asked if anyone had ever hurt him, he developed a vacant look and did not answer. He denied seeing strange things or hearing things that others may not see or hear, but did

say he sometimes had bad dreams in the daytime. He did not think he was asleep for these dreams but was unable to explain further.

Z. was diagnosed with ASD and rule-out diagnoses of child victim of physical abuse and child victim of neglect. He was started on risperidone 0.5 mg 45 minutes prior to once-daily dressing changes and 0.5 mg at bedtime. It was also requested that family visits occur at a consistent and predictable time, that Z. be made aware of such visits just before they were to occur, and that he have therapeutic activities to attend after family visits to assist him with expressing emotions. Twenty-four hours after starting risperidone, Z. slept approximately 6 hours, although he was still restless. He was much less tearful and worrisome and had eaten better at breakfast and lunch. He tolerated his dressing change much better that morning without his typical resistance, screaming, or need for restraint. The dosage of risperidone was increased to 0.75 mg prior to each dressing change and 1 mg nightly. By day 3 of risperidone, Z. was notably more calm but not sedated. No psychomotor agitation was noted. His affect was much brighter and he would smile and play by himself, as well as with others. He was able to sleep in his room throughout the night. There were no episodes of Z. appearing to be vacant or in a trance-like state. He was beginning to help with his baths and dressing changes and no longer appeared terrified in the tubroom. His dosage requirement for as-needed fentanyl and midazolam decreased significantly during dressing changes. He took in enough calories to avoid NG tube placement. He did continue to voice concerns over his siblings and would become upset if staff moved their picture. By day 5, he started to talk more with staff about his fear that someone would hurt his siblings.

CPS was contacted for permission to treat Z.'s anxiety and, because his symptoms had improved, he was interviewed a second time by law enforcement specialists. Neglect was substantiated with the mother as perpetrator and all of the children were removed from her care. On day 9 of risperidone therapy, Z. and his siblings were to be reunited in a safer environment at the time of his discharge. He progressed rapidly in his burn healing, nutritional status, and emotional stability. There were no adverse effects of risperidone seen throughout the course of treatment. He was referred for outpatient psychiatric care, but the foster parents did not follow through on this recommendation.

CASE 3

D. was a 25-month-old African-American (AA) male admitted to a tertiary-care children's hospital for the evaluation and treatment of 15% TBSA scald burns to his left foot, buttocks, and left hand. D.'s case was suspicious for nonaccidental trauma and neglect; therefore, county CPS was contacted at the time of his admission. CPS established limited visitation with the family with only supervised visits being allowed. The mother and her fiancé were both suspected of perpetrating abuse and neglect on D. CPS and the patient's mother provided written informed consent for treatment.

The burn unit staff were concerned that D. appeared extremely withdrawn and would not respond to them. He would lie in a transport wagon in the hallway and stare. Child psychiatry consultation was requested and completed 1 day after D.'s admission. Nursing staff reported that D. had not spoken to them. He would gaze at the ceiling and seemingly not blink for minutes at a time. He had not slept well and seemed to jerk awake as if terrified when he would fall asleep. He had great distress with baths and was struggling with burn dressing changes despite being premedicated with large doses of narcotics and sedatives. The nurses did find it unusual that D. did not seem to mind having other procedures done to him and tended to look very calm and quiet except during baths. He appeared to avoid looking at his wounds and notably tried to avoid his mother at visits by hiding under his covers and refusing to look at her. He was "fussy" much of the time when not staring away. The patient had not eaten and would require a Dobhoff tube if his oral nutrition did not begin to improve.

Initial mental status examination was carried out prior to the patient receiving larger doses of medicines for his dressing change and re-

vealed that D. was a relatively thin, 2-year-old AA male lying in a transport wagon with a limp posture and bandages covering his left hand and foot. He was looking toward the ceiling as if in a daze, but after repeated attempts to get his attention, did respond to verbal cues by looking toward the examiner and making eye contact. His affect was flat and he appeared frightened. He did not speak throughout the first contact, therefore thought processes and content were difficult to assess. He would startle with loud noises and with the sound of water running in the tubroom.

History was obtained from the mother regarding D.'s premorbid functioning. She stated that his only health issue was an undescended testis. He had normal hearing and had been developing speech with at least a 100- to 200-word vocabulary. She denied that D. had experienced any past traumas or emotional, behavioral, or developmental issues. He was described as a very quiet but affectionate child who did not typically require any discipline. D. had been living with his biological mother and her fiancé prior to his hospitalization. The biological father had never had contact with the patient.

On physical examination, D. was found to be a thin-appearing 2-year old male with 15% TBSA burns to his left foot, left hand, and buttocks believed to be consistent with immersion injury per the opinion of the child abuse specialist consulting on his case. Computerized tomography of the head and a skeletal survey were found to be normal, as were routine blood chemistries. Scheduled medications at the time of consultation included: Collagenase, silver sulfadiazine, bacitracin, vitamin C, and a multivitamin. Medications prescribed as needed included: Morphine sulfate, midazolam, diphenhydramine, odansetron, and acetaminophen with codeine.

D. was diagnosed with ASD and rule-out diagnoses of child victim of physical abuse and child victim of neglect. Risperidone 0.25 mg nightly was prescribed. Two days after starting risperidone, D. was sleeping better, but would still awaken in jerking motions as if startled and afraid. He would cry during baths, but was quiet during dressing changes. He seemed less dazed and began to show some interest in his surroundings. On day 5 of risperidone, D. continued to experience restless sleep and would periodically cry out in the night. He had begun to pay attention to television and movies. He would eat some food, but his oral nutrition remained overall poor and a Dobhoff tube was placed to help supplement calories and promote healing. D. continued to have an anxious affect, but he was not as detached as he had been initially. He was demonstrating less staring and would occasionally smile and use words. The risperidone was increased to 0.5 mg nightly and a speech and language consult was requested. Within 24 hours after the increased dose of antipsychotic, D. slept peacefully through the night. He had less crying and whining with his bath and tolerated the dressing change very well. He was smiling and playful with others. He ate more at meals and was verbally more responsive, although he still had a relative paucity of speech for his age. He was diagnosed by the speech pathologist as suffering from a receptive and expressive language disorder, but it was unknown if this was a baseline disorder or might be secondary to the trauma. He received speech therapy during the remainder of his stay. D. was able to tolerate baths and dressing changes with only oral narcotics and diphenhydramine from that point forth in his care. The intravenous narcotics were discontinued except for brief periods surrounding times he required debridement of a wound. Over the following 10 days of his hospital stay, D. continued to show a decrease in his level of anxiety. He was able to view his wounds without distress and tolerated his mother's visits with little affect, but would interact with her. He was able to have the feeding tube removed and was eating fairly well by the time of discharge. His behavior was more like that of a typical 2 year old. He was oppositional and make attempts to manipulate the staff. His affect appeared euthymic by the time of discharge, and he was using a number of words to communicate. His sleep had normalized, and he denied bad dreams. Some daytime drowsiness was noted when the dose of risperidone was increased to 0.5 mg nightly, but this dissipated after 3–4 days and he had no obvious adverse effects at the time of his discharge.

CPS substantiated abuse and neglect with the fiancé being the perpetrator of the abuse and mother being charged with neglect. No biological family member was believed to be fit to care for D. Thus, foster care was arranged, and he was discharged to his new foster family on day 15 of risperidone therapy.

D. was seen in outpatient psychiatric follow up 1 month after the date of his trauma. He was speaking in phrases, smiling, laughing, and playful in his interactions. He appeared to be physically healthy and his weight was good. He had been eating and sleeping well without evidence of restlessness or bad dreams. He talked about his burns and showed others his wounds, but not to excess. His affect was only irritable when he was tired, per report. He was tolerant of supervised visits with his mother, but still was not showing much affect when with her. D. was seen again 2 months after his trauma and had a very similar presentation to that seen at his 1-month follow up. He was starting to work on toilet training with his foster mother and his vocabulary continued to improve.

DISCUSSION

The children in these three cases were all diagnosed with ASD and successfully treated with the atypical antipsychotic risperidone. They all demonstrated an improvement in ASD symptoms defined as improved emotional responsiveness and reduced dissociative symptoms, less frequent and less intense episodes of reexperiencing of the trauma, diminished avoidance of stimuli that arouse recollections of the event, and a decrease in hyperarousal. Reduction of symptoms was rapid and occurred within the first 1–2 days after starting risperidone. Dosages of risperidone prescribed for these children (0.5–1.75 mg/day) were consistent with those seen in case reports of other agitated, medically ill preschoolers, studies of preschool children diagnosed with autism spectrum disorders, and those diagnosed with bipolar disorder (Bealke and Meighen 2005; Biederman et al. 2005; Luby et al. 2006). Sustained improvement in all ASD symptoms was seen throughout follow up, which ranged from

1.3 to 8 weeks. One child experienced brief, minor daytime drowsiness after a dosage increase of risperidone; otherwise, the medication was well-tolerated. No clinically significant changes in glucose, lipid values, vital signs, or weight were seen and no extrapyramidal side effects, including hypersalivation, were noted in these children during treatment with risperidone. The response seen in this set of preschool children is consistent with that seen in adults where 10 burn patients diagnosed with ASD were prescribed risperidone at an average daily dose of 1 mg per day (Stanovic et al. 2001). In that study, improvement in sleep disturbance, nightmares, flashbacks, and hyperarousal were noted within the first 1–2 days of treatment. Another report of 4 adults who were hospitalized secondary to physical trauma demonstrated effectiveness and safety of risperidone in rapidly relieving symptoms of ASD at an average dosage of 1.6 mg/day (Eidelman et al. 2000).

Each of the children in these cases suffered serious thermal burns. The treatment protocol for all of the children required daily bathing of their wounds with dressing changes. Due to the type of initial trauma sustained by each child these procedures could, themselves, also be highly stressful. They all had disturbed sleep and poor nutrition and were highly distressed or combative during necessary medical procedures. Risperidone was believed to be the best choice of medication for these severely impaired children on the basis of evidence from the adult literature of its ability to target all ASD symptom clusters, its rapid onset of action, and its favorable safety profile compared to conventional antipsychotic agents. There is preliminary evidence that treatment of children with certain psychotropic agents in the immediate peritraumatic period may prevent PTSD from developing (Saxe et al. 2001; Pitman et al. 2002; Vaiva et al. 2003). It was hypothesized that risperidone may not only provide reliable, immediate, and broad relief of ASD symptoms, but also may help to improve appetite and prevent the development of the disabling, potentially chronic disorder of PTSD in these children. Follow-up information beyond the initial 30-day period was only available for one child.

However, he and his caregivers denied significant PTSD symptoms at the time he was evaluated, 2 months posttrauma. All 3 children had been treated with benzodiazepines along with high doses of other sedating medications without significant impact on their anxiety. Risperidone was chosen over alternative psychotropic agents in each of these children due to the severity of their impairments and the urgent need for medication efficacy to reduce anxiety and the potential for further emotional trauma and physical complications during hospitalization.

It is difficult to diagnose ASD and PTSD in the preschool population with complete precision due to the subjectivity inherent in some of the required criteria. Children in this age group do not possess the verbal skills, abstract thought, or emotional processing necessary to accurately describe many of the symptoms of these disorders. Many preschool children are not able to relay specific events of the trauma. Preverbal children cannot report on their reaction at the time of a traumatic event. Clinicians have relied upon their interpretations of a child's behavior in many cases to make the diagnosis. Systematic interviews with caregivers can increase the potential to diagnose PTSD and ASD accurately in young children. Psychometrically sound measures of traumatic stress in preschool children are only now available (Scheeringa et al, 2001; Scheeringa et al. 2003). Alternative diagnostic criteria have been proposed for PTSD that are developmentally modified to be more sensitive to the lack of cognitive and verbal abilities of young children than the DSM-IV criteria. Children, ages 1–3 years, have been found to manifest higher rates of intrusive recollections of trauma, nightmares, separation anxiety, and major depressive symptoms than older children. In preschool children, recurrent and intrusive recollections of the event may not necessarily be distressing. Diminished interest in significant activities in young children is most often manifested as a constriction of play, and feelings of detachment or estrangement are mainly observed as social withdrawal. Alternative criteria for diagnosing PTSD do not require a description of the child's response to the traumatic event. Often adults have not witnessed the response and preschool children cannot provide a verbal description of their reactions. Alternative criteria only require one symptom of avoidance and numbing of general responsiveness to be present as opposed to the three symptoms that are required in the adult criteria (Scheeringa et al. 2003). If alternative criteria for young children are employed in determining a diagnosis in these cases, all 3 children could clearly be diagnosed with PTSD, except symptoms had been apparent for a period less than 30 days at the time of psychiatric evaluation.

The use of opiate and benzodiazepine medications, as well as diphenhydramine and ketamine, in these children in the medical setting can further complicate the clinical picture and make diagnosis challenging. Intoxication on or withdrawal from these medications can cause anxiety, agitation, and symptoms that look like dissociation. In these three cases, the children all had stable doses of these medications until risperidone treatment began to demonstrate clinical benefit. Their anxiety and dissociative symptoms improved before the doses of these medications were adjusted. After treatment with risperidone, dosages of opiates and sedatives needed to achieve adequate pain control were reduced. Other medical factors that may mimic symptoms of anxiety include infectious processes, fever, and pain. All of these factors remained stable, in all cases, during the initial treatment course with risperidone and did not appear to be contributing to the psychiatric presentation of these children.

All of these children are at risk for other types of anxiety and mood disorders because they have been physically abused and/or neglected, they are hospitalized, and they are separated from their families. Some symptoms of separation anxiety were noted in the children, but they did not meet full criteria for any DSM-IV anxiety or mood disorder diagnosis except ASD. Other premorbid diagnoses must also be entertained for these children, especially reactive attachment disorder, but none of the parents gave clear histories that would confirm this diagnosis.

A factor that could influence response to risperidone for these children was the fact that they were in a safe environment distanced from the perpetrator of any potential abuse or neglect. They received art therapy, music therapy, and opportunities for therapeutic play and to learn self-care techniques, as is standard protocol on the pediatric burn unit. These would be stable factors throughout the course of treatment, and in two of the cases, psychiatric consultation was not sought until several days after the patient's admission when accommodation to the hospital environment could have occurred. It was not until risperidone was initiated that any significant impact on anxiety symptoms was noted for the children. In Z.'s case, requesting that family visits only occur at predictable and consistent times with therapeutic activities scheduled for him after each visit may have contributed to a reduction in his anxiety level. However, once the antipsychotic was started, he immediately demonstrated an improvement in symptoms prior to the change in visitation schedule. Quality sleep and proper nutrition can help reduce anxiety symptoms but it was risperidone that helped provide the improvements in sleep and appetite initially. ASD symptoms can abate spontaneously, but each of these children had some residual symptoms within the first 1 month of treatment, making the possibility of spontaneous remission unlikely.

In summary, the child psychiatry consultation-liaison service of a tertiary-care children's hospital was able to implement treatment successfully with risperidone in 3 preschool children with severe thermal burn injuries and ASD. All 3 children had a rapid and sustained response to risperidone at moderate doses for their weight with only one mild, transient side effect. There are few reports in the literature regarding the use of atypical antipsychotic agents for ASD in adults, and there are no current reports of their use for ASD in children. As with all off-label uses of medications in this population, caution and vigilance should be exercised. Further studies are needed to assess the efficacy and safety of risperidone in the treatment of children with ASD and other anxiety disorders, especially those below the age of 6 years.

DISCLOSURES

The authors have no conflicts of interest to report.

REFERENCES

Altier N, Malenfant A, Forget R, Choiniere M: Long-term adjustment in burn victims: A matched-control study. Psychol. Med 32:677–685, 2002.

American Psychiatric Association: Diagnostic and Statistical Manual of Mental Disorders, 4th edition. Washington, D.C., American Psychiatric Association, 1994.

Bartzokis G, Lu PH, Turner J, Mintz J, Saunders CS: Adjunctive risperidone in the treatment of chronic combat-related posttraumatic stress disorder. Biol Psych 57:474–479, 2005.

Bealke JM, Meighen KG: Risperidone treatment of three seriously medically ill children with secondary mood disorders. Psychosom 46:254–258, 2005.

Biederman J, Mick E, Hammerness P, Harpold T, Aleardi M, Dougherty M, Wozniak J: Open-label, 8-week trial of olanzapine and risperidone for the treatment of bipolar disorder in preschool-age children. Biol Psych 58:589–594, 2005.

Donnelly CL: Pharmacologic treatment approaches for children and adolescents with posttraumatic stress disorder. Child Adolesc Psychiatr Clin N Am 12:251–269, 2003.

Donnelly CL, Amaya-Jackson L, March JS: Psychopharmacology of pediatric posttraumatic stress disorder. J Child Adolesc Psychopharmacol 9:203–220, 1999.

Eidelman I, Seedat S, Stein DJ: Risperidone in the treatment of acute stress disorder in physically traumatized in-patients. Depress Anxiety 11:187–188, 2000.

Horrigan JP, Barnhill LJ: Risperidone and PTSD in boys. J Neuropsychiatry Clin Neurosci 11:126–127, 1999.

Kant R, Chalansani R, Chengappa KN, Dieringer MF: The off-label use of clozapine in adolescents with bipolar disorder, intermittent explosive disorder, or posttraumatic stress disorder. J Child Adolesc Psyhcopharmacol. 14:57–63, 2004.

Luby J, Mrakotsky C, Stalets MM, Belden A, Heffelfinger A, Williams M, Spitznagel E: Risperidone in preschool children with autistic spectrum disorders: An investigation of safety and efficacy. J Child Adolesc Psychopharmacol 16:575–587, 2006.

Meyer WJ 3rd, Blakeney P, LeDoux J, Herndon DN: Diminished adaptive behaviors among pediatric survivors of burns. J Burn Care Rehabil 16:511–518, 1995.

Pitman RK, Sanders KM, Zusman RM, Healy AR, Cheema F, Lasko NB, Cahill L, Orr SP: Pilot study of secondary prevention of posttraumatic stress disorder with propranolol. Biol Psych 51:189–192, 2002.

Saxe G, Stoddard F, Courtney D, Cunningham K, Chawla N, Sheridan R, King D, King L: Relationship between acute morphine and the course of PTSD in children with burns. J Am Acad Child Adolesc Psychiatry 40:915–921, 2001.

Scheeringa MS, Peebles CD, Cook CA, Zeanah CH: Toward establishing procedural, criterion, and discriminant validity for PTSD in early childhood. J Am Acad Child Adolesc Psychiatry 40:52–60, 2001.

Scheeringa MS, Zeanah CH, Myers L, Putnam FW: New findings on alternative criteria for PTSD in preschool children. J Am Acad Child Adolesc Psychiatry 43:561–570, 2003.

Stanovic JK, James KA, Van Devere CA: The effectiveness of risperidone on acute stress symptoms in adult burn patients: A preliminary retrospective pilot study. J Burn Care Rehab 22:210–213, 2001.

Stathis S, Martin G, McKenna JG: A preliminary case series on the use of quetiapine for posttraumatic stress disorder in juveniles within a youth detention center. J Clin Psychopharmacol 25:539–544, 2005.

Stigler KA, Potenza MN, McDougle CJ: Tolerability profile of atypical antipsychotics in children and adolescents. Paediatric Drugs 3:927–942, 2001.

Stoddard F: Psychiatric management of the burned patient. In: Acute Care of the Burn Patient. Edited by Martyn JA. Orlando (Florida), Grune & Stratton, 1990, pp 256–272.

Vaiva G, Ducrocq F, Jezequel K, Averland B, Lestavel P, Brunet A, Marmar CR: Immediate treatment with propranolol decreases posttraumatic stress disorder two months after trauma. Biol Psychiatry 54:947–949, 2003.

ADVANCES IN PRESCHOOL PSYCHOPHARMACOLOGY
© 2009 Mary Ann Liebert, Inc.
140 Huguenot Street, 3rd Floor
New Rochelle, NY 10801-5215

Fluoxetine in Posttraumatic Eating Disorder in Two-Year-Old Twins

Gonca Celik, M.D.,[1] Rasim Somer Diler, M.D.,[2] Aysegul Yolga Tahiroglu, M.D.,[1]
and Ayşe Avci, M.D.[1]

ABSTRACT

Feeding disorders of infancy or early childhood are relatively uncommon in the pediatric population. In posttraumatic eating disorder, the infant demonstrates food refusal after a traumatic event or repeated traumatic events to the oropharynx or esophagus. We present case reports of 24-month-old twin girls, A and B, who presented to our clinic with food refusal and fear of feeding. Several invasive gastrointestinal procedures were performed when they were 3 months old, and they started to refuse all solid food and some liquids soon after hospitalization. Fluoxetine 0.3 mg/kg per day (5 mg/day) was started to target their anxiety and fear about feeding. In the second month of weekly follow up, the children began to be fed without a nasogastric catheter. A significant decrease in anxiety and fear was observed during feeding. Although the use of serotonin-selective reuptake inhibitors (SSRIs) in preschool children is controversial due to the lack of empirical data in this age group, we observed clinical improvements in anxiety in these two cases. Furthermore, fluoxetine was well tolerated and no side effects were observed.

INTRODUCTION

THE TERM "POSTTRAUMATIC EATING DISORDER" was first coined (Chatoor et al. 1988) in an article on food refusal in five latency-age children who experienced episodes of choking or severe gagging and refusal to eat any solid food following this traumatic event. If left untreated, this condition can impair physical and emotional development of the child (Chatoor 1991), but the treatment of this condition has not been well studied. Operational diagnostic criteria in posttraumatic food disorder (PTFD) of infancy

and early childhood are: (1) The infant demonstrates food refusal after a traumatic event or repeated traumatic events to the oropharynx or esophagus (e.g., choking, severe gagging, vomiting, reflux, insertion of nasogastric or endotracheal tubes, suctioning, force-feeding); (2) the event (or events) triggered intense distress in the infant; (3) the infant experiences distress when anticipating feedings (e.g., when positioned for feeding, when shown the bottle or feeding utensils, and/or when approached with food); (4) the infant resists feedings and becomes increasingly distressed when force-

---

[1]Department of Child and Adolescent Psychiatry, Cukurova University, Adana, Turkey 01330.
[2]Department of Child Psychiatry, Western Psychiatric Institute and Clinic, Pennsylvania, Pittsburgh, Pennsylvania.

fed. (Chatoor et al. 1988; Chatoor et al. 2001) The *Diagnostic and Statistical Manual of Mental Disorders*, 4th edition (DSM-IV) (American Psychiatric Association, 1994) describes Feeding Disorders of Infancy or Early Childhood in the pediatric population with an estimated prevalence rate of 1–5% of pediatric hospital admissions. According to DSM-IV and International Statistical Classification of Diseases and Related Health Problems (ICD-10) (1992) choking phobia is defined as a specific phobia. More broad diagnostic classification related to eating disorders in early childhood may be necessary due to insufficiencies in DSM-IV classification and lack of consensus with other diagnostic criteria and DSM-IV.

Three pediatric cases in 7- to 12-year-old children with choking phobia have been reported in the literature. It was reported that these children's anxiety symptoms during meal time were reduced by serotonin-selective reuptake inhibitor (SSRI) treatment (Banerjee et al. 2005). However, antidepressant administration is rare and controversial, especially in the preschool age group where no data on safety or efficacy to guide treatment practices are available. (Avci et al. 1998).

We present cases of 2-year-old twin girls who developed eating disorders soon after a medical procedure and who both responded well to fluoxetine treatment.

CASE REPORT

Parents brought their 24-month-old twin girls, A and B, to our clinic because of food refusal and fear of feeding. The parents consented to the treatment as well as to publishing the medical information about their children in a scientific journal. The girls were hospitalized with the diagnosis of gastroesophageal reflux (GER) when they were 3 months old. Several invasive gastrointestinal procedures were performed during GER treatment, and the twins started to refuse all solid food and some liquids soon after hospitalization. Feeding attempts without nasogastric catheter were unsuccessful, following which the children were fed only by nasogastric catheter.

At their first child psychiatric evaluation, behavioral interventions were recommended to the family, such as desensitization and feeding without nasogastric catheter by liquid food administration. Neurological and medical exams and routine blood tests were within normal limits. After these exams, both twins were started on haloperidol 0.03 mg/kg per day bid (0.5 mg units/day) because of feeding resistance in catheter absence, regression in toilet training, and anxiety symptoms (frequently crying, restlessness, fear of strangers, and separation anxiety). Neither extrapyramidal symptoms (EPS) nor other side effects were observed. The dose was not increased because of the risks of dyskinesia withdrawal and tardive dyskinesia risks from these drugs. There was no improvement after 1 month of combined medical and behavioral therapy. The parent's anxiety increased during feeding of their children and practicing of behavioral therapy. For this reason, haloperidol was stopped. Then fluoxetine 0.3 mg/kg per day (5 mg/day) was started to target their anxiety and fear of feeding. In approximately the second month of weekly follow up, the children began to be fed without nasogastric catheter. A significant decrease in anxiety and fear during feeding occurred and toilet training was regained. No side effects were seen during the 6-month therapy with fluoxetine. Because of the optimal therapeutic response, the dose was not increased. The fluoxetine was discontinued after 8 months of treatment, but follow-up visits were continued for 3 years, and the symtpoms did not recur. However, patient B presented with preschool separation anxiety according to DSM-IV diagnostic criteria after 3 years and regressed spontaneously. However, no psychopathology was seen in patient A.

DISCUSSION

These case studies build upon the clinical observation of infants and young children who have undergone traumatic experiences to the oropharynx or esophagus and subsequently refused to eat and demonstrated severe distress before feeding (Chatoor 1991; Chatoor et al. 2000a). The observation of infants with PTFD during feeding suggests that these infants are highly resistant to feedings and engage in intense conflict with their mothers. They show fear and become distressed when positioned for feedings and when presented with feeding utensils and food. They resist being fed by crying, arching, and refusing to open their mouth (Chatoor et al. 2001). The cases in our clinic presented very similarly. Twin girls A and B also refused to be fed by their mother, and they frequently cried during feeding time.

According to this classification, our cases meet criteria for choking phobia or PTFD. Because the eating disorder onset occurred after the esophagus operation, PTFD appeared to be the appropriate diagnosis. Choking phobia is characterized by difficulty swallowing solids and/or liquids without an underlying physiological cause and is accompanied by intense anxiety that results in restricted eating patterns or complete avoidance of eating (Chatoor et al. 1988).

Controlled, quantitative research is lacking in this area and to date literature discussing symptoms of choking phobia have focused on case studies demonstrating improvements following behavioral therapy and cognitive-behavioral therapy (Chatoor 1988; McNally 1994; Chorpita et al. 1997). We planned the use of behavioral techniques such as desensitization and a diet that gradually progressed from liquids to semisolid to solids without use of a catheter. However, these interventions resulted in increased rather than decreased anxiety. Resistance to behavioral treatment has also been described due to an earlier invasive medical procedure (Kerwin 1999). In keeping with these reports, our cases did not respond to behavioral treatment. The young age and poor verbal developmental level of the twins may also have contributed to the failure of CPT techniques. For this reason, drug treatment became necessary. Combination treatment, which included both behavioral and drug treatment, appeared to be more effective.

Anxiolytic effects have been described in low-dose neuroleptics (Hanna et al. 1999; Simeon et al. 2002). Berger-Gross et al. (2004) reported that risperidone was safe and effective in childhood eating disorders. Schwamm et al. (1998) reported that risperidone was safe and effective in a 3-year-old autistic child. Haloperidol at 0.5 mg was therefore used first in our cases due to its availability and apparent application. However, no therapeutic effects were observed after the 1 month of haloperidol. Neuroleptics have well-known risks, such as tardive dsykensia, EPS, new-onset diabetes mellitius, hypertriglycemia, withdrawal syndromes, and sedation, as well as other complications (Silva et al. 1993; Yoshida et al. 1993; Berger-Gross et al. 2004). Increases in the dose of haloperidol were not pursued because of the risks in the face of the lack of therapeutic effect.

It is now known that SSRIs are effective in a variety of childhood anxiety disorders (American Academy of Child and Adolescent Psychiatry 1997; Birmaher et al. 1998; Masi et al. 2001). The use of SSRI's in preschool-age childrem remains highly controversial because of the relatively higher neuroplasticity of brain during this developmental period and the lack of data on safety and efficacy. When choosing an SSRI, we found a published case on fluoxetine use in a 2.5-year-old child. It was reported that fluoxetine was well tolerated and did not produce any side effects (Avci et al. 1998).

Parents of children with eating disorders often have anxiety related to feeding. This parental anxiety may increase with insufficient feeding or aspiration. The child's anxiety can result from her/his parent's anxiety or be exacerbated by it. The mother of the twins spontaneously reported her anxiety about feeding her children insufficiently. For this reason, psychiatric treatment was suggested to the mother. In such cases, it is very important to identify and address family difficulties while treating the children's symptoms. Moreover, close clinical follow up and parental education about drug usage and family attitude are important (Chatoor 1988). Potentially related to this issue, Chatoor et al. (2000b) reported that mothers of infantile anorexics showed greater attachment insecurity.

Adolescents who failed to thrive as infants did not have more anxiety or depressive scores compared with healthy adolescents (Drewett et al. 2006); however, childhood feeding disorders may lead to later forms of psychiatric disorders, mainly increasing the risk for anxiety disorders (Cinemre 1999). Longitudinal clinical follow up is essential for children with eating disorders. The use of behavioral interventions and SSRIs in combination may be helpful in relieving anxiety and resolving fear of food. Our patients did not respond to behavioral and then combined behavioral and haloperidone treatment for 1 month. Their anxiety and feeding problems became significantly better a month after fluoxetine was initiated; however, the possibility of sponteneous response as a result of time passing or placebo effect on children or parents should also be taken into account when drawing conclusions. Controlled clinical research about the efficacy and safety of SSRI's in preschool children with eating disorders is now warranted.

DISCLOSURES

The authors have no conflicts of interest to disclose.

REFERENCES

American Academy of Child and Adolescent Psychiatry: Practice parameters for the assessment and treatment of children and adolescents with anxiety disorders. J Am Acad Child Adolesc Psychiatry 36 (Suppl. 10):69–84, 1997.

American Psychiatric Association: Diagnostic and Statistical Manual of Mental Disorders, 4th ed. (DSM-IV). Washington, D.C., American Psychiatric Association, 1994.

Avci A, Diler RS, Tamam L: Fluoxetine treatment in a 2.5 years old girl—a letter. J Am Acad Child Adolesc Psychiatry 37:901–902, 1998.

Banerjee S. Preeya, Bhandari Rashmi P, Rosenberg David R: Use of low-dose selective serotonin reuptake inhibitors for severe, refractory choking phobia in childhood. J Dev Behav Pediatr 26:123–127, 2005.

Berger-Gross P, Coletti DJ, Hirschkorn K, Terranova E, Simpser EF: The effectiveness of risperidone in the treatment of three children with feeding disorders. J Child Adolesc Psychopharmacol 14:621–627, 2004.

Birmaher B, Yelovich AK, Renaud J: Pharmacologic treatment for children and adolescents with anxiety disorders. Pediatr Clin North Am 45:1187–1204, 1998.

Chatoor I, Conley C, Dickson L: Food refusal after an incident of choking: A posttraumatic eating disorder. J Am Acad Child Adolesc Psychiatry 27:105–110, 1988.

Chatoor I: Eating and nutritional disorders of infancy and early childhood. In: Textbook of Child and Adolescent

Psychiatry. Edited by Wiener J. Washington, D.C., American Psychiatric Press, 1991, pp 351–361.

Chatoor I, Harrison J, Ganiban J, Hirsch R: A diagnostic classification of feeding disorders of infancy and early childhood. Presented at the Annual Conference of the Society for Research on Eating Disorders, Germany, Prien, 9–12, 2000a.

Chatoor I, Ganiban J, Hirsch R, Borman-Spurrell E, Mrazek D: Maternal characteristics and toddler temperament in infantile anorexia. J Am Acad Child Adolesc Psychiatry 39:743–751, 2000b.

Chatoor I, Ganiban J, Harrison J, Hirsch R: Observation of feeding in the diagnosis of posttraumatic feeding disorder of infancy. J Am Acad Child Adolesc Psychiatry 40:595–602, 2001.

Chorpita BF, Vitali AE, Barlow DH: Behavioral treatment of choking phobia in an adolescent: An experimental analysis. J Behav Ther Exp Psychiatry 28:307–315, 1997.

Cinemre B: Eating disorders. Ege Psychiatry Publication Series 4:137–154, 1999.

Drewett RF, Corbett SS, Wright CM: Physical and emotional development, appetite and body image in adolescents who failed to thrive as infants. J Child Psychol Psychiatry 47:524–531, 2006.

Hanna GL, Fluent TE, Fischer DJ: Separation anxiety in children and adolescents treated with risperidone. J Child Adolesc Psychopharmacol 9:277–283, 1999.

International Statistical Classification of Diseases and Related Health Problems, 10th revision. Geneva, Switzerland, World Health Organization, 1992.

Kerwin ME: Empirically supported treatments in pediatric psychology: Severe feeding problems. J Pediatric Psychol 24:193–214, 1999.

Masi G, Mucci P, Millepiedi S: Separation anxiety disorder in children and adolescents: epidemiology, diagnosis and management. CNS Drugs 15:93–104, 2001.

McNally RJ: Choking phobia: A review of the literature. Compr Psychiatry 35:83–89, 1994.

Schwam, Jeffrey S. MD; Klass, Emily MD: Alonso, Carmen MD; Perry, Richard MD Risperidone and refusal to eat. J Am Acad Child Adolesc Psychiatry 37:572–573, 1998.

Silva RR, Malone RP, Anderson LT, Shay J, Campbell M: Haloperidol withdrawal and weight changes in autistic children. Psychopharmacol Bull 29:287–291, 1993.

Simeon J, Milin R, Walker S: A retrospective chart review of risperidone use in treatment-resistant children and adolescents with psychiatric disorders. Prog Neuropsychopharmacol Biol Psychiatry 26:267–275, 2002.

Yoshida I, Sakaguchi Y, Matsuishi T, Yano E, Yamashita Y, Hayata S, Hitoshi T, Yamashita F: Acute accidental overdosage of haloperidol in children. Acta Paediatr 82:877–880, 1993.

ADVANCES IN PRESCHOOL PSYCHOPHARMACOLOGY
© 2009 Mary Ann Liebert, Inc.
140 Huguenot Street, 3rd Floor
New Rochelle, NY 10801-5215

Three Clinical Cases of DSM-IV Mania Symptoms in Preschoolers

Joan L. Luby, M.D., Mini Tandon, D.O., and Ginger Nicol, M.D.

ABSTRACT

Despite a growing body of empirical data describing the discriminant and longitudinal validity of mania in older children, little research has been conducted investigating the presence of mania symptoms in preschool-aged children. This report describes three cases of preschool children (ages 3.6 to 5.2) who presented to a subspecialty mental health clinic manifesting age-adjusted mania-like symptoms. Developmental manifestations of DSM-IV mania symptoms described include grandiosity, hypersexuality, elation, racing thoughts, and decreased need for sleep. These symptoms have been shown to be highly specific to distinguish bipolar disorder from attention deficit hyperactivity disorder (ADHD) in older children. Possible manifestations of mood cycling are also described. Clinical observations, parental reports, and related family mental health history are reviewed.

INTRODUCTION

A CONVERGING BODY of evidence has now established the discriminant validity and longitudinal stability of mania symptoms in school-aged children (Geller et al., 2002a; Geller et al., 2004; Biederman et al., 2005; Birmaher et al., 2006). Geller et al. (2002b) have also described age-adjusted manifestations of mania symptoms that are specific to bipolar disorder (BP) and distinct from the symptoms of ADHD in school-aged children. Despite these compelling findings of a specific and stable mania syndrome in children as young as 7 years, the question of whether mania symptoms can arise in even younger preschool-aged children has not yet been the focus of significant scientific study. This may be related to the longstanding assumption that preschool-aged children would be too developmentally immature to experience mood-disorder symptoms. Traditionally, developmentalists have theorized that preschoolers could not experience some of the key symptoms of mood disorders. Also, the assumption that many of the central emotions of mania, such as elation or grandiosity, might be indistinguishable from developmental norms during the preschool period has prevailed. However, recent advances in our understanding of the emotional and cognitive capacities of preschool-aged children have demonstrated that it is not developmentally impossible for children as young as 3 years of age to experience complex emotions such as guilt and shame (Zahn-Waxler et al., 1991; Zahn-Waxler and Robinson, 1995). Basic developmental research

Washington University School of Medicine, Department of Psychiatry, St. Louis, MO.

has also demonstrated that a stable self-concept arises during the preschool period, making it at least theoretically possible for a preschool child to display grandiosity (Thompson, 2006).

Whether clinically significant elated mood is possible during the preschool period cannot be addressed by studies of normative development. Several case studies and retrospective chart reviews have suggested that it is possible to manifest a bipolar syndrome during the preschool period (Mota-Castillo et al., 2001; Wilens et al., 2002, 2003; Tumuluru et al., 2003; Scheffer and Niskala, 2004; Biederman et al., 2005). However, the case studies available to date have focused predominantly on treatment and have not described age-specific symptom manifestations in detail. A recent exploratory investigation of mania symptoms in preschool children, part of a larger investigation focused on preschool depression, compared preschool children who met DSM-IV symptom criteria for bipolar disorder (BP)-I to those who were healthy. This study provided robust evidence that clinical elated mood, as defined by an age-appropriate preschool mania module of a larger preschool-aged diagnostic interview, is not a normative phenomenon (Luby and Belden, 2006). This investigation also demonstrated that "cardinal symptoms" of mania as previously described by Geller et al. (2002b), specifically clinical levels of elation and grandiosity, can also arise in preschool children between the ages of 3 and 6 years. Other symptoms useful to distinguish mania from other disruptive behavioral disorders, such as hypersexuality and decreased need for sleep described by Geller et al. (2002a) in older BP children, were also detected and served as markers of the disorder in preschool children (Luby and Belden, 2006). The clinical importance of this preschool syndrome is underscored by the finding that this group was significantly more impaired (according to both teachers and parents) than both healthy and disruptive groups (those who had DSM-IV ADHD, ODD, or CD) (Luby and Belden, 2006).

In addition to these highly suggestive findings, case studies that describe the clinical characteristics of preschool-aged children who seek mental health evaluation and receive a clinical diagnosis of presumptive BP are of interest.

They are of value in part due to the paucity of literature currently available on this issue. Also, the scant available empirical data do not elaborate on the details of how mania symptoms manifest in young children and how such symptoms might be distinguished from normative extremes and or other disruptive behavioral disorders, as outlined by Geller et al. (2002a, 2002b) for older children. Of particular interest is how these symptoms with known specificity for BP in older children, such as grandiosity, elation, hypersexuality, racing thoughts, and decreased need for sleep, would present in a preschooler. Such information about the course and duration of symptoms and potential manifestations of cycling would also be of interest. The increasing application of the BP diagnosis to younger children and the related use of mood-stabilizing medications for treatment also enhance the need for more detailed descriptions of age-adjusted symptom manifestations for use by clinicians to enhance diagnostic accuracy (Zito et al., 2000; Harpaz-Rotem and Rosenheck, 2004). Detailing the clinical characteristics of mania-specific symptoms is critically important due to the difficult distinction between the diagnosis of BP and the much more common and well-validated diagnostic categories, such as attention-deficit hyperactivity disorder (ADHD) and/or oppositional defiant disorder (ODD) in preschool-aged children.

Based on the preceding discussion, three clinical cases of presumptive BP arising in preschool-aged children evaluated at the Washington University School of Medicine (WUSM) Infant/Preschool Mental Health clinic are outlined. All cases were evaluated by the clinic director, an experienced infant–preschool psychiatrist specializing in mood disorders (JL) and a second-year child psychiatry fellow (MT or GN) over 4 sessions using standardized and age-appropriate clinical assessment techniques described in detail elsewhere (Luby and Morgan, 1997; Thomas et al., 1997). Initials will be used to protect the privacy of these patients; however, verbal consent to use patient information has been obtained from legal guardians of all patients.

PRESENTATION OF CASES

Case 1

LF first presented to the preschool clinic at the age of 5 years 2 months with a history of uncontrollable, silly laughing for "no apparent reason" noted by parents since the age of 4. Parents also indicated concern about the fact that "she thinks she is better than everyone else" at drawing, singing, ballet, and other activities. Parent's indicated that this sense of confidence was present even when she was not particularly talented in these areas. One example given was that after catching a fish during a fishing trip she declared proudly "nobody can do anything better than me." On another occasion, she demanded to be carried to the car after ballet practice since she was "the best dancer" and did not want to soil her shoes. When the family moved to a new home, she insisted that she have the master bedroom suite, despite parents' redirection on this issue (parents did not comply with this demand). She has difficulty with peer interactions because she often tells friends how to play and then leaves them behind if they will not conform to her rules.

Her grandiosity was routinely evident in the clinic setting. In the first clinical contact, this 5-year-old boldly teased the child psychiatry fellow about "having a crush" on the clinic secretary; she was clearly unintimidated and taking charge of the clinical setting. In subsequent follow-up office visits, the patient told the senior child psychiatrist, "You do not have me on the correct dosage. Let me help you because I know what it should be." In these visits, it is not uncommon for LF to storm out of the room, demanding that only she knows what pills should be taken. Of note is that she feels remorseful in the aftermath of these outbursts and at times returns to apologize after prompting by her mother. Along these lines, she will frequently tell teachers how to improve their skills.

LF's symptomotology and impairment in family functioning were further exacerbated by an ongoing decreased need for sleep. Parents report that she may awaken as early as 3 A.M. without fatigue episodically since very early childhood. She is easily angered at times and has become aggressive when her demands are not met, as evident when she once bit her mother, who had stated she could not watch a video at that particular time. Her brother has no known behavioral problems but has been victimized by her tantrums, which have lasted as long as 3 hours at a time. Another manifestation of her grandiose behavior in the sibling relationship is that she attempts to control her brother by requesting that he remain quiet during long car trips; but she talks incessantly herself and is unwilling or unable to be interrupted.

An extensive medical workup, including MRI of the brain, revealed no organic abnormalities. Interestingly, family history in this case was strongly suggestive of multiple members with mania-like symptoms. For example, a paternal grandmother apparently engaged in multiple new business ventures each year, was extremely social, and never seemed to tire despite sleeping little. A paternal aunt was described as having multiple marriages, extramarital affairs, and alcohol abuse. No formal psychiatric evaluations had been obtained for any of these family members. Of note is that LF has been followed in the clinic for >5 yr since her initial presentation at age 5. The symptoms have been managed on an outpatient basis with a combination of psychotherapy and mood-stabilizing medications. Despite some improvement in mood and, related to this, in her ability to be maintained in a regular classroom setting, she continues to be significantly socially impaired, and symptoms of grandiosity and irritability have been stable and unremitting over this period of time.

Case 2

MG was referred to the WUSM Infant/ Preschool clinic at age 3 years and 8 months due to parental concern about extreme "ups and downs" or "mood swings" first noted at the age of 2 years; however, MG was also described as emotionally labile and irritable even as an infant. He began to show signs of euphoria, described as being "excessively happy," at times with no apparent precipitant. He was noted to be overly amorous with older friends, relatives, and teachers. For example, when playing with peers, he was known to repeat "I love you" over and over, while hugging or licking their faces aggressively. This behavior was also displayed toward adult females, both known acquaintances and strangers. MG had reportedly been overly flattering and flirtatious with teachers and friends of his mother, who expressed discomfort at his displays of romanticism. He has also been known to point to strange women in public and shout, "I'm going to marry you!" MG was described as "overly friendly" with strangers in public settings and would not uncommonly convince them to buy him treats at a bakery as an example. Strangers as well as caregivers often found him to be "extremely charming."

Alternately, MG could become aggressive and at times violent with minimal or no obvious provocation and would state that he wanted to kill others or die himself. MG sometimes expressed to his parents the fear that strangers in public were talking about or laughing at him.

MG demonstrated an inflated sense of self, demanding always to be the leader or "in the front" during family outings and in preschool. He consistently commanded the undivided attention of adult family members during family get-togethers and seemed to prefer the company of adults to children. During clinical evaluation, MG repeatedly stated he knew things "because my mind is just made that way" and described himself as "the king." He was known to express the same kind of thoughts to the teachers at school and to peers, resulting in social problems in the preschool setting. In keeping with this, he attempted to take control of the preschool classroom, and his behavior in this setting was chronically problematic, resulting in dismissal from several preschool settings prior to the current placement.

There were also reports of decreased need for sleep. Since infancy, he seemed to need less sleep than his fraternal twin sister and reportedly had never slept through the night. He rarely took naps and had significant problems with initial insomnia. After being put to bed at night, MG's parents reported that he would bang his head repetitively on his pillow, sometimes into the early hours of the morning. Despite this relative lack of sleep, he was noted to arise early with "all kinds of energy." It is of note that MG demonstrated some insight into the consequences, stating "sometimes I get crabby when I don't sleep but my brain doesn't want to." In addition, MG demonstrated high levels of productive energy, often spending hours of undivided attention on a large building task. He was able to do this even after several nights of very few hours of sleep.

MG's medical history is significant for being a fraternal twin. He and his sister were born $8\frac{1}{2}$ weeks premature, and the first 5 weeks of life were spent in the neonatal intensive care unit without neurologic sequelae. Gross motor, speech, and language development was also reported as normal. The family history was positive for several maternal relatives, including the mother who was treated for anxiety disorders. Additionally, a great maternal uncle had been diagnosed with BP. No behavioral or emotional concerns were reported for MG's twin and younger sisters. The home and psychosocial environment appeared stable; both parents were well educated and productively employed and appeared to engage in appropriate parenting strategies. There was no suspected physical or sexual abuse or neglect.

Case 3

AF presented to the clinic at 4 years 6 months of age with intense irritability and mood lability, which were impairing his function both at home and preschool. He is reported to change his mood from one extreme to the other "on a dime" and for no apparent reason. He is described by parents as having moment to moment fluctuations in mood, in which he may appear "giddy" and "bouncing off the walls" and expresses that he is "very happy." These periods alternate with melancholia during which he seems listless and without energy and is readily tearful. These intense mood changes occurred daily and many times a day, and his mother found it exhausting to attempt to help him maintain his emotions at a socially appropriate level. He also becomes easily irritated with low frustration tolerance, as evidenced by his rolling his 2-yr-old brother down the stairs and poking his brother's eye with a pencil with no known provocation. This behavior resulted in a hospitalization prior to his presentation to our clinic.

He is described by his mother as often inconsolable and "clingy," with ongoing but episodic difficulty tolerating separation. He may become dysphoric when his mother leaves his side, after drop-off at school, or during bedtime separation. He readily attaches to the teacher's assistant at school, engaging her in charming ways, but then may have difficulty separating from her at the end of the school day as well. While he has been able to be maintained in a preschool setting for 2 hours a day, parents are unable to find a stable babysitter due to the difficulty of caring for AF. Baby sitters have generally refused to return after their first experience.

He has lived with his biological parents since birth and has one younger sibling. A complete medical workup was unremarkable. Of interest in this case is the fact that his mother receives treatment for depression and anxiety; the diagnosis of BP has not been made in any family member to date to the parent's knowledge.

DISCUSSION

These three cases provide examples of DSM-IV mania-like symptoms arising in preschool-aged children. These cases illustrate age-adjusted manifestations of those symptoms known to best differentiate BP from ADHD in older children (Geller et al., 2002a). The notion that these symptoms are also specific to distinguish BP from ADHD in preschool-aged children has also been suggested by an exploratory study (Luby and Belden, 2006). The symptom of grandiosity was manifested by two cases, one in a girl and the other in a boy. In the case of LF grandiosity was evident in the clinical evaluation based on the highly unusual precocious directive behavior toward the unfamiliar clinician authority figures. This kind of behavior toward the parents was also reported in the history, was observed in the clinic, and had been long-standing. This behavior arose in the context of competent parenting and a sibling without similar behavioral problems. In addition, the same grandiose behavior was observed by teachers and in church and was highly problematic in those contexts. This behavior was determined to be grandiose, rather than simply oppositional or defiant, based on the child's underlying belief that she could direct the interview, make decisions about treatment plans, and have authority over the doctors and teachers. The behavior also arose in the context of competent parenting and an appropriate and structured home environment, and in the absence of a pervasive angry emotional tone suggestive of oppositionality. The grandiose behavior of MG had a similar manifestation in that the child felt he had age-inappropriate stature and abilities which he believed in firmly even when pressed. Further, he believed he had an adult status in several circumstances and behaved persistently and in multiple contexts in a manner consistent with this belief.

A characteristic feature of the grandiosity manifested by both LF and MG was that it was pervasive in all environments, home, school, and clinic, and thus was not state or relationship specific. And quite importantly, it was a fixed and false belief that was held by the children even when pressed. That is, these children tenaciously asserted their belief about their status as "the best" at various skills, which empowered them to make executive decisions, even when attempts were made to dissuade them by parents and/or teachers. Confirmation that the inflated self-concept of these preschoolers represented a fixed false belief was evident not only by their verbal description of their own capacities (which could be developmentally discounted), but also more importantly by persistent inappropriate grandiose behaviors across contexts. These qualities are key to inferring delusional grandiosity in a young child for whom verbal description is less reliable. The absence of an underlying angry tone or oppositional behavior that arises only in reaction to demands or directives from authority figures is also key to distinguishing grandiosity from oppositionality.

Hypersexuality, or perhaps more accurately "hyper-romanticism," was also evident in the case of MG. MG displayed strong romantic inclinations that he acted on toward both adolescent girls and adult women. Of importance, a repetitive pattern of interest along these lines differentiated the behavior from a more intense attachment to one person, as can occur normatively (e.g., a young child who is "in love" with a particular teacher). In this case, MG found numerous older girls and/or women to be amorous figures to pursue. The behaviors went beyond early "crushes" and were clearly associated with a lot of emotion and outward expressions of affection and romanticism (such as wanting to send roses to a teenage girl and asking a teacher to marry him). The intensity of these amorous behaviors was evidenced by the adult women's expressions of discomfort. Again, these feelings are associated with an underlying fixed belief that these encounters are appropriate and will be requited. In this sense, hyper-romantic behavior also has a grandiose quality. This behavior arose in the absence of suspected sexual abuse or inappropriate exposure.

Decreased need for sleep is particularly poignant in the case of MG, but is also described in LF as well. In this case, MG's inability to sleep combined with his intense almost around the clock productive energy became highly impairing for the child's caregiver and family. In fact, this symptom was the single most difficult one for the family to deal with and is ultimately what led them to the use of medication in addition to the primary recommendation of psychotherapy. Notable is that MG did not sleep more than a few hours a night, but awoke the next morning full of energy and did not seem to tire. This produced significant family impairment, because his mother was too exhausted to perform other household activities due to her need to care for MG. MG also expressed some discomfort with this state of "hyper-awakeness," stating in one office visit, "I wish my brain would take a rest but it just doesn't want to." This patient also had an interesting form of hypersociability evidenced by his ability to engage and "charm" strangers in public places, often convincing them to buy him treats.

Elation associated with hyper-talkativeness was evident in several of the cases described. Parents reported elevated mood states that were sustained (lasting for hours or all day) and arising for no apparent reason. The child appeared giddy and was laughing inappropriately, described as "bouncing off the walls," and unable to calm down. These states appeared distinctive from normative silliness or a joyful mood often seen in young children, given its intensity, duration, contextually incongruent quality, and the child's inability to regulate or control the elevated mood and return to a euthymic state when socially required. In all cases, parents described this elevated mood as significantly impairing to the child and disruptive to family life. Also of note is the family history of affective disorders, in two cases diagnosed BP. Also notable was that in all cases siblings in the family did not manifest behavioral problems, confirming the clinical impression that the parenting environment was in general appropriate.

These case descriptions provide examples of our clinical experience of the manifestations of DSM-IV mania-like symptoms arising in preschool-aged children. Symptoms appear to be age-appropriate forms of DSM-IV mania and are not typical of symptoms found in other well-known disruptive behavioral disorders in young children. These clinical presentations appear to be age-adjusted manifestations of the symptoms previously described by Geller and colleagues (2002b), which also emerged as key differentiators between mania and ADHD in a large controlled investigation of slightly older school-aged samples (Geller et al., 2002a). Large-scale controlled systematic studies are now needed to determine the validity (e.g., specificity and longitudinal stability) of these symptom constellations in preschool-aged children. These investigations should also address the issue of specificity as well as impairment. Of central importance to the definition of the disorder in early childhood, longitudinal data are needed to inform the continuities and discontinuities between these early onset forms and later childhood phenotypes and course. The need for longitudinal follow-up in preschool-aged samples at school age is also underscored by reports of preschool onset of symptoms in several samples of school-aged bipolar children known to have stable symptoms in adolescence (Geller et al., 2002a; Geller et al., 2004; Biederman et al., 2005; Birmaher et al., 2006).

DISCLOSURES

Doctors Luby, Tandon, and Nicol do not have any conflicts of interest or financial relationships to disclose.

REFERENCES

Biederman J, Faraone SV, Wozniak J, Mick E, Kwon A, Clayton GA, Clark SV: Clinical correlates of bipolar disorder in a large, referred sample of children and adolescents. J Psychiatr Res 39:611–622, 2005.

Biederman J, Mick E, Hammerness P, Harpold T, Aleardi M, Dougherty M, Wozniak J: Open-label, 8-week trial of olanzapine and risperidone for the treatment of bipolar disorder in preschool-age children. Biol Psychiatry 58:589–594, 2005.

Birmaher B, Axelson D, Strober M, Gill MK, Valeri S, Chiappetta L, Ryan N, Leonard H, Hunt J, Iyengar S, Keller M: Clinical course of children and adolescents with bipolar spectrum disorder phenotype. Arch Gen Psychiatry 63:175–183, 2006.

Geller B, Zimerman B, Williams M, Bolhofner K, Craney JL, Frazier J, Beringer L: DSM IV mania symptoms in a prepubertal and early adolescent bipolar disorder phenotype compared to attention-deficit hyperactive and normal controls. J Child Adolesc Psychopharmacol 12:11–25, 2002a.

Geller B, Zimerman B, Williams M, DelBello MP, Frazier J, Beringer L: Phenomenology of prepubertal and early adolescent bipolar disorder: Examples of elated mood, grandiose behaviors, decreased need for sleep, racing thoughts and hypersexuality. J Child Adolesc Psychopharmacol 12:3–9, 2002b.

Geller B, Tillman R, Craney JL, Bolhofner K: Four-year prospective outcome and natural history of mania in children with a prepubertal and early adolescent bipolar disorder phenotype. Arch Gen Psychiatry 61:459–467, 2004.

Harpaz-Rotem I, Rosenheck R: Changes in outpatient psychiatric diagnosis in privately insured children and adolescents from 1995 to 2000. Child Psychiatry Hum Dev 34:329–340, 2004.

Luby J, Belden A: Defining and validating bipolar disorder in the preschool period. Dev Psychopathol 18:971–988, 2006.

Luby JL, Morgan K: Characteristics of an infant/preschool psychiatric clinic sample: Implications for clinical assessment and nosology. Infant Ment Health J 18:209–220, 1997.

Mota-Castillo M, Torruella A, Engels B, Perez J, Dedrick C, Gluckman M: Valproate in very young children: An open case series with a brief follow-up. J Affective Disord 67:193–197, 2001.

Scheffer RE, Niskala JA: The diagnosis of preschool bipolar disorder presenting with mania: Open pharmacological treatment. J Affective Disord 82:S25–S34, 2004.

Thomas JM, Benham AL, Gean M, Luby J, Minde K, Turner S, Wright HH: Practice parameters for the psychiatric assessment of infants and toddlers (0–36 months). J Am Acad Child Adolesc Psychiatry 36:21S–36S, 1997.

Thompson RA: The development of the person: Social understanding, relationships, self, conscience. In: Handbook of Child Psychology 6th ed., Vol. 3: Social, Emotional, and Personality Development. Edited by Damon W, Lerner RM, Eisenberg N. Wiley (New York), 2006, pp 24–98.

Tumuluru RV, Weller EB, Fristad MA, Weller RA: Mania in six preschool children. J Child Adolesc Psychopharmacol 13:489–494, 2003.

Wilens TE, Biederman J, Brown S, Monuteaux M, Prince J, Spencer T: Patterns of psychopathology and dysfunction in clinically referred preschoolers. J Dev Behav Pediatr 23:S31–S36, 2002.

Wilens TE, Biederman J, Forkner P, Ditterline J, Morris M, Moore H, Galdo M, Spencer TJ, Wozniak J: Patterns of comorbidity and dysfunction in clinically referred preschool and school-age children with bipolar disorder. J Child Adolesc Psychopharmacol 13:495–505, 2003.

Zahn-Waxler C, Cole P, Barrett K: Guilt and empathy: Sex differences and implications for the development of depression. In: The Development of Emotion Regulation and Dysregulation. Edited by Garber J, Dodge KA. Cambridge University Press (New York), 1991, pp. 243–272.

Zahn-Waxler C, Robinson J: Empathy and guilt: Early origins of feelings of responsibility. In: Self-Conscious Emotions: The Psychology of Shame, Guilt Embarrassment, and Pride. Edited by Tangney JP, Fischer KW. Guilford Press (New York), 1995, pp 143–173.

Zito JM, Safer DJ, dosReis S, Gardner JF, Boles M, Lynch F: Trends in the prescribing of psychotropic medications to preschoolers. JAMA 283:1025–1030, 2000.

ADVANCES IN PRESCHOOL PSYCHOPHARMACOLOGY
© 2009 Mary Ann Liebert, Inc.
140 Huguenot Street, 3rd Floor
New Rochelle, NY 10801-5215

Risperidone in Preschool Children with Autistic Spectrum Disorders: An Investigation of Safety and Efficacy

Joan L. Luby, M.D.,[1] Christine Mrakotsky, Ph.D.,[2] Melissa Meade Stalets, M.A.,[1] Andy Belden, Ph.D.,[1] Amy Heffelfinger, Ph.D.,[3] Meghan Williams, B.A.,[1] and Edward Spitznagel, Ph.D.[4]

ABSTRACT

Introduction: Early intervention in autism spectrum disorders (ASDs) appears promising and may represent a window of opportunity for more effective treatment. Whereas the safety and efficacy of risperidone have been established for children aged 5 and older, they have not been adequately tested in preschool children.

Methods: A randomized placebo-controlled study of risperidone in preschool children was conducted in a sample of young children, most of whom were also undergoing intensive behavioral treatment.

Results: Preschool children tolerated low-dose risperidone well with no serious adverse effects observed over a 6-month treatment period. Weight gain and hypersalivation were the most common side effects reported, and hyperprolactinemia without lactation or related signs was observed. Significant differences between groups found at baseline complicated the analyses; however, controlling for some of these differences revealed that preschoolers on risperidone demonstrated greater improvements in autism severity. The change in autism severity scores from baseline to 6-month follow up for the risperidone group was 8% compared to 3% for the placebo group. Notably, both groups significantly improved over the 6-month treatment period.

Conclusions: Study findings suggest that risperidone is well tolerated in preschoolers over a 6-month period, but that only minimally greater improvement in target symptoms was evident in the risperidone group, possibly due to the differences between groups at baseline or due to the small sample size. Although these findings are not sufficient to direct treatment, they suggest that larger-scale, double-blind, placebo-controlled investigations of risperidone in preschoolers with ASDs should now be conducted.

[1]Department of Psychiatry, Washignton University School of Medicine, St. Louis, Missouri.
[2]Department of Psychiatry, Children's Hospital/Harvard Medical School, Boston, Massachusetts.
[3]Department of Neurology, Medical College of Wisconsin, Milwaukee, Wisconsin.
[4]Department of Mathematics, Washington University, St. Louis, Missouri.

INTRODUCTION

Autism Spectrum Disorders (ASDs) are a group of chronic disorders characterized by early childhood onset of profound impairment in social relatedness, delayed and deviant communication, and a markedly restricted repertoire of behavior and interests. These core symptoms are often accompanied by behavior disturbances, including hyperactivity, poor adaptability, anxiety, aggression, irritability, sterotypies, and self-injurious behavior. These nonspecific behavioral problems are disruptive, impeding remediation of core symptoms as well as daily living skills. A recent epidemiological study reported a prevalence rate for ASD of 4 cases per 1,000 children (Bertrand et al. 2001). Substantially higher rates, 6.7 cases per 1,000, are reported when milder forms of ASDs are accounted for. Because autism can be diagnosed in early childhood and autistic individuals are expected to have a normal life span, Gerlai and Gerlai (2004) recently noted that the number of 'patient years' associated with autism is second only to Alzheimer's disease.

The mainstay treatment for autism for more than a decade has been intensive behavioral intervention. A number of treatment programs based on this fundamental approach are available and have demonstrated effectiveness (for review, see Schreibman, 2000). Importantly, several studies now suggest that intensive intervention before the age of 5 years provides a window of opportunity for more effective treatment using this modality (for review, see Dawson et al., 2000). Early intervention during the preschool period (or earlier) appears to be the most promising, resulting in substantially better outcomes than later intervention (Faja and Dawson, 2006). This finding, taken together with basic neurodevelopmental research demonstrating greater neuroplasticity during the first 5 years of life, suggest that a similar window of opportunity might exist for pharmacologic interventions as well.

Pharmacological treatment of autism has been guided by the demonstrated effectiveness of medications in the treatment of psychiatric symptoms exhibited by individuals with ASDs. Along these lines, treatment to date has targeted the reduction of specific associated behavioral problems such as aggression and hyperactivity as opposed to improving the core deficits of autism. Typical antipsychotics were among the first medications to be studied systematically in autistic children and have been widely used for the control of agitation, aggression, and self-harming behaviors (McDougle et al. 2003). A suboptimal risk–benefit ratio related to untoward side effects, such as sedation, weight gain, and the risk of tardive dyskinesia, has catalyzed the search for new and better medications in this class.

Newer atypical antipsychotics have been used effectively in the treatment of adults and older children with autism (McCracken et al. 2002). Compared to conventional antipsychotics, these medications have a reduced risk of extrapyramidal and sedating side effects. The latter is particularly important when treating children for whom social learning is still actively developing, albeit atypically. Among atypical antipsychotics used for the treatment of ASDs, risperidone has been the most well-studied agent. Studies have demonstrated that children with ASDs treated with risperidone display decreased aggression and self-injurious behavior (e.g., McCracken et al. 2002). As a result, risperidone has now been identified as the only evidence-based pharmacological treatment for autism (McClellan and Werry 2003). Although multiple studies have demonstrated decreases in impulsivity, aggression, and self-harm (and even stereotypic behavior) with use of risperidone, there is considerably less evidence that the core social impairments of autism can be reduced through the use of risperidone or similar agents in children over 6 years old (McCracken et al. 2002; Shea et al. 2004; McDougle et al. 2005).

Despite lack of controlled data supporting their safety and efficacy, preschool age children in general (and presumably those with ASDs) are being treated with antipsychotics at very high rates in the community (Zito et al. 2000). Witwer and Lecavalier (2005) reported that nearly 10% of children with ASDs under the age of 7 were treated with antipsychotic medications in the previous year. Pharmacologic treatment at this early point in development could pose unique promise or unique risk on the basis of greater neuroplasticity of the brain during the preschool period (Vitiello 1998). For this reason, as well as known high rates of prescribing in this age group, studies focusing on the safety and efficacy of atypical antipsychotics specifically in preschool age children are needed.

Despite the promising findings on early intervention in ASDs, information on the effectiveness of risperidone in the treatment of ASDs among preschool age children is limited to case descriptions and open-label studies. Masi and colleagues (2001) conducted the largest available open-label trial of risperidone for preschool children aged 3.9–6.6 years with ASDs and found improvement in the global severity of autistic symptoms. Notably, the core social impairments of the disorder improved, with gains seen in the ability to relate to people, increased verbal and nonverbal communication, and reduced social withdrawal. The authors hypothesized that the unique and promising improvements in social behaviors, which most previous studies in school age samples had failed to demonstrate, may have been related to the subjects having received treatment earlier in life. These findings, while promising, are limited by the use of an open-label design and the inherent lack of a control group.

To date, only two double blind, placebo-controlled studies investigating the efficacy of risperidone for the treatment of ASDs are available (McCracken et al. 2002; Shea et al. 2004). Although findings from both studies demonstrated efficacy for the amelioration of disruptive symptoms of the disorder in children ranging in age from 5 to 17 years, the study by Shea and colleagues also found improvements in scales measuring inappropriate speech and lethargy/social withdrawal. Another limitation of the available database is that the treatment duration of most trials is relatively short, typically 8–16 weeks. Longer duration of treatment is desirable for mimicking real-life practice and providing a more rigorous test for placebo effects, which may occur early and appear robust and sustained over the short term, particularly in this population, but do not endure over time (Sandler and Bodfish 2000). In addition, longer treatment dura-

tion is necessary to monitor for adverse effects such as weight gain, metabolic changes, and tardive dyskinesias.

The goal of the present study was to examine the safety and effectiveness of risperidone in the treatment of preschool children with ASDs over a 6-month period. Of interest was whether the medication was safe and well tolerated and whether it ameliorated the associated disruptive behavioral features and/or the core social deficits of the disorder when this early intervention was applied. Unique features of this investigation were the very young sample and the implementation of a randomized, double blind, placebo-controlled design for an extended duration of treatment. The majority of the study sample was receiving varying amounts of Applied Behavior Analysis (ABA) because it is a mandated treatment through the local public school district for eligible children. Therefore, the efficacy of risperidone was tested in the context of a population in which many children were undergoing an intensive behavioral intervention. To our knowledge, this investigation is the first double-blind, placebo-controlled trial in a preschool-age ASD population, including preschoolers with Pervasive Developmental Disorder Not Otherwise Specified (PDD-NOS). The inclusion of those with PDD-NOS and those undergoing behavioral treatments have been noted to be particularly important because they mimic real world practice (Troost et al. 2005).

MATERIALS AND METHODS

Setting and patients

This 6-month, randomized, double blind, placebo-controlled trial was conducted in a psychiatric outpatient clinic at Washington University School of Medicine (WUSM) in St. Louis between November, 1999, and November, 2002. The study protocol was approved by the WUSM Institutional Review Board, and written informed consent was obtained from a parent or legal guardian prior to enrollment. Parents were specifically informed about the experimental use of the drug for ASDs, as well as the lack of data on safety in younger children (e.g., effects on growth and development).

Twenty four (*n* = 24) preschool children between the ages of 2.5 and 6.0 years who met *Diagnostic and Statistical Manual of Mental Disorders*, 4th edition (DSM-IV) criteria for autism or PDD-NOS (American Psychiatric Association 1994), previously diagnosed and referred by a clinician, were recruited for participation. Subjects were ascertained from the child psychiatry outpatient clinic, offices of pediatricians and neurologists, and the special education department of local public school districts. All subjects were randomized, *n* = 12, to each treatment group. Other inclusion criteria at the time of enrollment included: (1) absence of other known significant central nervous system (CNS) disorders; and (2) absence of significant medical problems or other psychiatric disorders requiring pharmacotherapy. A complete physical exam was performed on all study participants by a board-certified pediatrician to rule out neurological and medical illness. In addition, participating families were strongly encouraged to minimize the use of adjunctive medications and/or supplements (hormones, vitamins, diets) over the duration of treatment.

Protocol schedule and design

Patients were consecutively assigned by an unblinded child psychiatrist (J.L.) to risperidone or placebo treatment using a randomization table obtained from the WUSM pharmacy and derived using a standard software package. Parents and raters who conducted all standardized assessments were blind to treatment group. Due to the exploratory nature of this study and to assure safety in this very young study population, the treating child psychiatrist (J.L.) was unblended and conducted regular clinical assessments over the 6-month period as follows: A baseline visit, weekly visits during the first study month, biweekly visits during the second month, followed by monthly visits for months 3–6. A thorough psychiatric and medical history, mental status exam, as well as physical exam were conducted at baseline.

Structured diagnostic assessments of autism symptoms were conducted at baseline, 2 months,

4 months, and 6 months. Standardized measures were used to assess general cognitive and socio-emotional functioning at baseline and after 6 months. Assessments were completed over 2 half-day periods, including multiple breaks and rewards to elicit maximum performance from children. Due to limited data regarding the effects of risperidone on growth and development in young children, height and weight and potential adverse events were carefully monitored at each study visit. In addition, electrocardiograms and a battery of laboratory tests (including prolactin and leptin) were performed at baseline, 2 months, and 6 months. Data about other medical, educational and developmental interventions (including hours of ABA weekly) were obtained through parental interview or the child's medical record.

Baseline assessment and efficacy measures

The central diagnostic outcome measures included the Childhood Autism Rating Scale (CARS) (Schopler et al. 1988), a 15-item behavior rating on a 7-point Likert scale based on clinician observation of the core social and behavioral symptoms of autism; and the Gilliam Autism Rating Scale (GARS) (Gilliam 1995), a rating scale completed by the clinician based on parent report and direct observation of the child's behavior that assessed frequency of DSM-IV autistic symptoms, including communication, social interaction, stereotypical behavior, and developmental regression, all yielding a total Autism Quotient. These were administered at baseline 2, 4, and 6 months by raters blinded to treatment group status.

The following measures were administered at baseline and 6-month endpoint. Socialization and general adaptive development were assessed with the Vineland Adaptive Behavior Scales, Interview Edition (VABS) (Sparrow et al. 1984), a semistructured parent interview assessing communication, social skills, daily living skills, and motor development. The Childhood Behavior Checklist 1.5–5 (CBCL) (Achenbach and Edelbrock 1995) was completed by parents to assess behavior and emotion problems. Patients completed the Preschool Language Scale, Third Edition (PLS-3) (The Psychological Corporation, 1992), a standardized measure to assess receptive and expressive language development. Patients underwent an additional comprehensive developmental assessment using standardized and experimental cognitive, neuropsychological, and observational measures.

Medication dosing

Risperidone was administered in low doses and titrated by the unblinded child psychiatrists on the basis of the individual subject's progress and side-effect profile. The dosing range used in the study population was narrow and low (0.5–1.5 mg total daily dose). Medication was administered twice daily when doses greater than 0.5 mg were administered. Adjustments in dose were made as needed, depending upon treatment response and side effects, based on the clinical judgment of the unblinded child psychiatrist. Placebo dosing was also "titrated" to better maintain the blind design.

Most patients in the active medication group (90.9%) started risperidone at 0.5 mg once daily (91.7% of placebo patients were dispensed 0.5-mg daily doses) and mean starting dose was 0.03 mg/kg/day. Mean starting dose in the risperidone and placebo group were similar [0.50 mg (SD 0.15) risperidone versus 0.54 mg (SD 0.14) placebo]. With weekly dose escalation, 81.8% of risperidone and 66.7% of placebo patients took 1 mg (0.5 mg twice daily) after 4 weeks; 27.3% of risperidone and 33.3% of placebo patients were dispensed total daily doses of 1.5 mg after 8 weeks (2 months), whereas all others received total daily doses of 1 mg. Most patients were maintained on this schedule for the remainder of the study. Only 1 patient in the risperidone group was tapered from 1 mg at 4 months to 0.5 mg at 6-month endpoint. The final risperidone mean dose was 0.50 mg/kg/day. Mean daily final dose was 1.14 mg (SD 0.32) risperidone versus 1.38 mg (SD 0.57) placebo, which was comparable.

Safety monitoring

Treatment and side effects, including any occurrences of adverse events, were monitored at each study visit by the child psychiatrist who was not blind to the treatment condition, to assure safety in this very young study sample. All standardized baseline and outcome assessments were, however, administered by raters blind to the treatment conditions as described above. Physical and physiological parameters potentially affected by treatment were assessed including height, weight, and serum leptin and prolactin levels (known to be elevated in older children and adults on this medication).

Data analyses

Preliminary analyses were conducted to examine the possibility of differences between the two study groups (i.e., treatment and control groups) in relation to several demographic variables. To test for these differences, t tests, Mann–Whitney U tests, or Chi-square analyses were performed. To test for the effects of treatment over the course of four time points as well as the potential interactions between treatment and time, repeated measures analyses of variance (ANOVA) were conducted. Because the study groups significantly differed in autism severity at baseline, several methods were used to adjust for these differences. Specifically, covariates were entered into factorial or repeated measures ANOVAs to reduce the effect of the differences in autism severity between the two groups at baseline. To account further for the differences in autism severity at baseline, in several analyses CARS change scores were used as the dependent variable. CARS change scores were created by subtracting a child's baseline CARS score from their final CARS score obtained during the last assessment. The overall treatment effects were then estimated by comparing change scores between the risperidone and placebo groups with independent t-tests or Mann–Whitney U tests (for ordinal scale data). Additional analyses using covariates in these nonparametric tests were also conducted.

RESULTS

Sample characteristics

Twenty four children 2.5–6 years of age with a diagnosis of an ASD participated in a 6-

month treatment trial; $n = 23$ of these children were included in the analyses that follow. One child did not meet the threshold for an ASD on the CARS or GARS at baseline, despite having been referred with a clinical diagnosis, and was excluded from analyses. From the total sample, $n = 11$ children were randomly assigned to the risperidone [mean age 49.0 months (4.1 years), SD 10.9 months] treatment group and $n = 12$ preschool-age children were assigned to the placebo group [mean age 48.1 months (4 years), SD 13.2]. The demographic and clinical characteristics of the sample at baseline are illustrated in Table 1. The two groups did not differ significantly in age, gender, or maternal education. The groups did also not differ significantly with regard to the ABA treatment. The mean number of weekly ABA treatment hours was 21.2 for the risperidone group and 11.3 for the placebo group. This different in

treatment intensity was, however, not significant ($p = 0.13$).

Baseline differences between study groups

Despite using conventional methods (e.g., random digits table) to randomize the assignment of children to each treatment group, preschoolers in the risperidone group displayed significantly greater severity of autism symptoms at baseline as measured by the CARS ($t = -2.34$, df = 21, $p = 0.03$). In addition, the risperidone group had significantly poorer language skills as measured by the PLS-3 and poorer motor skill development as measured by the VABS Motor Skills Scale (see Table 1). To account for these baseline differences in symptom severity and developmental impairment between groups, these key developmental variables were entered as covariates in sub-

TABLE 1. BASELINE CHARACTERISTICS OF PRESCHOOL STUDY SAMPLE: RISPERIDONE VERSUS PLACEBO GROUP

	Risperidone (n = 11)	Placebo (n = 12)	Test of significance
Age in months: Mean (SD)	49.0 (10.9)	48.1 (13.2)	$p = 0.86$, $t = -0.18$, df = 21
Gender (M/F)	9/2	8/4	$p = 0.64$, Fisher's exact
Weight in kg: Mean (SD)	19.2 (3.3)	18.1 (4.2)	$p = 0.49$, $t = -0.70$, df = 21
Ethnicity-Caucasian	91%	92%	$p = 0.37$, $\chi^2 = 2.01$, df = 2
Household income: Median[a]	2.0	3.0	$p = 0.09$, U = 43.00,
>$60,000	46%	83%	$p = 0.12$, $\chi^2 = 4.30$, df = 2
Maternal Education: Median[b]	6.0	6.0	$p = 0.66$, U = 59.00
range	4–8	4–8	
ABA hours per week	21.2 (14.8)	11.3 (15.1)	$p = 0.13$, $t = -1.60$, df = 21
CARS Total Score: Mean (SD)*	37.6 (4.0)	33.3 (4.9)	$p = 0.03$, $t = -2.34$, df = 21
CARS Category: Median	2.0	1.0	$p = 0.15$, U = 44.5
Nonautistic (Cat 1)	0 (0%)	3 (25%)	$p = 0.19$, $\chi^2 = 3.36$, df = 2
Mild-moderate (Cat 2)	5 (46%)	5 (42%)	
Severe (Cat 3)	6 (56%)	4 (33%)	
GARS Autism Quotient SS[c]	91.6 (9.5)	91.3 (9.3)	$p = 0.94$, $t = -0.08$, df = 21
Object Assembly Scaled Score:			
>3 years Mean (SD) (n = 10/10)	5.5 (3.8)	8.1 (4.6)	$p = 0.19$, $t = 1.38$, df = 18
PLS-3 Total SS*	57.3 (10.1)	73.5 (19.4)	$p = 0.02$, $t = 2.48$, df = 21
VABS Communication SS	65.5 (18.5)	73.2 (8.8)	$p = 0.23$, $t = 1.26$, df = 21
VABS Daily Living Skills SS	64.7 (14.8)	74.6 (15.9)	$p = 0.14$, $t = 1.54$, df = 21
VABS Socialization SS	66.3 (16.3)	72.0 (16.4)	$p = 0.41$, $t = 0.84$, df = 21
VABS Motor Skills SS	73.1 (18.7)	86.9 (13.4)	$p = 0.05$, $t = 2.05$, df = 21

CARS = Childhood Autism Rating Scale; GARS = Gilliam Autism Rating Scale: PLS-3 = Preschool Language Scale, Third Edition; VABS = Vineland Adaptive Behavior Scales, Interview Edition.
[a]1 = $0–$29,999, 2 = $30,000–$59,999, 3 = ≥$60,000.
[b]1 = some grade school, 2 = completed grade school, 3 = some high school, 4 = high school diploma, 5 = some college or 2-year degree, 6 = 4-year college degree, 7 = some years beyond college, 8 = graduate or professional degree.
[c]SS = Standard Score (mean 100, SD 15).
*$p < 0.05$.

sequent analyses as appropriate. It should be noted that treatment groups did not differ significantly in autism severity on the GARS or IQ as measured by a nonverbal reasoning and problem-solving task (Wechsler Preschool and Primary Scale of Intelligence-Revised (WPPSI-R) Object Assembly). Thus, it was not necessary to control for the effects of these variables in the analyses that follow.

Safety of risperidone

No deaths or serious treatment-related adverse events occurred during the 6-month study period for any subject. Risperidone was well tolerated at the low doses administered. No clinically significant changes in EKG were detected for any subject from baseline to follow-up. The most common adverse events that occurred were transient sedation ($n = 5$), increased appetite ($n = 6$), and hypersalivation ($n = 2$). Constipation was reported by the parent of one study participant taking risperidone. Notably, no dystonic or dyskinetic movements were observed over the 6-month period for any participant on risperidone.

One participation on risperidone demonstrated transient staring spells (lasting several seconds) and periods of apparent waxy flexibility. These episodes were described by the parent and teacher and reportedly occurred over a 48-hour period after a minor head injury with visible bruising on her head but without loss of consciousness. An additional clinic visit was scheduled, during which time the subject was afebrile and no abnormalities were observed on AIMS evaluation. Although the episode was not deemed attributable to the medication, the dose was lowered as a precautionary measure and a pediatric exam was recommended. The episodes spontaneously resolved within 48 hours.

It was notable that subjects on placebo also were reported by their parents to be experiencing transient sedation ($n = 4$) and increased appetite ($n = 3$). One subject on placebo dropped out of the study after 5 days due to a parental report of severe hyperactivity after placebo was started.

Physiologic findings

Changes in physiological measures within study groups and analyses of group differences in change scores are summarized in Table 2. Increases in prolactin serum levels were noted for both study groups from baseline to endpoint, with changes significantly higher [$\lambda = 0.66$, $F (1, 15) = 7.61$, $p < 0.05$] in the risperidone group from mean baseline levels of 8.11 ng/ml (SD 4.56 ng/ml) to mean endpoint levels of 41.49 ng/ml (SD 18.30 ng/ml) [vs. from 9.29 ng/ml (SD 4.06 ng/ml) to 20.40 ng/ml (SD 18.09 ng/ml) in the placebo group]. There was a trend ($p = 0.05$) for a higher increased in mean leptin serum levels in the risperidone group from 3.09 mg/L (SD 0.79) at baseline to 5.16 mg/L (SD 4.21) at 6 months versus from 4.34 mg/L (SD 2.75) to 3.81 mg/L (SD 2.18) in the placebo group. Most notably, children on risperidone gained significantly more, $F (1, 21) = 8.67, p < 0.01$, weight than children in the placebo group, with a mean weight gain of 2.96 kg from baseline versus 0.61 kg in the placebo group.

Effectiveness in amelioration of autism symptoms: Comparing the risperidone and placebo groups at four time points

Results of primary outcome measures during all four assessment points (baseline 2, 4, and 6 months) are provided in Table 3. A repeated measures ANOVA across all four time points

TABLE 2. MEAN CHANGE SCORES OF PHYSIOLOGICAL MEASURES FROM BASELINE TO ENDPOINT

Measure	Risperidone		Placebo		Statistics	
	M	SD	M	SD	t (df)	p
Weight change in kg	2.96	2.53	0.61	1.10	−2.94 (21)	0.008
Leptin change in mg/L	0.66	0.97	−0.35	0.91	−2.15 (14)	0.050
Prolactin change in ng/ml	33.38	14.48	11.11	18.74	−2.76 (15)	0.015

indicated that all participants' CARS Total Scores improved significantly over time within the risperidone and placebo groups combined [$\lambda = 0.37$, F (3, 19) = 10.61, $p < 0.001$]. However, the degree of improvement was not statistically different between the risperidone and placebo groups. To minimize the potential effect of group differences in autism symptom severity at baseline, the two developmental variables that differed between groups at baseline (PLS-3 Total Language and VABS Motor Skills scores) were used as covariates in follow-up analyses. Results from the repeated measures ANCOVA revealed no significant differences between the risperidone and placebo groups when the effects of preschoolers' language and motor development were controlled for statistically (see Table 3).

Effectiveness in treatment of autism symptoms: Risperidone versus placebo at baseline and 6-month follow up

When differences in baseline developmental characteristics were accounted for, results indicated no statistically significant differences between the risperidone and placebo groups on any of the outcome measures of interest when examining all four time points. However, when the total number of intervals being examined was reduced from four to two points (i.e., baseline and final assessment), and when baseline differences in motor development between groups were accounted for, repeated measures analyses of autism symptom scores on the CARS over these two time points (baseline to 6-month study endpoint) revealed significant differences between the study groups [$\lambda = 0.74$, F (1,21) = 6.92, $p < 0.05$] with a large effect size of $d = 0.95$. Specifically, children treated with risperidone demonstrated greater improvement in autism symptom ratings when compared to placebo controls (see Table 4). Accordingly, the risperidone group mean CARS Total scores dropped from the "Severely Autistic" to the "Mildly to Moderately Autistic" range at endpoint, whereas severity classification did not change in the placebo group. The change in CARS total scores from baseline to 6-month follow up for the risperidone group was 8% compared to 3% for the placebo group.

In addition, results from a repeated measures ANCOVA revealed a significant difference [$\lambda = 0.78$, F (1,20) = 5.50, $p < 0.05$] between the risperidone and placebo groups on the CARS Emotional Response subscale when VABS Motor Skills was included as a covariate (see Table 4).

Additional related outcome measures of interest (e.g., CARS Adaptation, CARS Fear and Nervousness, GARS Total, and VABS Socialization scores), expected to differ significantly between the groups, revealed no significant time-by-treatment interaction, even when baseline language and motor development were included in the equations as covariates.

Effectiveness of risperidone versus placebo on anxiety: Baseline to 6-month follow up

A trend toward differences in change of anxiety symptoms was found between the risperidone and placebo groups using the CBCL. This trend emerged despite a smaller sample size due to missing data at follow up. Although no differences were found between the groups in the CBCL Internalizing T composite scores, results from an ANOVA indicated that differences between the two study groups' mean scores on the CBCL Anxious/Depressed subscale approached significance [F (1,13) = 4.42, $p = 0.056$]. Covariates were not included in these analyses because there were no differences between the study groups in these areas (e.g., motor skills, CARS scores, etc.) when only the means for the reduced number of subjects included in the analyses were calculated (the sample sizes were reduced due to missing data as described above).

DISCUSSION

The current study aimed to determine whether risperidone was well tolerated and safe in preschool aged children with ASDs. It also aimed to investigate the short-term and 6-month efficacy of low-dose risperidone in the early treatment of ASDs during the preschool period of development. The findings demonstrated that risperidone appeared safe and well tolerated in this young sample over a 6-month

TABLE 3. TREATMENT EFFECTS AND COVARIATES OVER FOUR TIME POINTS ON PRIMARY OUTCOME MEASURES

Outcome	Baseline		Week 8		Week 16		Week 24		Time		Time × treatment interaction		Between subjects	
	M	SD	M	SD	M	SD	M	SD	F	p	F	p	F	p
CARS Total[a]									10.61	<0.01*	1.43	0.26	3.99	0.059
Risperidone	37.6	4.0	32.6	4.8	32.6	4.3	33.0	4.0						
Placebo	33.3	4.9	29.6	3.4	29.6	3.9	31.5	5.1						
With VABS motor covariate									0.233	0.87	0.85	0.49	2.76	0.12
With PLS-3 language covariate									0.213	0.89	1.37	0.19	0.299	0.67

CARS = Childhood Autism Rating Scale; VABS = Vineland Adaptive Behavior Scales; PLS = Preschool Language Scale.
[a]CARS total score: 15–29.99 "Non Autistic"; 30–36.99 "Mildly-Moderately Autistic"; 37.0–60 "Severely Autistic."
*p < 0.05

TABLE 4. EFFICACY OF PRIMARY AND SECONDARY OUTCOMES FROM BASELINE TO 6-MONTH FOLLOW UP

| | Baseline | | Endpoint | | Time × treatment interaction | |
Outcome	Mean	SD	Mean	SD	F	p
CARS total[a]						
Risperidone (n = 11)	37.6	4.0	33.0	4.0	2.73	0.114
Placebo (n = 12)	33.3	4.9	31.5	5.1		
With VABS Motor					6.92	0.16*
With PLS-3 Language					2.82	0.109
CARS Emotional Response						
Risperidone (n = 11)	3.0	0.6	2.4	0.8	2.16	0.157
Placebo (n = 12)	2.3	0.8	2.2	0.5		
With VABS Motor					5.50	0.029*
With PLS-3 Language					1.24	0.278

CARS = Childhood Autism Rating Scale; VABS = Vineland Adaptive Behavior Scales; PLS = Preschool Language Scale.
[a]CARS Total Score: 15–29.99 "Non Autistic"; 30–36.99 "Mildly-Moderately Autistic"; 37.0–60 "Severely Autistic."
*$p < 0.05$.

treatment period, with the most common enduring side effects including weight gain, hypersalivation, and elevations in prolactin levels (with no clinical lactation in any study subject). Low levels of sedation were observed; however, all observed sedation was transient and spontaneously resolved after several days. It was notable that no serious adverse side effects deemed attributable to the medication were observed during the 6-month trial. There were no occurrences of extrapyramidial movements, and no subjects dropped out due to side effects of risperidone. There was a trend toward greater elevations in leptin levels among subjects on risperidone. All of these side effects are well known from investigations of risperidone in older children and adults. These data suggest that low-dose risperidone can be given over a 6-month period and is well tolerated by preschool children.

The finding that differences between the study groups were detected in the baseline to 6 month comparison and not in the four time point repeated measures comparison is based on the fact that the former tests are specific to a single change, namely 6-month improvement. By comparison, the repeated measures tests involving all four time points are sensitive to many possible differences across time and therefore are less powerful at detecting any specific change.

The etiology of the weight gain as well as potential remedies, which could be used to min-imize this, should be the focus of future study. The use of an unblinded clinician may have diminished the occurrence of adverse events; however, the fact that medication dosage was lowered for only 1 subject at only one study visit minimizes this possibility.

Study findings suggest that preschool children treated with low-dose risperidone displayed greater improvements in global measures of autism symptoms compared to those treated with placebo. These findings emerged only when baseline differences in development between the two study groups were accounted for. Specifically, differences between study groups in CARS autism symptom scores of a large effect size became evident when baseline differences in motor skills were controlled. Although these findings were statistically significant, the possibility of a Type I (or Type II) error cannot be ruled out due to the small sample size and the severity differences between groups at baseline that complicated the analyses. Therefore, although findings overall are promising and suggestive of treatment effects, we do not believe they should be used for direct clinical practice. Instead, these study findings suggest that further study with larger samples and longer treatment durations is warranted.

The original study hypothesis was that risperidone, when used at very early points in development, would allow for greater improvements in the core symptoms of autism, including communicative language, restricted interests, stereotypies, as well as social competence and reciprocity. Although global autism scores appeared to improve, this study did not detect evidence of more specific improvement in autism core symptoms as a function of treatment group. This finding is consistent with results from double-blind treatment trials of risperidone in older children with ASDs, which demonstrated that despite improvements in nonspecific disruptive behavior and autism-related stereotypic behavior, the core social and language impairments were not affected by medication treatment (McCracken et al. 2002). More recently available data from the multisite trial (Research Units on Pediatric Psychopharmacology Autism Network, RUPP) of older autistic children has also shown that whereas improvements in restricted, repetitive, and stereotypic behaviors were detected, no significant improvement in social skills or communication emerged (McDougle et al. 2005).

In contrast to the current findings, Shea and colleagues (2004) found children treated with risperidone for 8 weeks showed greater improvement in the core symptoms of inappropriate speech and lethargy/social withdrawal in addition to decreases in stereotypic and disruptive behaviors. Given that the final mean dose of both the Shea et al. study and the current study were similar (0.05 mg/kg/day), and the fact that the current study was of longer duration, suggests that the failure of the current study to detect differences in core autistic features could be due to lack of statistical power related to the relatively small sample size.

Although parents and treatment providers have held out great hope that a medication such as risperidone might have a primary ameliorating effect on the core symptoms of autism, the more restricted improvements observed could be expected based on the fact that the medication was developed as an antipsychotic to treat debilitating impairments in emotional and behavioral control. These symptoms, while viewed as more peripheral to autism, are still quite disabling, and therefore, an important treatment target.

It was notable that both study groups improved significantly over the study period, a finding that could have been related to the on-going developmental therapies in both groups applied during this young age. Furthermore, positive effects of both medication and placebo were evident in both groups early in the study; however, notably, the risperidone treated group sustained gains over the 6-month period. The important clinical implication here is that, if monitored adequately, the beneficial effects of risperidone over placebo should be evident after 6 months of treatment. Although this study was only continued for 6 months, the effects gained were maintained throughout that time. Pertinent to and extending this finding, a blinded discontinuation arm of the RUPP Autism Network demonstrated that risperidone showed sustained efficacy and tolerability over a 6-month treatment period and that discontinuation resulted in a reversal of these gains (RUPP Autism Network 2005). Further studies are needed to address whether or not there are ongoing improvements in behavior symptoms over longer durations in autism samples treated during the preschool period.

When baseline differences between groups were controlled, some significant differences in symptom improvement were evident between groups. Although the findings are not robust, they must be viewed in light of the fact that many study subjects also were undergoing an intensive behavioral intervention. This would suggest that differences between groups could have been more pronounced in a similar study group that was not also undergoing this intensive treatment. Whereas these findings may reflect some level of improvement among all children receiving risperidone, another possibility is that only a small number of children treated with risperidone demonstrated improvement in symptoms beyond those resulting from intensive intervention. Thus, one interpretation of the findings might be that risperidone would be most judiciously used in those children who fail to make significant gains despite intensive psychosocial and educational treatment. Additional double-blind, placebo-controlled treatment trials in larger samples of preschool children with ASDs, including careful safety monitoring, are necessary before clinical use in this age group can be recommended with confidence.

Limitations

The clinical significance of the changes observed are difficult to determine on the basis of the lack of any objective measures of functioning beyond symptom manifestations. Therefore, further study is still needed to determine if the benefits outweigh the risks of this medication in preschool aged children with ASDs. These investigations should make direct comparisons of preschoolers in ABA treatment with and without medication augmentation. It is also unclear whether the dosing schedules used by the unblinded clinician were comparable to those implemented in similar studies of this medication in older children or were too low to produce more detectable changes.

The findings of greater severity of ASD symptoms and greater developmental impairments in the risperidone treatment group were limitations of the study. This, as well as the relatively small sample size, increases the possibility of Type I and/or Type II errors. Furthermore, the absence of corrections for multiple tests for outcome analyses are another clear limitation of the findings. The lack of a more comprehensive observational assessment and structured clinical interview of autism, such as the Autism Diagnostic Observation Schedule (ADOS) and Autism Diagnostic Interview-Revises (ADI-R), was also a study limitation. In addition, although safety of the medication over the 6-month period was established on the basis of measures of growth and development and physiology used, the longer-term effects of the medication on the developing brain remain unknown and should be the focus of future studies. Furthermore, other metabolic measures such as insulin resistance, now known to be important in atypical antipsychotic medications, were not measured in this investigation and should be included in future clinical trials of risperidone in children.

ACKNOWLEDGMENT

This study was funded by Janssen Pharmaceutica as an investigator initiated project to Dr. Luby.

DISCLOSURES

Drs. Luby, Mrakotsky, Belden, Heffelfinger, and Spitznazel and Ms. Stalets and Williams have no conflicts of interest or financial relationships to disclose.

REFERENCES

Achenbach T, Edelbrock C: Manual for the Child Behavior Checklist and Revised Behavior Profile. Burlington (Vermont), University of Vermont, Department of Psychiatry, 1995.

American Psychiatric Association. Diagnostic and Statistical Manual of Mental Disorders, 4th ed. (DSM-IV). Washington, DC: American Psychiatric Association, 1994.

Bertrand J, Mars A, Boyle C, Bove F, Yeargin-Allsopp M, Decoufle P: Prevalence of autism in a United States population: The Brick Township, New Jersey, investigation. Pediatrics 108:1155–1161, 2001.

Dawson G, Ashman SB, Carver LJ: The role of early experience in shaping behavioral and brain development and its implications for social policy. Dev Psychopathol 12:695–712, 2000.

Faja S, Dawson G: Early Intervention for autism. In: Handbook of Preschool Mental Health: Development Disorders and Treatment. Edited by Luby JL. New York, Guilford Press, 2006.

Gerlai R, Gerlai J: Autism: A target of pharmacotherapies? Drug Discov Today 9:366–374, 2004.

Gilliam J: The Gilliam Autism Rating Scale. Austin (Texas), Pro-Ed, Inc., 1995.

Masi G, Cosenza A, Mucci M, Brovedani P: Open trial of risperidone in 24 young children with pervasive developmental disorders. J Am Acad Child Adolesc Psychiatry 40:1206–1241, 2001.

McClellan JM, Werry JS: Evidence-based treatments in child and adolescent psychiatry: an inventory. J Am Acad Child Adolesc Psychiatry 42:1388–1400, 2003.

McCracken JT, McGough J, Shah B, Cronin P, Hong D, Aman MG, Arnold LE, Lindsay R, Nash P, Hollway J, McDougle CJ, Posey D, Swiezy N, Kohn A, Scahill L, Martin A, Koenig K, Volkmar F, Carroll D, Lancor A, Tierney E, Ghuman J, Gonzalez NM, Grados M, Vitiello B, Ritz L, Davies M, Robinson J, McMahon D: Risperidone in children with autism and serious behavioral problems. N Engl J Med 347:314–321, 2002.

McDougle CJ, Scahill J, Aman MG, McCracken JT, Tierney E, Davies M, Arnold LE, Posey DJ, Martin A, Ghuman JK, Shah B, Chuang SZ, Swiezy NB, Gonzalez NM, Hollway J, Koenig K, McGough JJ, Ritz L, Vitiello B: Risperidone for the core symptom domains of autism: Results from the study by the autism network of the Research Units on Pediatric Psychopharmacology. Am J Psychiatry 162:1142–1148, 2005.

McDougle CJ, Stigler KA, Posey DJ: Treatment of aggression in children and adolescents with autism and conduct disorder. J Clin Psychiatry 64 Suppl 4:16–25, 2003.

Sandler A, Bodfish J: Placebo effects in autism: lessons from secretin. J Dev Behav Pediatr 21:347–350, 2000.

Schopler E, Reichler RJ, Rochen RB: The Childhood Autism Rating Scale. Los Angeles (California), Western Psychological Services, 1988.

Schreibman L: Intensive behavioral/psychoeducational treatments for autism: Research needs and future directions. J Autism Dev Disord 30:373–378, 2000.

Shea S, Turgay A, Carroll A, Schulz M, Orlik H, Smith I, Dunbar F: Risperidone in the treatment of disruptive behavioral symptoms in children with autistic and other pervasive developmental disorders. Pediatrics 114:634–641, 2004.

Sparrow S, Balla D, Cicchetti D: Vineland Adaptive Behavior Scales-Interview Edition, Survey for Manual. American Guidance Service, 1984.

The Psychological Corporation: Preschool Language Scale-3, San Antonio (Texas), 1992.

The Research Units on Pediatric Psychopharmacology Autism Network: Risperidone treatment of autistic disorder: Longer-term benefits and blinded discontinuation after 6 months. Am J Psychiatry 162:1361–1369, 2005.

Troost PW, Lahuis BE, Steenhuis MP, Ketelaars CE, Buitelaar JK, van Engeland H, Scahill L, Minderaa RB, Hoekstra PJ: Long-term effects of risperidone in children with autism spectrum disorders: A placebo discontinuation study. J Am Acad Child Adolesc Psychiatry 44:1137–1144, 2005.

Vitiello B: Pediatric psychopharmacology and the interaction between drugs and the developing brain. Canad J Psychiatry 43:582–584, 1998.

Witwer A, Lecavelier L: Treatment incidence and patterns in children and adolescents with autism spectrum disorders. J Child Adolesc Psychopharmacol 15:671–681, 2005.

Zito J, Safer D, dosReis S, Gardner J, Boles M, Lynch F: Trends in the prescribing of psychotropic medications to preschoolers. JAMA 283:1025–1030, 2000.

PART 2

Psychopharmacologic Treatment of Preschool
Attention-Deficit/Hyperactivity Disorder

ADVANCES IN PRESCHOOL PSYCHOPHARMACOLOGY
© 2009 Mary Ann Liebert, Inc.
140 Huguenot Street, 3rd Floor
New Rochelle, NY 10801-5215

Introduction

New Findings from the Preschoolers with Attention-Deficit/Hyperactivity Disorder Treatment Study (PATS)

Mark A. Riddle, M.D.

T HE FIRST SEVEN PAPERS in Part Two of this book report new findings from the 6-site Preschoolers with Attention-Deficit/Hyperactivity Disorder Treatment Study (PATS). The PATS was designed to assess the efficacy and safety of short-term methylphenidate (MPH) and the effectiveness and tolerability of long-term MPH in 3-to 5-year-old children with attention-deficit/hyperactivity disorder (ADHD). The design of PATS was complex, reflecting input from multiple government agencies and scientific review in addition to the investigators, and included 8 phases: 1) screening/enrollment, 2) 10-week, uncontrolled parent training, 3) baseline assessment, 4) 1-week, open-label, safety lead-in, 5) 5-week, random sequence (doses = 1.25 mg, 2.5 mg, 5 mg, 7.5 mg, and placebo, administered tid), double-blind, crossover titration, 6) 4-week, optimal dose, double-blind, placebo-controlled parallel phase, 7) 10-month, open-label maintenance, and 8) 6-week, placebo-substitution discontinuation. Informed consent was obtained at each phase (Kollins et al., 2006).

The first 5 papers from PATS were published in 2006. The primary outcome results from Phase 5 crossover titration (n = 165 of 303 enrolled) were: Compared to placebo, significant differences were found for tid MPH doses of 2.5 mg, 5 mg and 7.5 mg, but not for 1.25 mg (p < .06). Of participants (n = 114) randomized into

the parallel-design, best-dose, Phase 6, only 21% on MPH and 13% on placebo achieved remission (Greenhill et. al., 2006). Also, of note, only 7% of 261 who completed Phase 2 parent training showed significant improvement (Greenhill et al., 2006).

Safety and tolerability data for the entire study was described in a paper by Wigal and colleagues (2006). For Phases 4 to 7 combined, parents reported moderate or severe adverse events (AEs) in 30% of participants. The most common were: emotional outbursts, difficulty falling asleep, repetitive behaviors/thoughts, appetite decrease, and irritability. During Phase 5 titration, decreased appetite, trouble sleeping and weight loss occurred more frequently on MPH than on placebo. During Phase 7 maintenance, trouble sleeping and appetite loss persisted. Eleven percent of participants discontinued because of MPH-attributed AEs.

The impact of MPH on growth was presented in a paper by Swanson and colleagues (2006). Of note, the preschoolers with ADHD began the PATS study at significantly greater average heights and weights than established norms. During treatment, there was a significant decrement in growth: height = -1.38 cm/yr, weight = -1.32 kg/yr. These decrements in preschoolers were greater than those observed in school-aged children in the Mul-

Division of Child and Adolescent Psychiatry, Johns Hopkins University School of Medicine, Baltimore, Maryland.

timodal Treatment of ADHD (MTA) Study (MTA 2004).

Finally, McGough and colleagues (2006) reported on the pharmacogenetics of MPH in the PATS sample. The primary analysis did not indicate significant genetic effects. In secondary analyses, associations were seen between symptom response and variants at the dopamine receptor (DRD4) promoter and synaptosomal-associated protein 25 (SNAP25) alleles *T1065G* and *T1069C*. SNAP25 variants were also associated with tics, buccal-lingual movements, and irritability. DRD4 variants were associated with picking.

In the first paper in Part Two of this volume, Posner and colleagues (2007) elaborate on the clinical presentation of the PATS sample. Younger children (within the 3.0- to 5.5-year age range at enrollment) had greater severity of ADHD symptoms. Approximately 70% had comorbid disorders, most commonly oppositional defiant disorder (ODD), communication disorders, and anxiety disorders. Those with comorbid communication disorders were more anxious and depressed. Finally, ADHD severity correlated with more internalizing symptoms and lower functioning.

Ghuman and colleagues (2007) assessed predictors of treatment response using exploratory moderator analyses of the Phase 5 crossover titration data. They found a significant interaction of number of comorbid disorders and treatment response. Specifically, participants with 3 or more comorbid disorders did not respond to MPH, while those with 0, 1, or 2 comorbidities did respond. The effect size for response of those with 0 or 1 comorbidities was quite robust (Cohen's $d = .89$ and 1.0, respectively), and comparable to effect sizes for school-aged children with ADHD (MTA 1999). Of note, in the group with 1 comorbidity, by far the most common disorder was oppositional defiant disorder (ODD).

Abikoff and colleagues (2007) examined the effects of MPH on functional outcomes during the 4-week, parallel groups Phase 6. The primary finding was that medication effects on functional outcomes varied by informant and outcome measure. This is not surprising given that several weeks of medication treatment would not be expected to consistently change

such outcomes as social skills, classroom behavior, emotional status, or parenting stress.

Vitiello and colleagues (2007) examined the effects of MPH during the 10-month, open-label, continuation Phase 7. In the 95 participants who completed Phase 7, improvements were observed in measures of ADHD global severity, global functioning, and social skills. Measures of specific ADHD symptom severity remained stable. Forty-five participants discontinued for various reasons, 7 for AEs, 7 for behavior worsening, 7 to switch to a long-acting stimulant, 3 for inadequate benefit, and 21 for other reasons. The mean MPH daily dose increased from about 14 mg to about 20 mg.

Murray and colleagues (2007) assessed parent-teacher concordance on ratings of DSM-IV (APA, 1997) ADHD symptoms in preschoolers referred for the PATS study. Interestingly, correlations between parent and teacher ratings were low for both Inattentive ($r = .24$) and Hyperactive-Impulsive ($r = .26$) symptom domains. Teachers were moderately likely to agree with parents on the presence or absence of symptoms. Parents were quite likely to agree with teachers' endorsement of symptoms, but much less likely to agree with teachers when symptoms were not endorsed.

Hardy and colleagues (2007) assessed 1- and 2-factor models of ADHD using the 18 DSM-IV symptoms in the entire cohort of 533 preschoolers referred, but not necessarily recruited into, the PATS study. They found that for parent ratings, the 2-factor model was minimally acceptable while the 1-factor model was not. For teachers, neither model was acceptable. After excluding several symptoms, the 2-factor model was satisfactory for both parents and teachers. These results suggest that for preschoolers, the symptom criterion set for ADHD may need to be modified in DSM-V.

Swanson and colleagues (2007) assessed the effect of the source of DNA (from buccal or blood cells) on genotyping success rate and allele percentages for candidate genes assessed in the PATS (see McGough et al., 2006). Interestingly, using methods available in 2004, the genotyping success rate was much higher for DNA from blood cells (91%) vs. buccal cells (54%). Also, for some polymorphisms, allele proportion varied by source of cells. These results illuminate a major methodological issue in pediatric pharmacogenetics: How does the investigator balance the advantage of obtaining buccal cells (more children will likely participate) versus the disadvantage (lower genotyping success rate and altered allele frequencies).

Wigal and colleagues (2007) examined the pharmacokinetics of MPH in preschoolers with ADHD and compared them with school-aged children. The main findings were that preschoolers had a significantly higher peak plasma concentration (C_{max}) and slower clearance of MPH than school-aged children.

Taken together, the results of the PATS provide important new evidence regarding the treatment of preschoolers with ADHD. Clearly, MPH is an effective short-term and long-term (up to 10 months) treatment. The best total daily MPH dose in preschoolers (mean = about 14 mg/day) is considerably lower than that in school-aged and older youngsters. With long-term treatment, somewhat higher total daily MPH doses are needed (mean = 20 mg/day). Side effects are generally tolerable. However, decrements in height and weight during long-term treatment are a potential concern. The most likely nonresponders are those with multiple comorbidities. Functional improvement, particularly in global function and social skills, emerges during long-term treatment.

The PATS data set also reveals interesting findings about ADHD in preschoolers. The most common comorbidities are ODD, communication disorders, and anxiety disorders. Parent and teacher agreement on symptom ratings is poor. A 2-factor model (inattention and hyperactivity/impulsivity) fits the data only after several DSM symptoms are removed, suggesting that the DSM symptoms for ADHD need to be modified for preschoolers. Finally, the PATS data sheds important light on the issue of using buccal vs. blood samples for genotyping.

Where next with interventions research in preschoolers with ADHD? It will be useful for the PATS group to publish the findings from the 10-week parent training. To date, what is known is that only 7% of the preschoolers of the participating families improved sufficiently to no longer meet study entry criteria. Why was the response rate so low? What can the data teach us about psychosocial treatment for preschoolers with ADHD?

The PATS group is conducting a 5-year follow-up study of 202 of the 303 participants in the original PATS sample. Data from this study will be important regarding long-term stability of ADHD presenting in preschoolers, the effectiveness and tolerability of MPH in this age group, as well as the impact of MPH on growth at this stage in development.

Hopefully, future studies will compare the best medication treatments available with the best psychosocial treatments available, separately and in combination. The MTA study provided such data for school-age children with ADHD, but such a study is needed to inform treatment in preschoolers.

DISCLOSURE

Dr. Riddle has no conflict of interest or financial ties to disclose for the past 2 years.

REFERENCES

Abikoff HB, Vitiello B, Riddle MA, Cunningham C, Greenhill LL, Swanson JM, Chuang SZ, Davies M, Kastelic E, Wigal SB, Evans L, Ghuman JK, Kollins SH, McCracken JT, McGough JJ, Murray DW, Posner K, Skrobala AM, Wigal T: Methylphenidate effects on functional outcome in preschoolers with attention deficit/hyperactivity disorder: Results from the National Institute of Mental Preschoolers with Attention Deficit/Hyperactivity Disorder Treatment Study (PATS). J Child Adolesc Psychopharm 17:581–592, 2007.

Ghuman JK, Riddle MA, Vitiello B, Greenhill LL, Chuang SZ, Wigal SB, Kollins SH, Abikoff HB, McCracken JT, Kastelic E, Scharko AM, McGough JJ, Murray DW, Evans L, Swanson JM, Wigal T, Posner K, Cunningham C, Davies M, Skrobala AM: Comorbidity moderates response to methylphenidate in the Preschoolers with Attention-Deficit/Hyperactivity Disorder Treatment Study (PATS). J Child Adolesc Psychopharm 17:563–579, 2007.

Greenhill LL, Kollins SH, Abikoff H, McCracken J, Riddle M, Swanson J, McGough J, Wigal S, Wigal T, Vitiello B, Skrobala A, Posner K, Ghuman J, Cunningham C, Davies M, Chuang S, Cooper T: Efficacy and safety of immediate-release methylphenidate treatment for preschoolers with ADHD. J Am Acad Child Adolesc Psychiatry 45:1284–1293, 2006.

Hardy KK, Kollins SH, Murray DW, Riddle MA, Greenhill LL, Cunningham C, Abikoff HB, McCracken JT, Vitiello B, Davies M,, McGough JJ, Posner K, Skorbala AM, Swanson JM, Wigal T, Wigal SB, Ghuman JK, Chuang SZ: Factor structure of parent- and teacher-rated attention-deficit/hyperactivity disorder symptoms in the Preschoolers with Attention-Deficit/Hyperactivity Disorder Treatment Study (PATS). J Child Adolesc Psychopharm 17:621–633, 2007.

Kollins SH, Green L, Swanson J, Wigal S, Abikoff H, McCracken J, Riddle M, McGough J, Vitiello B, Wigal T, Skrobala A, Posner K, Ghuman J, Davies M, Cunningham C, Bauzo A: Rationale, design, and methods of the Preschool Attention-Deficit/Hyperactivity Disorder Treatment Study (PATS). J Am Acad Child Adolesc Psychiatry 45:1275–1283, 2006.

McGough J, McCracken J, Swanson J, Riddle M, Kollins S, Greenhill L, Abikoff H, Davies M, Chuang S, Wigal T, Wigal S, Posner K, Skrobala A, Cunningham C, Shigawa S, Moyzis R, Vitiello B: Pharmacogenetics of methylphenidate response in preschoolers with ADHD. J Am Acad Child Adolesc Psychiatry 45:1314–1322, 2006.

MTA Cooperative Group: A 14-month randomized clinical trial of treatment strategies for attention-deficit/hyperactivity disorder. Arch Gen Psychiatry 56:1073–1086, 1999.

MTA Cooperative Group: National Institute of Mental Health Multimodal Treatment Study of ADHD followup: Changes in effectiveness and growth after the end of treatment. Pediatrics 113:762–769, 2004.

Murray D, Kollins SH, Hardy KK, Abikoff HB, Swanson JM, Cunningham C, Vitiello B, Riddle MA, Davies M, Greenhill LL, McCracken JT, McGough JJ, Posner K, Skrobala AM, Wigal T, Wigal SB, Ghuman JK, Chuang SZ: Parent versus teacher ratings of attention-deficit/hyperactivity disorder symptoms in the Preschoolers with Attention-Deficit/Hyperactivity Disorder Treatment Study (PATS). J Child Adolesc Psychopharm 17:605–619, 2007.

Posner K, Melvin GA, Murray DW, Gugga SS, Fisher P, Skrobala AM, Cunningham C, Vitiello B, Abikoff HB, Ghuman JK, Kollins SH, Wigal SB, Wigal T, McCracken JT, McGough JJ, Kastelic E, Boorady R, Davies M, Chuang SZ, Swanson JM, Riddle MA, Greenhill LL: Clinical presentation of attention-deficit/hyperactivity disorder in preschool children: The Preschool Attention-Deficit/Hyperactivity Disorder Treatment Study (PATS). J Child Adolesc Psychopharm 17:547–562, 2007.

Swanson J, Greenhill L, Wigal T, Kollins S, Stehli A, Davies M, Chuang S, Vitiello B, Skrobala A, Posner K, Abikoff H, Oatis M, McCracken J, McGough J, Riddle M, Ghuman J, Cunningham C, Wigal S: Stimulant-related reductions of growth rates in the PATS. J Am Acad Child Adolesc Psychiatry 45:1304–1313, 2006.

Swanson JM, Moyzis RK, McGough JJ, McCracken JT, Riddle MA, Kollins SH, Greenhill LL, Abikoff HB, Wigal T, Wigal SB, Posner K, Skrobala AM, Ghuman JK, Cunningham C, Vitiello B, Stehli A, Smalley SL, Grady D: Effects of source of DNA on genotyping success rates and allele percentages in the Preschoolers with Attention-Deficit/Hyperactivity Disorder Treatment Study (PATS). J Child Adolesc Psychopharm 17:635–645, 2007.

Vitiello B, Abikoff HB, Chuang SZ, Kollins SH, McCracken JT, Riddle MA, Swanson JM, Wigal T, McGough JJ, Ghuman JK, Wigal SB, Skrobala AM, Davies M, Posner K, Cunningham C, Greenhill LL: Effectiveness of methylphenidate in the 10-month continuation phase of the Preschoolers with Attention-Deficit/Hyperactivity Disorder Treatment Study (PATS). J Child Adolesc Psychopharm 17:593–603, 2007.

Wigal SB, Gupta S, Greenhill LL, Posner K, Lerner M, Steinhoff K, Wigal T, Kapelinski A, Martinez J, Modi NB, Stehli A, Swanson J: Pharmacokinetics of Methylphenidate in Preschoolers with Attention-Deficit/Hyperactivity Disorder. J Child Adolesc Psychopharm 17:153—164, 2007.

Wigal T, Greenhill L, Chuang S, McGough J, Vitiello B, Skrobala A, Swanson J, Wigal S, Abikoff H, Kollins S, McCracken J, Riddle M, Posner K, Ghuman J, Davies M, Thorp B, Stehli A: Safety and tolerability of methylphenidate in preschool children with ADHD. J Am Acad Child Adolesc Psychiatry 45: 1294–1302, 2006.

ADVANCES IN PRESCHOOL PSYCHOPHARMACOLOGY
© 2009 Mary Ann Liebert, Inc.
140 Huguenot Street, 3rd Floor
New Rochelle, NY 10801-5215

Clinical Presentation of Attention-Deficit/Hyperactivity Disorder in Preschool Children: The Preschoolers with Attention-Deficit/Hyperactivity Disorder Treatment Study (PATS)

Kelly Posner, Ph.D.,[1] Glenn A. Melvin, Ph.D.,[1] Desiree W. Murray, Ph.D.,[2]
S. Sonia Gugga, M.S.,[1] Prudence Fisher, Ph.D.,[1] Anne Skrobala, M.A.,[1]
Charles Cunningham, Ph.D.,[3] Benedetto Vitiello, M.D.,[4] Howard B. Abikoff, Ph.D.,[5]
Jaswinder K. Ghuman, M.D.,[8] Scott H. Kollins, Ph.D.,[2,7] Sharon B. Wigal, Ph.D.,[6]
Tim Wigal, Ph.D.,[6] James T. McCracken, M.D.,[7] James J. McGough, M.D.,[7]
Elizabeth Kastelic, M.D.,[9] Roy Boorady, M.D.,[5] Mark Davies, M.P.H.,[1]
Shirley Z. Chuang, M.S.,[10] James M. Swanson, Ph.D.,[6] Mark A. Riddle, M.D.,[9]
and Laurence L. Greenhill, M.D.[1]

ABSTRACT

Objective: The aim of this study was to describe the clinical presentation of preschoolers diagnosed with moderate to severe attention-deficit/hyperactivity disorder (ADHD) recruited for the multisite Preschool ADHD Treatment Study (PATS). The diagnosis and evaluation process will also be described.

Method: A comprehensive multidimensional, multi-informant assessment protocol was implemented including the semistructured PATS Diagnostic Interview. Parent- and teacher-report measures were used to supplement information from interviews. Consensus agreement by a cross-site panel on each participant's diagnoses was required. Analyses were conducted to describe the sample and to test associations between ADHD severity and demographic and clinical variables.

Results: The assessment protocol identified 303 preschoolers (3–5.5 years) with moderate to severe ADHD Hyperactive/Impulsive or Combined type. The majority of participants (*n* = 211, 69.6%) experienced co-morbid disorders, with oppositional defiant disorder, communication disorders, and anxiety disorders being the most common. Participants with co-morbid

[1]New York State Psychiatric Institute/Columbia University, New York, New York.
[2]Duke University Medical Center, Durham, North Carolina.
[3]McMaster University, Hamilton, Ontario, Canada.
[4]National Institute of Mental Health, Bethesda, Maryland.
[5]New York University Child Study Center, New York, New York.
[6]University of California Irvine, Irvine, California.
[7]University of California Los Angeles, Los Angeles, California.
[8]University of Arizona, Tucson, Arizona.
[9]Johns Hopkins University, Baltimore, Maryland.
[10]Formerly at New York State Psychiatric Institute/Columbia University.
Statistical consultant: S. Sonia Gugga, M.S.

communication disorders were found to be more anxious and depressed. ADHD severity was found to correlate with more internalizing difficulties and lower functioning. Although boys and girls had similar symptom presentations, younger children had significantly higher ADHD severity.

Conclusions: Preschoolers with moderate to severe ADHD experience high co-morbidity and impairment, which have implications for both assessment and treatment.

INTRODUCTION

ATTENTION-DEFICIT/HYPERACTIVITY DISORDER (ADHD) in preschool-aged children is a significant public health challenge affecting as many as 6% of community samples (Campbell and Ewing 1990; Lavigne et al. 1996; Angold et al., submitted). The rate of diagnosis has been increasing as symptoms and impairment are now detected as early as 2 years of age (Campbell and Ewing 1990; Lavigne et al. 1996; Egger and Angold 2006). Furthermore, in a cross-sectional study of children aged 3–18 years, severity of ADHD experienced by preschoolers was found to be greater than that experienced by school-aged children with the disorder (Nolan et al. 2001). Preschool-onset ADHD has been shown to be chronic and stable over time, as well as being a strong risk factor for ongoing behavioral problems during the school-age period (Campbell et al. 1986; McGee 1991; Lahey et al. 1998; Pierce et al. 1999).

Although the onset of impairing ADHD, predominately overactive-impulsive type is most likely to occur during the preschool years (Connor et al. 2003), limited descriptive information is available about the disorder in this age group. It is known that ADHD significantly impairs a young child's functioning in multiple domains, including home, school, and social settings, as well as his/her physical safety (Posner and Greenhill, in press). For example, a community study found that 15% of preschoolers with ADHD (versus 0.4% of controls without ADHD) had been suspended from day care and 7.8% had been expelled (versus 0.8% of controls without ADHD; Angold et al., submitted). In addition to functional impairment, children with ADHD exhibit an increased chance of physical injury related to impulsive behavior, with more reported accidents, unintentional injuries, and visits to emergency departments than children without ADHD (Di-

Scala et al. 1998; Lam 2002; Schwebel et al. 2002). Impairment from ADHD in the preschool years underscores the need for accurate and early diagnosis, in turn enabling appropriate treatment and potentially improved developmental trajectories.

Similar to their older counterparts, co-morbidity with other disorders appears to be common among preschoolers with ADHD, with previous studies reporting that 64% (Angold et al., submitted) to 74% (Wilens et al. 2002) of 2- to 6-year-old children with ADHD met criteria for at least one additional disorder. Oppositional defiant disorder (ODD), conduct disorder (CD), generalized anxiety disorder (GAD), and mood disorders (Angold et al., submitted; Lavigne et al. 1996; Wilens et al. 2002) are most commonly reported, suggesting vulnerability to both internalizing and externalizing disorders. Internalizing symptoms in children aged 4–6 years with ADHD have been significantly associated with reading and math underachievement (Lahey et al. 1998). Co-morbidity can also predict future impairment. Speltz et al. (1999) found that preschool boys with both ADHD and ODD were significantly more likely to have psychiatric diagnosis at a 2-year follow up than those with ADHD alone. Diagnosis and identification of co-morbidities informs treatment and can, in turn, potentially influence prognosis. Therefore, a better understanding of co-morbid conditions in this age group is critical.

The extant literature also provides limited data regarding clinical presentation and correlates of different diagnostic subtypes for ADHD in preschoolers. Although all three subtypes have demonstrated diagnostic validity in preschoolers, the combined type (C) and hyperactive/impulsive type (H/I) are most common (Lahey et al. 1998). Moreover, the H/I type does not appear to be stable across time, with most children with the H/I type later meeting criteria for C (Lahey et al. 2005).

There are challenges to the early identification of preschool-onset ADHD, including the impact of the numerous developmental changes that occur during the preschool years and the high base rates of ADHD behaviors in normal children of this age. Preschool-aged children are just beginning to develop the capacity to sustain attention and inhibit impulses, thus deficits in these areas may be hard to identify. They are simultaneously developing self-awareness, engaging in more goal-directed behavior, and experiencing a desire for increased independence. This contributes to normative resistance to following directions and rules that can be perceived as difficulty listening and following instructions. Moreover, some ADHD symptoms are commonly endorsed by parents of preschoolers. In their review of four community studies of preschoolers, Egger and Angold (2006) report that several ADHD symptoms were identified by more than 10% of parents, including leaving seat, talking excessively, being on the go, fidgeting, having difficulty waiting, interrupting, and distractibility. Lower rates of inattentive symptoms must also be considered in the context of developmental constraints such that there may be limited opportunity for young children to exhibit some symptoms. For example, most preschool children are not expected to independently keep track of many belongings.

Although the *Diagnostic and Statistical Manual of Mental Disorder*, 4th edition, Text Revision (DSM-IV-TR) (APA 2000) acknowledges the difficulty of distinguishing ADHD symptoms from age-appropriate behaviors and requires that the symptoms must be inconsistent with developmental level, it provides no guidance on how to consider the symptoms in very young children. Determining when such behaviors meet criteria for the full disorder requires specific developmentally based decisions that have not yet been operationalized in evidence-based publications. There is, however, a small but important body of work on the diagnosis of other disruptive disorders in preschoolers that is relevant to consider. Keenan and colleagues demonstrate that oppositional defiant and conduct disorder can be validly differentiated in preschool children when some developmental modifications to

the DSM framework are made (Keenan and Wakschlag 2004; Keenan et al. 2007). These modifications include assessing children's developmental levels to interpret any behavioral deviance, defining "often" in more specific frequency terms, and considering qualitative aspects of the behavior such as the context in which it occurs and the constraints on symptom manifestation (Keenan and Wakschlag 2002). Additional descriptive information on the manifestation of symptoms in a clinical sample of preschoolers with ADHD may inform the development of such guidelines for this disorder as well.

The present study reports on the ADHD symptoms, impairment, and associated characteristics in the current largest clinical sample of preschool children rigorously diagnosed with ADHD. The sample was recruited for a randomized clinical trial, the National Institute of Mental Health (NIMH)-funded Preschoolers with ADHD Treatment Study (PATS; Greenhill et al. 2006). The purpose of this paper is three-fold: (1) to describe the diagnostic process used in PATS, (2) to examine the relationship between ADHD symptom severity and demographic and other clinical measures, and (3) to describe the rate of co-morbidity and clinical characteristics in the PATS sample.

METHOD

Diagnostic process

The PATS study was a six-site randomized clinical trial of methylphenidate (MPH). The criteria for ADHD were modified to prevent the inclusion of preschoolers with symptoms of ADHD that were subthreshold, transient, and/or more likely associated with another condition. Preschoolers were required to meet criteria for DSM-IV (APA 2000) ADHD, Combined or Hyperactive-Impulsive type, for 9 months duration (versus the 6 months required by the DSM-IV). As described below, children had to be between 3 and 5.5 years of age, meet unanimous approval of their diagnosis during a consensus conference call, have a *T*-score higher than 65 on both parent and teacher DSM-IV subscale of the Conners' Parent Rating Scale (CPRS:R-L; Conners 2000) and Teacher Rating Scale (CTRS:R-L; Conners 2000), have an impairment rating of 55 or lower on the Children's Global Assessment Scale (C-GAS; Shaffer et al. 1983), score above 70 (full scale) on the Differential Ability Scale (DAS; Elliott 1990), a measure of cognitive ability and achievement, live with the caretaker for at least 6 months, and be enrolled in a school or day-care program with 8 same-aged peers for at least 2 half-days a week (Kollins et al. 2006). Children were also excluded if during assessment there was current evidence of pervasive developmental disorders, psychosis, significant suicidality, or other psychiatric disorder that required treatment with additional medication, or history of bipolar disorder in both biological parents. Further details on selection criteria can be found in Kollins et al. (2006). The procedure used to assess for ADHD and other diagnoses is now described.

Following telephone screening with the inclusion and exclusion criteria, eligible prospective participants (child and parent) were invited to the site's research clinic and given a thorough explanation of the PATS study, followed by an informed consent procedure. Once the parent signed a consent form, the family participated in a multidimensional assessment to determine diagnosis and assess selection criteria. Assessment was conducted by a child psychiatrist or child psychologist following a comprehensive clinical protocol that included a battery of instruments. Evaluation commenced with a review of the inclusion and exclusion criteria and collection of demographic information. This was followed by computer administration of the parent report Diagnostic Interview Schedule for Children–Version 4.0 (DISC-IV; Shaffer et al. 1996) for screening purposes and included the anxiety, mood, elimination and disruptive behavior disorder and pica, tic disorder, and trichotillomania modules. The Diagnostic Interview Schedule for Children–Young Child (Lucas et al. 1998) and the Preschool Age Psychiatric Assessment (Egger and Angold 2004) would have been considered as alternative age-appropriate measures but were still under development at the time of study commencement. Parents were given a narrow-band standardized measure of

ADHD symptoms (CPRS-R:L; Conners 2000) and a broadband measure of child problem behaviors (Child Behavior Checklist, CBCL; Achenbach and Edelbrock 1983). With parental consent, the child's preschool or day-care teacher was contacted and asked to complete the corresponding versions of these scales—CTRS-R:L (Conners 2000) and Teacher Report Form (TRF; Achenbach et al. 1991).

The semistructured PATS Diagnostic Interview (PDI) was specifically developed for the study (contact author for a copy). The PDI interview includes age-appropriate probes, administered to the preschooler's main caretaker, to aid in the determination of symptom presence and severity. Probes for each ADHD symptom were developed and agreed upon by an expert panel. For example, parents were specifically asked if their child rolls around during "circle time" rather than sitting still (preschool equivalent for "difficulty remaining seated") or if the child loses interest easily while listening to a story or gives up quickly if unable to learn how to do something immediately (for difficulty concentrating). The 18 ADHD symptoms were rated on a scale of 0 (never) to 5 (always) by the evaluator, with a 3 representing a behavior that occurs "at least often," considered a symptom. Thus, parental report of frequencies of each symptom was collected on the PDI. Teacher report of symptom frequencies came from the CTRS-R:L. Parent and teacher symptom frequencies were then integrated by the clinician to render a final composite summary rating, documented in the PDI ADHD checklist. The PDI ADHD Checklist's internal consistency was $\alpha = 0.838$. The PDI systematically assessed all areas of ADHD impairment, including home, school, peer relations, other settings, and physical risk and injury. Anecdotal examples of the most severe types of impairment experienced by the PATS sample are presented in Table 1. In addition, the table also contains the various types of impairment to be assessed.

In addition to ADHD, the PDI used DSM-IV criteria to assess systematically for ODD, CD, depressive and bipolar disorders, tic disorders, psychotic disorders, and anxiety disorders. The PDI gathered information on disorders not assessed by the DISC-IV including learning,

TABLE 1. AREAS OF IMPAIRMENT: ANECDOTAL EXAMPLES OF SEVERE IMPAIRMENT REPORTED BY THE PATS SAMPLE

Physical injury

Fractured collarbone after running off a bed into the dresser. Pulled a heavy rope from a pole, hitting her in the head. She fell and hit head on table while climbing on her grandmother's sofa.

By the age of four, he has had stitches over right eye due to falling off the sofa onto the fish tank which cut him; fell and cut his head requiring stitches; climbed on shower rod and fell to floor, also requiring stitches; and collided with his babysitter requiring stitches over his eyebrow.

He stood up in stroller before age 2, fell backwards, and injured his ribs. He almost fell out of a window attempting to check out a noise he had heard below.

Risk behaviors

Child was found hanging halfway out of a window. Mother also found him lying across electric burners after turning on the stove. He runs into traffic if his hand is not held.

He climbed into his mother's car when it was parked in the driveway. Sat in driver's seat, turned key, put gear into neutral. The car rolled down the driveway, across the street, and crashed into a fence.

She poured bleach over her entire body.

He has stuck things into electrical sockets and has jumped out of the window onto fire escape.

She is always unbuckling car seat restraints and once stood up in the car. Mother bought a special five-point harness, which child learned to unfasten after 4 months.

Home

Mother has to lock herself in the bathroom to use the phone because child will not stop talking to her.

Child often pours shampoo or lotion over herself and smears it on the bathroom floor.

It takes her 4 hours to do homework because she is so distractible and cannot stop talking.

School

Disruptive in class

Child described as often going from the desk to tabletop to climbing bookcase and getting other children to follow her.

He has been singled out to a desk in a separate area due to frequently being out of his seat and disrupting the class.

Father lost his job as a cab driver because he often had to pick up his son early from school due to disruptive behavior.

He knocks people over and is unaware of the children around him. Teacher suggests that he wear a weight jacket.

The child has been expelled from five day-care programs or preschools.

Impairs academic progress

The child attends to a page in a book fleetingly, though she is smart and could do so much better if not for inattention.

Peers

According to teacher, child has inability to function appropriately with peers and adults in class. She distracts other children and adults and they become extremely frustrated, resulting in losing friends and being disliked by teachers.

Teacher notes that she gets picked last for teams because she does not pay attention to the game.

Other settings

Mother cannot take child out of house anymore because he is so disruptive in any setting.

The child could not be brought to church and related activities due to incessant talking and inability to remain seated.

PATS = Preschoolers with Attention-Deficit/Hyperactivity Disorder Treatment Study.

speech and language, and pervasive developmental disorder (PDD). The PDI also included a clinical interview and mental status observation with the preschooler to supplement the diagnostic information given by the child's caretaker.

Using a written template developed by the study team, each site's clinicians integrated and summarized all assessment information into a comprehensive written diagnostic report including a profile of DSM-IV multiaxial diagnoses (Axes I–IV) and presence and severity ratings for symptoms of ADHD. Furthermore, the template required the clinician to elucidate all differential diagnosis considered as well as the criteria or diagnoses the subject did or did not meet. Thus, all diagnostic criteria for each disorder were clearly delineated. This report summary included information on social adjustment, family psychiatric history, treatment history, significant medical history, and mental status.

Each case was then anonymously presented to a cross-site panel by the site clinician during a weekly national consensus teleconference. Prior to the teleconference call, all clinicians reviewed the case diagnostic report. Both present and lifetime diagnoses and diagnoses considered but ruled out were discussed. All diagnoses were voted on and a unanimous consensus was required prior to inclusion into the study.

Measures

Although the full set of baseline measures for the PATS study has been presented elsewhere (Kollins et al. 2006), certain measures of interest are presented in detail below to highlight their suitability for use in the preschool age range.

The DISC-IV–Parent Version (Shaffer et al. 1996) is a structured diagnostic instrument for children aged 6–17 years. The interview has demonstrated reliability and validity (Shaffer et al. 2000). Given the age of the sample, slight modifications were made to some items to ensure that they were developmentally appropriate, based on a review of the DISC–Young Child Version.

The C-GAS (Shaffer et al. 1983) is a 100-point clinician rating scale of a child's overall function across settings. A single score is given with higher scores reflecting better functioning. The scale has demonstrated that it can discriminate between levels of functioning in children (Bird et al. 1990; Weissman et al. 1990), but has not been studied in preschoolers.

The CBCL (Achenbach and Edelbrock 1983) is a widely used measure of behavioral competencies and problems experienced by children in the preschool age range as reported by parents. Similarly, the TRF (Achenbach et al. 1991) is the teacher-completed measure of a child's behavioral/emotional problems, academic performance, and adaptive functioning. These measures have established reliability and validity in the preschool ages (Achenbach and Edelbrock, 1983; Achenbach et al. 1991).

The Conners' Rating Scales (Conners et al. 1998a; Conners et al. 1998b) are research and clinical tools widely used to assess hyperactivity-impulsivity, attentional problems, and oppositional behavior in youths aged 3–17 years. The parent version has 80 items comprising 14 subscales and the teacher version has 59 items and 13 subscales (psychosomatic subscale omitted). The psychometric properties of the scales have been demonstrated in children as young as 3 years of age (Conners et al. 1998a; Conners et al. 1998b). Each scale is able to correctly classify more than 85% of children as having ADHD or not. Ratings of a 2 or 3 (representing "often" or "very often") were considered to indicate symptoms, an approach that has been used previously (Pelham et al. 1992; Lahey et al. 2005).

Data analyses

The present report includes only data from measures collected before treatment to obtain baseline ratings. Prior to conducting any analyses, distributional characteristics were examined, and variance on all measures was considered appropriate for examination despite some restriction of range of scores due to selection criteria. Eight participants had been expelled from school and were missing teacher report measures; however, these participants did not significantly differ from the rest of the sample on demographic or diagnostic variables.

Initial analyses were descriptive in nature. Prevalence rates for co-morbid diagnoses as determined by the cross-site consensus described above were calculated. Frequencies of individual ADHD and ODD symptoms, as reported on the CPRS-R:L, CTRS-R:L, and the PDI ADHD Checklist, are presented. Frequencies of ADHD symptoms were then examined for each ADHD type (Combined type versus Hyperactive/Impulsive type) and chi-square analyses were performed to evaluate any group differences.

Next, the relationships between ADHD severity and age, gender, impairment ratings, and number of co-morbid diagnoses were examined.

ADHD severity was measured by the ADHD DSM-IV Symptoms (Total) subscales from the CPRS-R:L and CTRS-R:L. Simple regression analyses were performed to indicate the correlation between age and ADHD severity. *T*-tests for independent groups were performed with both raw and *T*-scores on teacher and parent rating scales to examine the relationship between gender and ADHD severity. Boys' and girls' scales are normed separately, so comparison of *T*-scores does not assess the absolute difference between ADHD severity of boys and girls. Rather, this analysis more accurately compares the relative difference on the ADHD subscale between PATS boys and the Conners' normative sample of boys to the difference between PATS girls and the Conners' normative sample of girls. Furthermore, multiple regression analyses tested the unique contribution of ADHD severity to measures of internalizing and externalizing problems (CBCL and TRF), general functioning (C-GAS), and number of co-morbidities. ADHD severity, CBCL/TRF subscales, and presence of specific co-morbid conditions were examined using independent-groups *t*-tests of means. Given the symptom overlap between ODD and internalizing problems and to control for the effect of ODD, it was included in a multiple regression analysis in order to ascertain the unique effect of co-morbid communication disorder on internalizing problems. For all analyses, statistical significance was evaluated using the appropriate Bonferroni corrections.

RESULTS

Characteristics of the sample

The preschool sample comprised 303 children aged 3–5.5 years ($M = 4.41$ years, 76% male) who had a diagnosis of ADHD, Combined or Hyperactive-Impulsive type, and met all other selection criteria for the PATS. Sample characteristics are summarized in Table 2. Participants were recruited at six academic sites (Columbia University, Duke University, Johns Hopkins University, New York University, University of California, Irvine, and University of California, Los Angeles) via infor-

mation at local clinics and paid and public advertising.

Mean *T*-scores on selected measures before treatment are reported in Table 3. The proportion of participants at or above the clinical range is also reported.

As can be seen, the sample mean score was in the clinical range (>98th percentile) for all ADHD-related and externalizing subscales on the CPRS-R:L and CTRS-R:L. Similarly, on the CBCL overall externalizing scale and on the Aggression subscales, the sample mean score was elevated and almost half of the sample was above the clinical threshold. Also of note, given the subtype requirement of Combined or Hyperactive-Impulsive type in this study, clinically significant elevations were also seen on scales assessing inattention (CPRS-R:L and CTRS-R:L Cognitive Problems/Inattention and CBCL Attention scale).

In contrast, mean *T*-scores on parent and teacher rating scales reflecting internalizing symptoms (CPRS-R:L and CTRS-R:L Anxious/Shy, CPRS-R:L Psychosomatic, CBCL and TRF withdrawn and anxious/depressed) fell within the normal range. A relative minority of participants (8–11%) were above the clinical threshold on these scales (Achenbach et al. 1991).

Co-morbidity with ADHD

Co-morbid diagnoses were highly prevalent in this sample (Table 4). Only 30.4% (92/303) of participants had no co-morbid diagnoses at

TABLE 2.   DESCRIPTIVE CHARACTERISITICS OF THE SAMPLE

Demographics	Total n = 303
Age, mean (SD)	4.41 (0.70)
Gender, *n* (%)	
Male	229 (75.6)
Female	74 (24.4)
Ethnicity, *n* (%)	
White	190 (62.7)
Black or African American	58 (19.1)
Hispanic or Latino	47 (15.5)
Asian	6 (2.0)
American Indian or Alaskan Native	2 (0.7)
C-GAS, mean (SD)	47.3 (4.07)
Differential Abilities Scale, mean (SD)	96.06 (18.30)

SD = standard deviation; C-GAS = Children's Global Assessment Scale.

TABLE 3.   MEAN SCORES AND PROPORTION ABOVE CLINICALLY-RELEVANT THRESHOLD FOR SELECTED PARENT AND TEACHER REPORT MEASURES

	Informant			
	Parent		Teacher	
	T-score mean (SD)	Above clinical cutoff n (%)	T-score mean (SD)	Above clinical cutoff n (%)
	CPRS-R:L n = 303		CTRS-R:L n = 295	
Oppositional	70.68 (12.8)	204 (67.3)	71.86 (14.6)	204 (69.2)
Cognitive problems/Inattention	75.17 (12.7)	234 (77.2)	70.37 (14.5)	168 (57.3)
Anxious/Shy	53.36 (11.3)	55 (18.2)	58.59 (11.5)	98 (33.2)
Perfectionism	54.69 (11.8)	58 (19.1)	59.16 (14.2)	91 (31.1)
Social Problems	64.20 (16.5)	123 (40.6)	67.93 (16.7)	167 (56.6)
Psychosomatic	55.79 (14.3)	73 (24.1)	—	—
Global Index: Restless/Impulsive	75.35 (7.0)	133 (43.9)	75.38 (9.0)	263 (89.2)
Global Index: Emotional Lability	62.66 (12.0)	272 (89.8)	71.09 (14.6)	193 (65.4)
Global Index: Total	75.02 (8.5)	267 (88.1)	77.34 (9.5)	269 (91.2)
DSM-IV: Inattentive	79.15 (11.1)	267 (88.1)	72.34 (11.5)	218 (73.9)
DSM-IV: Hyperactive/Impulsive	78.62 (7.7)	300 (99.0)	76.63 (7.6)	291 (98.6)
DSM-IV: Total ADHD	78.35 (8.5)	284 (93.7)	76.09 (8.9)	268 (90.8)
	CBCL, n = 288		TRF n = 263	
Total Behavior Problems	65.10 (8.5)	85 (29.5)	64.82 (10.2)	68 (25.9)
Internalizing Problems	56.55 (10.5)	34 (11.8)	59.94 (9.3)	28 (10.6)
Externalizing Problems	68.48 (9.6)	140 (48.6)	69.94 (9.5)	112 (42.6)
Withdrawn	59.16 (8.9)	47 (16.3)	60.81 (8.0)	26 (9.9)
Anxious/Depressed	56.33 (7.9)	20 (6.9)	57.08 (8.0)	23 (8.7)
Attention Problems	68.02 (6.7)	130 (45.1)	69.51 (11.1)	126 (47.9)
Aggressive Behavior	69.30 (11.3)	128 (44.4)	67.63 (10.8)	88 (33.5)
Emotionally Reactive	—	—	60.61 (9.2)	41 (15.6)

SD = standard deviation; ADHD = attention-deficit/hyperactivity disorder; CPRS-R:L = Conners' Parent Rating Scale-Revised: Long Version; CTRS-R:L = Conners' Teacher Rating Scale-Revised: Long Version; CBCL = Child Behavior Checklist; TRF = Teacher Report Form; DSM-IV = *Diagnostic and Statistical Manual of Mental Disorders*, 4th edition.
— indicates that subscale is not assessed by form.

baseline. More than half (52.1%) were diagnosed with ODD, with an additional 7 subjects diagnosed with CD. More than one fifth of children ($n = 68$, 22.4%) were diagnosed with a communication disorder (phonological disorder, expressive language disorder, communication disorder not otherwise specified (NOS), mixed expressive-receptive language disorder, stuttering). Anxiety disorders were found in 14.5% of children, with specific phobias present in 22 children and separation anxiety disorder in 20 children. The other anxiety disorders represented were anxiety disorder NOS, obsessive compulsive disorder, GAD, social phobia, acute stress disorder, and posttraumatic stress disorder. As illustrated in Fig. 1, 65.3% (198/303) of children in this sample have one or more co-morbid diagnoses belonging to these three classes of disorders. Other less common co-morbidities are listed in Table 4.

Participants with co-morbid diagnoses to ADHD had lower C-GAS scores than those with none ($t = -5.25$, $p < 0.001$), indicating that children with co-morbidity are rated by clinicians as functioning more poorly than children with ADHD alone. Further, controlling for ODD, because of overlap with internalizing problems, subjects with co-morbid communication disorders were rated by their teachers as significantly more anxious/depressed on the TRF (partial $t = 3.106$, $p = 0.002$). No other significant relationships were found between number of co-morbidities and clinician, parent, or teacher ratings.

Prevalence of ADHD symptoms: Overall and by subtype

ADHD symptom frequencies by measurement method (e.g., teacher ratings, parent rat-

TABLE 4. PATS DIAGNOSTIC INTERVIEW DSM-IV DIAGNOSES CO-MORBID
WITH ATTENTION-DEFICIT/HYPERACTIVITY DISORDER

Diagnosis	n (%)
No co-morbid disorder	92 (30.4)
Disruptive disorders	
Oppositional defiant disorder	158 (52.1)
Conduct disorder	7 (2.3)
Communication disorders	
Phonological disorder	31 (10.2)
Expressive language disorder	24 (7.9)
Communication disorder NOS	12 (4.0)
Mixed receptive-expressive language disorder	7 (2.3)
Stuttering	1 (0.3)
Anxiety disorders	
Specific phobia	22 (7.3)
Separation anxiety disorder	20 (6.6)
Anxiety disorder NOS	3 (1.0)
Reactive attachment disorder	3 (1.0)
Obsessive compulsive disorder	2 (0.6)
Generalized anxiety disorder	1 (0.3)
Social phobia	1 (0.3)
Acute stress disorder	1 (0.3)
Posttraumatic stress disorder	1 (0.3)
Elimination disorders	
Enuresis	14 (4.6)
Encopresis	8 (2.6)
Encopresis with constipation and overflow incontinence	1 (0.3)
Other disorders	
Developmental coordination disorder	10 (3.3)
Pica	6 (1.8)
Adjustment disorder	4 (1.2)
Sleep disorder	1 (0.3)

PATS = Preschoolers with Attention-Deficit/Hyperactivity Disorder Treatment Study; DSM-IV = *Diagnostic and Statistical Manual of Mental Disorders*, 4th edition; NOS = not otherwise specified.

ings, and clinician composite) are presented in Table 5. The severity of this sample is evident in that, according to the clinician-completed PDI ADHD checklist, eight of eighteen symptoms were identified for more than 90% of the sample. The two least-frequent symptoms were "loses things necessary for activities" and "forgetful in daily activities." There is some variability in the number of participants identified as having symptoms across the measurement method, although this generally falls within 10–15% for most symptoms. There appears to be greater variability across measurement method for the inattentive symptoms relative to hyperactive-impulsive symptoms, most notably for difficulty following instructions, avoiding tasks requiring sustained attention, losing things, and forgetfulness. Overall, teachers tended to report fewer symptoms than parents. Also of note, more participants were iden-

tified as having symptoms on the PDI ADHD checklist than by either parent or teacher rating alone, with only a few exceptions, as was expected given that the checklist integrates information from both sources. As assessed by the CPRS, the first four ODD symptoms, "often loses temper," "often argues with adults," "often defies adults' requests and rules," and "often deliberately annoys people" were endorsed for more than two thirds of the sample.

Both combined type (75.2%) and H/I type (24.8%) of ADHD were represented in the sample. For those with H/I type, four inattentive symptoms were evident in more than 50% of the sample. The frequency of both "distracted by extraneous stimuli" (82.9%) and "does not seem to listen" (75.0%) suggest that moderate-to-severe cases of ADHD H/I would commonly also experience some inattention symptoms. No difference was found in the pro-

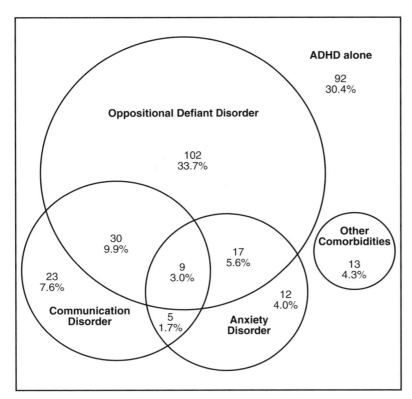

FIG. 1. Most prevalent comorbidities with preschool Attention-Deficit/Hyperactivity Disorder and their overlap.

portion of children in the H/I and Combined groups that experienced hyperactive and impulsive symptoms, although the differences between groups on "difficulty playing quietly" and "always on the go" approached statistical significance, with a higher number of combined-type children having the symptom.

Age, gender, and severity of ADHD

Age was inversely correlated with severity on the CTRS-R:L ADHD DSM-IV Symptoms (Total) subscale ($r = -0.319$, $p < 0.001$) such that older participants' ADHD was judged by teachers to be less severe than younger participants. Age was also correlated with a number of other measures, including C-GAS ($r = 0.183$, $p < 0.001$), and the aggression ($r = -0.330$, $p < 0.001$) and total problems ($r = -0.313$, $p < 0.001$) scales on the TRF. Interestingly, however, these age differences were not found by parent report. In sum, younger subjects were found to have poorer functioning and more aggression than older subjects in this sample by teacher report and clinician rating but not parent report.

There were no differences between boys and girls using raw scores of the CPRS-R:L and CTRS-R:L. Using *T*-scores, however, girls' be-

havior was more deviant relative to same-aged and gender peers than were boys' behavior on both the CPRS-R:L ($t = -9.862$, $p < 0.001$) and the CTRS-R:L ADHD DSM-IV Symptoms (Total) subscale ($t = -12.723$, $p < 0.001$) and CBCL inattention subscale ($t = 3.42$, $p < 0.001$). There was no gender effect on child functioning as measured by C-GAS, or child behavior as measured by TRF and all other CBCL subscales.

Severity of ADHD and other measures of functioning

ADHD severity as rated by parents on the CPRS-R:L ADHD DSM-IV Symptoms (Total) subscale was associated with decreased functioning on the C-GAS ($r = -0.175$, $p < 0.001$). This measure of ADHD severity was also significantly associated with parent CBCL ratings in the areas of anxious/depressed ($r = 0.299$, $p < 0.001$) and withdrawn ($r = 0.218$, $p < 0.001$), indicating more internalizing problems with increasing ADHD severity. Teacher ratings of ADHD severity on the CTRS-R:L were significantly correlated with TRF scales for emotional problems ($r = 0.198$, $p < 0.001$), anxious/depressed ($r = 0.174$, $p < 0.001$), and withdrawn ($r = 0.299$, $p < 0.001$).

TABLE 5. DSM-IV SYMPTOM FREQUENCIES AS REPORTED BY REVISED CONNERS' PARENT AND
TEACHER RATING SCALES AND THE ADHD CHECKLIST

	Conners' Parent Rating Scale n = 303 n (%)	Conners' Teacher Rating Scale n = 291 n (%)	ADHD checklist (clinician-completed)		
			n = 303 n (%)	ADHD C n = 228 (%)	ADHD H/I n = 75 (%)
Inattention					
1. Makes careless mistakes	175 (58.3)	147 (53.1)	197 (64.9)	77.5	28.0
2. Difficulty sustaining attention	236 (78.1)	227 (78.0)	268 (88.5)	96.1	66.7
3. Does not seem to listen	277 (91.7)	230 (78.8)	277 (91.4)	96.9	76.0
4. Does not follow instructions	219 (72.8)	164 (56.9)	258 (85.1)	95.6	54.7
5. Difficulty organizing tasks	168 (57.5)	156 (56.5)	180 (59.4)	74.1	14.7
6. Avoids sustained mental effort	191 (63.9)	160 (56.3)	233 (76.9)	86.0	49.3
7. Loses things necessary for activities	80 (26.8)	49 (19.3)	125 (41.2)	50.0	14.7
8. Distracted by extraneous stimuli	269 (90.6)	251 (86.9)	282 (93.1)	96.5	84.0
9. Forgetful in daily activities	134 (44.2)	72 (25.5)	124 (40.9)	53.1	4.0
Hyperactive					
1. Fidgets or squirms in seat	275 (90.8)	250 (85.0)	290 (95.7)	96.5	94.7
2. Often leaves seat	279 (92.4)	241 (82.8)	294 (97.0)	98.7	93.3
3. Runs about or climbs excessively	279 (92.1)	228 (77.3)	287 (94.7)	95.2	94.7
4. Difficulty playing quietly	221 (73.4)	208 (71.0)	231 (76.2)	80.7	64.0
5. Often on the go	291 (96.0)	265 (89.8)	297 (98.0)	99.6	94.7
6. Often talks excessively	250 (82.5)	218 (74.1)	239 (78.8)	79.8	77.3
Impulsivity					
1. Often blurts out answers	197 (65.0)	180 (62.3)	205 (67.6)	68.4	66.7
2. Often has difficulty awaiting turn	281 (93.4)	251 (85.1)	279 (92.0)	93.4	89.3
3. Often interrupts or intrudes on others	287 (94.7)	246 (83.7)	294 (97.1)	97.8	96.0

DSM-IV = *Diagnostic and Statistical Manual of Mental Disorders*, 4th edition; ADHD C = Attention-Deficit/Hyperactivity Disorder Combined type; ADHD H/I = Attention-Deficit/Hyperactivity Disorder Hyperactive/Impulsive type.
On the Connors' Parent Rating Scale-Revised: Long Form and Connors' Teacher Rating Scale-Revised: Long Form, endorsement of a symptom is indicated by a score of 2 ("often") or 3 ("very often").

DISCUSSION

This paper describes the symptom presentation, clinical correlates, and co-morbidity of PATS participants. Overall, results resemble those seen for smaller clinical samples of preschoolers and school-aged children with ADHD (DuPaul et al. 2001; Gadow and Nolan 2002; Wilens et al. 2002). Seventy percent of the sample presented with co-morbid diagnoses, most frequently ODD (52.1%), communication disorders (24.7%), and anxiety disorders (17.7%). These rates are comparable to co-morbidity in clinical samples of school-aged children with ADHD (Biederman et al. 1991; Spencer 2006) and are broadly consistent with previous research with children aged 2–6 years in terms of the frequency and types of co-morbidity (Wilens et al. 2002; Angold et al. submitted). Similar findings were also seen on more dimensional measures

of symptoms, with clinically significant elevations on externalizing scales of the CPRS-R:L/CTRS-R:L and CBCL/TRF and significant correlations between ADHD-related symptom scales and scales assessing aggression and oppositionality.

Notably, ADHD severity was significantly associated with higher ratings on anxiety/depression symptom subscales, highlighting internalizing problems as a potential area of clinical attention. Anxiety was of particular concern in this sample given its rate of co-morbidity with ADHD, as well as its relationship with ADHD severity. Rates of co-morbid anxiety disorder were consistent with previous studies documenting higher-than-expected levels of co-morbid anxiety in preschoolers (Angold et al., submitted) and school-aged children with ADHD (MTA Cooperative Group 1999; Schatz and Rostain 2006). This is an important finding given that anxiety appears to influence treatment outcomes and approaches (March et al. 2000) and suggests that additional investigation of anxiety interventions for younger children is needed. Follow-up evaluation of the PATS data will allow us to determine if anxiety serves a similar moderating role in preschool-aged children. Although anxiety was common, no participant was diagnosed with co-morbid depression, similar to the MTA study (another large referred sample), where only of 3.8% of school-aged children with ADHD had co-morbid major depressive disorder (MTA Cooperative Group 1999). The findings on high rates of co-morbid communication disorders contribute to a limited body of data on this clinical presentation. Previous studies of school-aged children with ADHD have similarly found to have elevated rates of communication disorders. For example, Hinshaw (2002) identified 25% of girls with ADHD as having speech and language problems, and Tirosh et al. (1998) diagnosed language deficit in 45% of children with ADHD. These findings highlight the importance of communication disorders in ADHD research and clinical practice.

Participants with moderate-to-severe ADHD were found to exhibit high frequencies of hyperactive and impulsive symptoms in addition to several inattentive symptoms, and these symptoms were related to clinician-rated impairment. More than 90% of participants met the cardinal symptoms of ADHD routinely reported in school-aged children with the disorder: Not listening, distractibility, fidgeting, leaving seat, running about or climbing excessively, being often on the go, having difficulty waiting their turns, and interrupting. Four inattentive symptoms were present in over 50% of those with the H/I type, suggesting that these children may be at risk of shifting to the Combined type, as was reported by Lahey et al. (2005). The inattention symptoms of "difficulty organizing tasks" and "loses things necessary for activities" had the lowest frequency of all ADHD symptoms, which is predictable given they may not be age appropriate for preschool-aged children. Developmentally, preschoolers will lack the opportunity to display these symptoms. This potential mismatch between diagnostic criteria and developmental level has implications for symptom and diagnostic prevalences.

With regard to age and gender effects, there was some indication that teachers perceived younger children to be more severe in their behavioral difficulties, consistent with clinician perception, although the same was not true for parents. Overall, there appeared to be few differences in the presentation of symptoms and pattern of impairment by gender, although girls appeared relatively more severe compared to their peers than did boys. ADHD severity correlated negatively with functioning; while significant, this relationship was modest, suggesting that other factors, such as co-existing co-morbid disorders, contribute to assessment of global functioning.

The methods of diagnostic evaluation were exceptionally rigorous in this study, requiring high symptom scores on both standardized parent and teacher reports as well as semi-structured clinical interviews and clinical consensus for all diagnoses rendered. The key elements were inclusion of both parent- and teacher-report threshold measures for inclusion and the careful review of symptoms and all diagnostic criteria by a developmentally trained clinician considering age-appropriate manifestations of symptoms. This multi-method and multistep approach is important, given that parents and teachers observe children with ADHD in different social and emotional contexts, so that concordance between parents and teachers on symptom ratings is expectably quite poor (e.g., Murray et al., this issue). Clinician-identified symptoms and diagnoses represent an integration of parent- and teacher-identified symptoms, as is consistent with the DSM-IV field trials of child and adolescent ADHD (Lahey et al. 1994). Furthermore, the PDI's developmentally specific probes assisted clinicians to detect age-appropriate symptoms. In addition, it operationalized age-appropriate manifestations and areas of impairment. Future revisions of diagnostic manuals would benefit from the incorporation of developmentally specific age-appropriate examples of the manifestation of ADHD symptoms and impairment.

Implications for clinical practice

Clinicians evaluating preschoolers with ADHD should routinely assess for the presence of ODD, communication disorders, and anxiety disorders, given the high prevalence of these disorders in this population. This is particularly important given the finding that high levels of co-morbidity negatively impacts upon MPH treatment outcome (Ghuman et al., 2007). Improved attention to communication and language difficulties may be useful, because this area may be overlooked. As with anxiety, co-morbid communication difficulties may moderate treatment outcomes and may require additional interventions. As an additional area of impairment clinicians should assess for the presence of physical injury and high-risk behaviors, such as running into streets, wandering away from parents in public places, or jumping from tall heights, that entail considerable danger to physical safety. One in four participants in PATS was female, which suggests that young girls can experience considerable hyperactivity that impairs functioning and warrants early interventions.

Limitations

As the inclusion criteria limited study entry to preschool-aged children with moderate-to-severe ADHD, H/I or C, this reduced the range of scores on assessment measures analyzed. These findings will be less applicable to preschoolers with mild or subthreshold ADHD. Moreover, the present results did not address clinical characteristics of those preschoolers who may meet criteria for ADHD, Predominantly Inattentive type. Since the current study was designed, others have investigated the utility of developmentally modified DSM-IV criteria when assessing preschool internalizing disorders (e.g., Scheeringa et al. 2001; Luby et al. 2002; Warren et al. 2006). It is possible that use of these proposed modified criteria in the present study may have resulted in greater identification of co-morbid disorders.

Second, although standardized rating scales were included as one method of identification of symptoms and disorders, neither the DISC-P nor the semistructured clinical interview and PDI ADHD checklist developed for this study have been validated for this age group. Therefore, it is possible that some measurement error may have been introduced into the re-

sults. However, there was general concordance across measures of ADHD symptoms, at least at the level at which diagnoses were to be determined. Future research examining the reliability and validity of different methodological approaches for diagnosis in this age range is warranted

Conclusions

This paper contributes to knowledge of the clinical presentation of ADHD in this preschool age group. Preschool-aged children with moderate-to-severe ADHD present with many symptoms, co-morbid disorders, and substantial impairment, which appear to justify interventions such as those provided in PATS. Improved descriptive information will help to refine assessment procedures and can inform treatment in clinical settings, as well as future research directions.

DISCLOSURES

The following financial disclosures indicate potential conflicts of interest among the PATS investigators and industry sources for the period 2000–2007, inclusive. [1]Honoraria/consultant, [2]research support, [3]speaker's bureau, [4]significant equity (>$50,000). Dr. Murray: Eli Lilly,[2] Pfizer.[2] Dr. Kollins: McNeil,[1,2,3] Shire,[1,2] Eli Lilly,[1,2] Pfizer,[2] New River Pharmaceuticals,[2] Psychogenics,[2] Athenagen,[1,2] Cephalon.[1] Dr. Greenhill: Celltech,[1,2] Cephalon,[1,2] Eli Lilly,[1,2] Janssen,[1] McNeil,[1,2] Medeva,[2] Novartis Corporation,[1,2] Noven,[1,2] Otsuka,[1,2] Pfizer,[1] Sanofi,[1] Shire,[1,2] Solvay,[1,2] Somerset,[2] Thomson Advanced Therapeutics Communications.[1] Dr. Swanson: Alza,[1,2] Celgene,[1,2] Celltech,[1,2,3] Cephalon,[1,2,3] Eli Lilly,[1,2] Gliatech,[1,2] Janssen,[1,2,3] McNeil,[1,2,3] Organon,[1] Novartis,[1,2] UCB, Shire.[1,2] Dr. Sharon Wigal: Celltech,[1,2,3] McNeil,[1,2,3] Cephalon,[1,2,3] Novartis,[1,2,3] Shire,[1,2,3] New River Pharmaceuticals,[2] Janssen,[3] Eli Lilly.[2] Dr. Abikoff: Abbot Labs,[1] Cephalon,[1] McNeil,[1,2] Shire,[1,2] Eli Lilly,[1,2] Pfizer,[2] Celltech,[2] Novartis.[2] Dr. McCracken: Abbott, UCB, Novartis, Johnson & Johnson, Eli Lilly,[1,2,3] Gliatech,[2] Shire,[1,2] Pfizer,[1,2] McNeil,[1,2] Noven,[1] Bristol Meyers Squibb,[1] Janssen,[1,3] Wyeth.[1] Dr. Riddle: Shire,[1] Janssen,[1] Glaxo-Smith-Kline,[1] Astra-Zeneca,[1] Pfizer.[2] Dr. McGough: Eli

Lilly,[1,2,3] McNeil,[1,2,3] Novartis,[1,2,3] Shire,[1,2,3] Pfizer,[1,2,3] New River Pharmaceuticals.[2] Dr. Posner: As part of an effort to help execute the FDA suicidality classification mandates, Dr. Posner has had research support (2) from GlaxoSmithKline, Forest Laboratories, Eisai Inc., Astra Zeneca Pharmaceuticals, Johnson and Johnson, Abbott Laboratories, Wyeth Research, Organon USA, Bristol Meyers Squibb, Sanofi-Aventis, Cephalon, Novartis, Shire Pharmaceuticals, and UCB Pharma; Shire.[1,2] Dr. Tim Wigal: Celltech,[2] Cephalon,[2] Eli Lilly,[2,3] Janssen,[2] McNeil,[2,3] Novartis,[2] Shire.[2,3] Mr. Davies: Merck,[4] GlaxoSmithKline,[4] Amgen,[4] Bard,[4] Pfizer,[4] Amgen,[4] Johnson & Johnson,[4] Wyeth.[4] Dr. Ghuman: Bristol Myers-Squibb.[2] Drs. Boorady, Cunningham, Fisher, Kastelic, Melvin, and Vitiello, Ms. Chuang, Gugga, and Skrobala have no conflicts of interest or financial ties to report.

REFERENCES

Achenbach TM, Edelbrock C: Manual for the Child Behavior Checklist and Revised Child Behavior Profile. Burlington (Vermont), Queen City Printers, 1983.

Achenbach TM, Howell CT, Quay HC, Conners CK: National survey of problems and competencies among four- to sixteen-year-olds: Parents' reports for normative and clinical samples. Monogr Soc Res Child Dev 56:1–131, 1991.

American Psychiatric Association: Diagnostic and Statistical Manual of Mental Disorders, Fourth Edition, Text Revision. Washington, D.C., American Psychiatric Publishing, 2000.

Biederman J, Newcorn J, Sprich S: Comorbidity of attention-deficit/hyperactivity disorder with conduct, depressive, anxiety, and other disorders. Am J Psychiatry 148:564–577, 1991.

Bird HR, Yager TJ, Staghezza B, Gould MS, Canino G, Rubio-Stipec M: Impairment in the epidemiological measurement of childhood psychopathology in the community. J Am Acad Child Adolesc Psychiatry 29: 796–803, 1990.

Campbell SB, Breaux AM, Ewing LJ, Szumowski EK: Correlates and predictors of hyperactivity and aggression: A longitudinal study of parent-referred problem preschoolers. J Abnorm Child Psychol 14:217–34, 1986.

Campbell SB, Ewing LJ: Follow-up of hard-to-manage preschoolers: Adjustment at Age 9 and predictors of continuing symptoms. J Child Psychol Psychiatry 31: 871–889, 1990.

Connor D, Edwards G, Fletcher K, Baird J, Barkley R, Steingard R: Correlates of comorbid psychopathology

in children with ADHD. J Am Acad Child Adolesc Psychiatry 42:193–200, 2003.

Conners CK: Conners' Rating Scales-Revised: Technical Manual. North Tonawanda (New York), Multi-Health Systems, 2000.

Conners CK, Sitarenios G, Parker JD, Epstein JN: The Revised Conners' Parent Rating Scale (CPRS-R): Factor structure, reliability, and criterion validity. J Abnorm Child Psychol 26:257–268, 1998a.

Conners CK, Sitarenios G, Parker JD, Epstein JN: Revision and restandardization of the Conners' Teacher Rating Scale (CTRS-R): Factor structure, reliability, and criterion validity. J Abnorm Child Psychol 26:279–291, 1998b.

DiScala C, Lescohier I, Barthel M, Li G: Injuries to children with attention-deficit/hyperactivity disorder. Pediatrics 102:1415–1421, 1998.

DuPaul GJ, McGoey KE, Eckert TL, Van Brakle J: Preschool children with attention-deficit/hyperactivity disorder: Impairments in behavioral, social, and school functioning. J Am Acad Child Adolesc Psychiatry 40:508–515, 2001.

Egger HL, Angold A: The Preschool Age Psychiatric Assessment (PAPA): A structured parent interview for diagnosing psychiatric disorders in preschool children. In: Handbook of Infant, Toddler, and Preschool Mental Assessment. Edited by DelCarmen-Wiggins R, Carter A, New York, Oxford University Press, 2004, pp. 223–243.

Egger HL, Angold A: Common emotional and behavioral disorders in preschool children: Presentation, nosology, and epidemiology. J Child Psychol Psychiatry 47:313–337, 2006.

Elliott CD: Differential Ability Scales (DAS). San Antonio (Texas), Psychological Corporation, 1990.

Gadow KD, Nolan EE: Differences between preschool children with ODD, ADHD, and ODD + ADHD symptoms. J Child Psychol Psychiatry 43:191–201, 2002.

Ghuman JK, Riddle MA, Vitiello B, Greenhill LL, Chuang SZ, Wigal SB, Kollins SH, Abikoff HB, McCracken JT, Kastelic E, Scharko AM, McGough JJ, Murray DW, Evans L, Swanson JM, Wigal T, Posner K, Cunningham C, Davies M, Skrobala AM: Comorbidity moderates response to methylphenidate in the Preschoolers with Attention-Deficit/Hyperactivity Disorder Treatment Study (PATS). J Child Adolesc Psychopharmacol 17:563–579, 2007.

Greenhill L, Kollins S, Abikoff H, McCracken J, Riddle M, Swanson J, McGough J, Wigal S, Wigal T, Vitiello B, Skrobala A, Posner K, Ghuman J, Cunningham C, Davies M, Chuang S, Cooper T: Efficacy and safety of immediate-release methylphenidate treatment for preschoolers with ADHD. J Am Acad Child Adolesc Psychiatry 45:1284–1293, 2006.

Hinshaw SP: Preadolescent girls with attention-deficit/hyperactivity disorder: I. Background characteristics, comorbidity, cognitive and social functioning, and parenting practices. J Consult Clin Psychol 70:1086–1098, 2002.

Keenan K, Wakschlag LS: Can a valid diagnosis of disruptive behavior disorder be made in preschool children? Am J Psychiatry 159:351–358, 2002.

Keenan K, Wakschlag LS: Are oppositional defiant and conduct disorder symptoms normative behaviors in preschoolers? A comparison of referred and nonreferred children. Am J Psychiatry 161:356–358, 2004.

Keenan K, Wakschlag LS, Danis B, Hill C, Humphries M, Duax J, Donald R. Further evidence of the reliability and validity of DSM-IV ODD and CD in preschool children. J Am Acad Child Adolesc Psychiatry 46:457–468, 2007.

Kollins S, Greenhill L, Swanson J, Wigal S, Abikoff H, McCracken J, Riddle M, McGough J, Vitiello B, Wigal T, Skrobala A, Posner K, Ghuman J, Davies M, Cunningham C, Bauzo A: Rationale, design, and methods of the Preschool ADHD Treatment Study (PATS). J Am Acad Child Adolesc Psychiatry 45:1275–1283, 2006.

Lahey BB, Applegate B, McBurnett K, Biederman J, Greenhill L, Hynd GW, Barkley RA, Newcorn J, Jensen P, Richters J: DSM-IV field trials for attention-deficit/hyperactivity disorder in children and adolescents. Am J Psychiatry 151:1673–1685, 1994.

Lahey BB, Pelham WE, Stein MA, Loney J, Trapani C, Nugent K, Kipp H, Schmidt E, Lee S, Cale M, Gold E, Hartung CM, Willcutt E, Baumann B: Validity of DSM-IV attention-deficit/hyperactivity disorder for younger children. J Am Acad Child Adolesc Psychiatry 37:695–702, 1998.

Lahey BB, Pelham WE, Loney J, Lee SS, Willcutt E: Instability of the DSM-IV subtypes of ADHD from preschool through elementary school. Arch Gen Psychiatry 62:896–902, 2005.

Lam LT: Attention Deficit Disorder and hospitalization due to injury among older adolescents in New South Wales, Australia. J Atten Disord 6:77–82, 2002.

Lavigne JV, Gibbons RD, Christoffel KK, Arend R, Rosenbaum D, Binns H, Dawson, N, Sobel H, Isaacs C: Prevalence rates and correlates of psychiatric disorders among preschool children. Am Acad Child Adolesc Psychiatry 35:204–214, 1996.

Luby JL, Heffelfinger AK, Mrakotsky C, Hessler MJ, Brown KM, Hildebrand T: Preschool major depressive disorder: Preliminary validation for developmentally modified DSM-IV criteria. J Am Acad Child Adolesc Psychiatry 41:928–937, 2002.

Lucas C, Fisher P, Luby J: Young-Child DISC-IV Research Draft: Diagnostic Interview Schedule for Children. New York, Columbia University, Division of Child Psychiatry, Joy and William Ruane Center to Identify and Treat Mood Disorders, 1998.

March JS, Swanson JM, Arnold LE, Hoza B, Conners CK, Hinshaw SP, Hechtman L, Kraemer HC, Greenhill LL, Abikoff HB, Elliott LG, Jensen PS, Newcorn JH, Vitiello B, Severe J,Wells KC, Pelham WE: Anxiety as a predictor and outcome variable in the Multimodal Treatment Study of Children with ADHD (MTA). J Abnorm Child Psychol 28:527–541, 2000.

McGee R, Partridge F, Williams S, Silva, PA: A twelve-year follow-up of preschool hyperactive children. J Am Acad Child Adolesc Psychiatry 30:224–232, 1991.

MTA Cooperative Group: A 14-month randomized clinical trial of treatment strategies for attention-deficit/hyperactivity disorder. Arch Gen Psychiatry 56:1073–1086, 1999.

Murray DW, Kollins SH, Hardy KK, Abikoff HB, Swanson JM, Cunningham C, Vitiello B, Riddle MA, Davies M, Greenhill LL, McCracken JT, McGough JJ, Posner K, Skrobala AM, Wigal T, Wigal SB, Ghuman JK, Chuang SZ: Parent–teacher agreement in preschool children at risk for ADHD. J Child Adolesc Psychopharmacol 17:605–619, 2007.

Nolan EE, Gadow, KD, Sprafkin, J: Teacher Reports of DSM-IV ADHD, ODD, and CD symptoms in school-children. J Am Acad Child Adolesc Psychiatry 40:241–249, 2001.

Pelham WE Jr, Gnagy EM, Greenslade KE, Milich R: Teacher ratings of DSM-III-R symptoms for the disruptive behavior disorders. J Am Acad Child Adolesc Psychiatry 31:210–218, 1992.

Pierce EW, Ewing LJ, Campbell SB: Diagnostic status and symptomatic behavior of hard-to-manage preschool children in middle childhood and early adolescence. J Clin Child Psychol 28:44–57, 1999.

Posner K, Greenhill LL: Attention deficit/hyperactivity disorder in preschool children. In: Attention Deficit Disorder and Comorbidities in Children, Adolescents and Adults, 2nd Edition. Edited by Brown TE. Washington, D.C., American Psychiatric Publishing, in press.

Schatz DB, Rostain AL: ADHD With comorbid anxiety: A review of the current literature. J Atten Disord 10:141–149, 2006.

Scheeringa MS, Peebles CD, Cook CA, Zeanah CH: Toward establishing procedural, criterion and discriminant validity for PTSD in early childhood. J Am Acad Child Adolesc Psychiatry 40:52–60, 2001.

Schwebel DC, Speltz ML, Jones K, Bardina P: Unintentional injury in preschool boys with and without early onset of disruptive behavior. J Pediatr Psychol 27:727–737, 2002.

Shaffer D, Gould MS, Brasic J, Ambrosini P, Fisher P, Bird H, Aluwahlia S: A children's global assessment scale (CGAS). Arch Gen Psychiatry 40:1228–1231, 1983.

Shaffer D, Fisher P, Dulcan MK, Davies M, Piacentini J, Schwab-Stone ME, Lahey BB, Bourdon K, Jensen PS, Bird HR, Canino G, Regier DA: The NIMH Diagnostic Interview Schedule for Children Version 2.3 (DISC-2.3): Description, acceptability, prevalence rates, and performance in the MECA Study. J Am Acad Child Adolesc Psychiatry 35:865–877, 1996.

Shaffer D, Fisher P, Lucas CP, Dulcan MK, Schwab-Stone ME: NIMH Diagnostic Interview Schedule for Children Version IV (NIMH DISC-IV): Description, differences from previous versions, and reliability of some common diagnoses. J Am Acad Child Adolesc Psychiatry 39:28–38, 2000.

Speltz M, McClellan J, DeKlyen M, Jones K: Preschool boys with oppositional defiant disorder: Clinical presentation and diagnostic change. J Am Acad Child Adolesc Psychiatry 38:838–845, 1999.

Spencer TJ: ADHD and comorbidity in childhood. J Clin Psychiatry 67(Suppl 8):27–31, 2006

Tirosh E, Cohen A: Language deficit with attention-deficit disorder: A prevalent comorbidity. J Child Neurol 13:497–497, 1998.

Warren SL, Umylny P, Aron E, Simmens, SJ: Toddler anxiety disorders: A pilot study. J Am Acad Child Adolesc Psychiatry 45:859–866, 2006.

Weissman MM, Warner V, Fendrich M: Applying impairment criteria to children's psychiatric diagnosis. J Am Acad Child Adolesc Psychiatry 29:789–795, 1990.

Wilens T, Biederman J, Brown S, Tanguay S, Monuteaux MC, Blake C, Spencer TJ: Psychiatric Comorbidity and functioning in clinically referred preschool children and school-age youths with ADHD. Am Acad Child Adolesc Psychiatry 4:262–268, 2002.

ADVANCES IN PRESCHOOL PSYCHOPHARMACOLOGY
© 2009 Mary Ann Liebert, Inc.
140 Huguenot Street, 3rd Floor
New Rochelle, NY 10801-5215

Comorbidity Moderates Response to Methylphenidate in the Preschoolers with Attention-Deficit/Hyperactivity Disorder Treatment Study (PATS)

Jaswinder K. Ghuman, M.D.,[1] Mark A. Riddle, M.D.,[2] Benedetto Vitiello, M.D.,[3]
Laurence L. Greenhill, M.D.,[4] Shirley Z. Chuang, M.S.,[4] Sharon B. Wigal, Ph.D.,[5]
Scott H. Kollins, Ph.D.,[6] Howard B. Abikoff, Ph.D.,[7] James T. McCracken, M.D.,[8]
Elizabeth Kastelic, M.D.,[2] Alexander M. Scharko, M.D.,[9] James J. McGough, M.D.,[8]
Desiree W. Murray, Ph.D.,[6] Lori Evans, Ph.D.,[7] James M. Swanson, Ph.D.,[5]
Tim Wigal, Ph.D.,[5] Kelly Posner, Ph.D.,[4] Charles Cunningham, Ph.D.,[10]
Mark Davies, M.P.H.,[4] and Anne M. Skrobala, M.A.[4]

ABSTRACT

Objective: The aim of this study was to examine whether demographic or pretreatment clinical and social characteristics influenced the response to methylphenidate (MPH) in the Preschoolers with ADHD Treatment Study (PATS).

Methods: Exploratory moderator analyses were conducted on the efficacy data from the PATS 5-week, double-blind, placebo-controlled six-site titration trial. Children ($N = 165$, age 3–5.5 years) were randomized to 1 week each of four MPH doses (1.25, 2.5, 5, and 7.5 mg) and placebo administered three times per day (t.i.d.). We assessed the fixed effects on the average slope in the regression outcome on moderators, weight-adjusted dose, and the moderator-by-dose interaction using SAS PROC GENMOD.

[1]University of Arizona, Tucson, Arizona.
[2]Johns Hopkins University, Baltimore, Maryland.
[3]National Institute of Mental Health, Bethesda, Maryland.
[4]New York State Psychiatric Institute/Columbia University, New York, New York.
[5]University of California Irvine, Irvine, California.
[6]Duke University Medical Center, Durham, North Carolina.
[7]New York University Child Study Center, New York, New York.
[8]University of California Los Angeles, Los Angeles, California.
[9]University of Wisconsin, Milwaukee, Wisconsin.
[10]McMaster University, Hamilton, Ontario, Canada.

Statistical consultants: Shirley Z. Chuang, M.S., Mark Davies, M.P.H. Ms. Chuang has no current affiliation; she was formerly at New York State Psychiatric Institute/Columbia University. Mr. Davies is affiliated with New York State Psychiatric Institute/Columbia University.

This research was supported by a cooperative agreement grants between the National Institute of Mental Health and the following institutions: Johns Hopkins University (U01 MH60642), NYSPI/Columbia University (U01 MH60903), University of California, Irvine (U01 MH60833), Duke University Medical Center (U01 MH60848), New York University Child Study Center (U01 MH60943), and University of California, Los Angeles (U01 MH60900); and by NIMH K23 MH01883-01A1 and Arizona Institute of Mental Health Research to J.K.G.

The opinions and assertions contained in this report are the private views of the authors and are not to be construed as official or as reflecting the views of the Department of Health and Human Services, the National Institutes of Health, or the National Institute of Mental Health.

Results: A significant interaction effect was found for a number of co-morbid disorders diagnosed in the preschoolers at baseline ($p = 0.005$). Preschoolers with three or more co-morbid disorders did not respond to MPH (Cohen's d at 7.5 mg dose relative to placebo $= -0.37$) compared to a significant response in the preschoolers with 0, 1, or 2 co-morbid disorders (Cohen's $d = 0.89$, 1.00, and 0.56, respectively). Preschoolers with more co-morbidity were found to have more family adversity. No significant interaction effect was found with the other variables.

Conclusions: In preschoolers with ADHD, the presence of no or one co-morbid disorder (primarily oppositional defiant disorder) predicted a large treatment response at the same level as has been found in school-aged children, and two co-morbid disorders predicted moderate treatment response; whereas the presence of three or more co-morbid disorders predicted no treatment response to MPH.

INTRODUCTION

ATTENTION-DEFICIT/HYPERACTIVITY DISORDER (ADHD) is the most prevalent psychiatric disorder of childhood; prevalence of ADHD in preschool-aged children is estimated to range from 2% to 5.7% (Lavigne et al. 1996; Egger and Angold 2006). Preschool children with ADHD are impaired in many functional domains (Lahey et al. 1998; DuPaul et al. 2001; Wilens et al. 2002a) and continue to have impairment and behavior problems later in childhood (Campbell 1987; Campbell and Ewing 1990; Lahey et al. 1998; Pierce et al. 1999; DuPaul et al. 2001; Wilens et al. 2002a; Lahey et al. 2004). More than 250 randomized clinical trials (RCTs) in school-aged children (Greenhill et al. 2002; Schachar et al. 2002; Wilens et al. 2002b) and 13 in preschool children provide evidence for short-term efficacy of psychostimulants for treatment of ADHD (Connors 1975; Barkley et al. 1984; Barkely et al. 1985; Cunningham et al. 1985; Barkley et al. 1988; Fischer and Newby 1991; Mayes et al. 1994; Musten et al. 1997; Handen et al. 1999; Short et al. 2004; Chacko et al. 2005; Greenhill et al. 2006). However, there is great variability in treatment response among the study participants and many children do not respond to psychostimulants or experience less than optimal symptomatic improvement (McCracken et al. 2000; Swanson et al. 2001; Greenhill et al. 2006).

RCTs are generally powered to compare the average efficacy results of all the study participants receiving the targeted treatment (treatment group) versus all of the study participants receiving treatment with the control condition (control group). However, there is variability in treatment response within each treatment group and applying group mean findings to the treatment of individual patients in clinical practice can be challenging. Therefore, it would be helpful to identify the factors that account for variability in treatment response among the study participants. Are there clinical subgroups among the study participants that might benefit most from the treatment employed in the RCT? Are there certain conditions that might optimize treatment effects? Moderator analyses can help advance our understanding of the factors contributing to treatment response variability. This understanding can aid in translation of the research findings from the RCT to clinical practice and start to bridge the gap that currently exists between research and clinical application.

In a RCT, the qualitative or quantitative factors that occur prior to randomization and influence the direction or magnitude of the relationship between these independent factors and treatment outcome are considered moderators of treatment response (Baron and Kenny 1986; Kraemer et al. 2002). Factors, such as gender, socioeconomic status (SES), severity of initial psychopathology, co-morbidity, and intelligence can function as moderators if they identify patient subgroups with different treatment effect sizes.

The Multimodal Treatment Study of Children with ADHD (MTA; MTA 1999a) provided evidence of moderators of treatment response in school-aged children with ADHD (MTA

1999b; Owens et al. 2003). In comparing treatment response across four treatment conditions in 579 school-aged children with ADHD, four moderators were identified: (1) co-morbid anxiety disorder in the child, (2) initial severity of the child's ADHD, (3) child's intelligence quotient (IQ), and (4) presence of high depressive symptoms in the parents (MTA 1999b; Owens et al. 2003).

The short-term crossover efficacy trial of the National Institute of Mental Health (NIMH)-sponsored multisite, randomized, double-blind Preschoolers with ADHD Treatment Study (PATS) provided evidence of methylphenidate (MPH) efficacy for preschoolers with ADHD (Greenhill et al. 2006). The intent-to-treat analysis revealed significant decreases in ADHD symptoms with three MPH doses—2.5, 5.0, and 7.5 mg three times per day (t.i.d.)—but not with the lowest 1.25-mg t.i.d. dose. The 7.5-mg t.i.d. dose was found to be the most effective in improving the primary outcome measure scores with an effect size of 0.72 relative to placebo. At the end of the efficacy trial, blinded raters classified 7 (4%) preschoolers as nonresponders; 14 (8%) as placebo responders; 24 (15%) as best responding to 1.25 mg t.i.d. (0.2 mg/kg per day); 26 (16%) as best responding to 2.5 mg t.i.d. (0.4 mg/kg per day); 30 (18%) as best responding to 5 mg t.i.d. (0.8 mg/kg per day); 36 (22%) as best responding to 7.5 mg t.i.d. (1.2 mg/kg per day); and 7 (4%) as best responding to 10 mg t.i.d. (1.3 mg/kg per day) (Greenhill et al. 2006). However, the intent-to-treat group mean efficacy findings did not offer any information about whether there were subgroups in the PATS intent-to-treat sample that might benefit the most or the least from MPH. We conducted secondary analyses on the short-term (5-week) efficacy data from the PATS to explore moderators of MPH treatment response in preschool children with ADHD. We identified potential moderators based on both theoretical grounds and empirical data from previous studies. Treatment response can vary by demographic characteristics, such as age (due to developmental differences in pharmacokinetics and pharmacodynamics influencing medication tolerability and efficacy; Ryan and Varma 1998; Vitiello et al. 1999), gender (Martenyi et al. 2001), ethnicity (Wood 1998),

and/or family socioeconomic status. Treatment may be less efficacious in more severe forms of illness or co-morbid conditions; type of disorder can also affect treatment response (MTA 1999b). Pharmacological effect can also vary by child's IQ (Kazdin and Mazurick 1994; Aman et al. 2003).

The objective of these exploratory (secondary) analyses was to examine whether certain prerandomization variables (i.e., age, ethnicity, gender, level of mother's education, family composition, referral source, child's IQ and adaptive functioning, ADHD subtype, severity of illness, and number of co-morbid disorders) moderated the efficacy of MPH. Specifically we hypothesized that younger age, lower IQ, greater baseline severity of illness, greater number of co-morbid disorders, and greater family adversity (lower SES, lower level of mother's education, parental unemployment, unmarried parents, living in a single-parent home) would be associated with lower MPH response.

METHODS

Study design

Moderator analyses were conducted using the MPH short-term efficacy data from the PATS. The study design, methods, and inclusion/exclusion criteria are detailed in Greenhill et al. (2006) and Kollins et al. (2006). Briefly, 3- to 5.5-year-old children with a *Diagnostic and Statistical Manual of Mental Disorders*, 4th edition (DSM-IV; American Psychiatric Association, 1994) diagnosis of ADHD, combined or predominantly hyperactive subtype; Children's Global Assessment Scale (C-GAS; Shaffer et al. 1983) impairment score of <55; hyperactive-impulsive subscale T score of 65 (1.5 SDs above the age- and sex-adjusted means) on both the parent and teacher Conners' Rating Scales–Revised (CRS-R; Conners 2001); and attending a preschool or day-care group program, were included in the PATS. Children with a diagnosis of adjustment disorder, pervasive development disorders, mental retardation (IQ of <70), bipolar disorder, psychosis, or significant suicidality were excluded. The

DSM-IV diagnoses of ADHD and co-morbid disorders were established using a multimethod and multistep approach. For screening purposes, parents completed the Autism Screener Questionnaire (Berument et al. 1999) and a computer-assisted structured diagnostic interview, the Diagnostic Interview Schedule for Children Version 4.0–Parent Version (DISC-IV-P; Shaffer et al. 1996) conducted by a research assistant. The DISC-IV-P was followed by a semistructured clinical interview with the parent conducted by a child psychiatrist or a child psychologist. A unanimous consensus vote of the PATS cross-site diagnostic panel was required to confirm the DSM-IV diagnosis of ADHD and co-morbid disorders. The institutional review boards at all the six participating sites approved the PATS protocol. The PATS study was monitored by the NIMH Data and Safety Monitoring Board. The caregivers/ legal guardians provided written informed consent at study entry and were reconsented at each phase of the study.

The eligible preschoolers with a DSM-IV diagnosis of ADHD were randomized to receive 1 week each of four MPH doses (1.25, 2.5, 5.0, and 7.5 mg) and 1 week of placebo administered three times daily. The primary outcome measure, parent and teacher Conners, Loney, and Milich (CLAM) and Swanson, Conners, Milich, and Pelham (SKAMP) ratings (Wigal et al. 1998), and parent and teacher Side Effect Rating scales were collected at the end of each week. The primary outcome measure for the study and for the moderator analysis was a composite formed by standardizing and then combining parent and teacher CLAM and SKAMP rating scales (Swanson 1992) to reflect overall medication response for each dose across settings.

Subjects

A total of 165 children (74% boys, $n = 122$) between 3 and 5 years of age (mean age = 4.7 ± 0.69 years), with a DSM-IV diagnosis of ADHD, entered the 5-week crossover titration phase. Baseline characteristics of the children are presented in Table 1. Oppositional defiant disorder (ODD) was the most common co-morbid disorder and was present in 90 preschoolers

(54.5%). An additional 5 children (3%) had conduct disorder (CD). Communication disorders were present in 33 children (20%), anxiety disorders in 17 children (10.3%), elimination disorders in 13 children (8%), specific phobia in 11 children (6.7%), developmental coordination disorder in 7 children (4.2%); and 3 children (1.8%) each had pica or reactive attachment disorder. Obsessive compulsive disorder, adjustment disorder, or sleepwalking disorder was present in 1 child (0.6%) each.

The PATS sample had a high rate of co-morbidity; 118 of the participants (71.5%) had at least one or more co-morbid disorders. There were no co-morbid disorders present in 47 (28.5%) children (no co-morbidity subgroup); 69 (41.8%) children had one co-morbid disorder (low co-morbidity subgroup); 34 (20.6%) children had two co-morbid disorders (moderate co-morbidity subgroup); 12 (7.3%) children had three co-morbid disorders; and three children (1.8%) had four co-morbid disorders. Because there were so few children with four co-morbid disorders, we grouped them together with the children with three co-morbid disorders to form a three or four co-morbid disorders group (high co-morbidity subgroup) with 15 (9%) children. The details of the co-morbid disorders present in each of the co-morbid subgroups are presented in Table 1.

Measures

The following potential moderator variables were assessed at baseline prior to randomization.

Baseline demographic variables were obtained from the demographic form completed by the caregivers at study entry. Age was examined as a continuous and categorical variable; dose–response slope estimates were compared for 3, 4, and 5 year olds. Gender comparisons were made for boys and girls. Race/Ethnicity comparisons were made for Caucasian, African-American, and Hispanic children. Hollingshead SES was examined as a continuous variable and dose–response slope estimates were compared for high and low SES. Welfare status comparisons were made for families receiving welfare versus families not receiving welfare. Parents' marital status com-

TABLE 1. CHARACTERISTICS OF THE CROSSOVER TITRATION SAMPLE

Subject variables (n = 165)		
Demographic variables		
Age,[a] year, mean (SD) [range]	4.74 (0.69)	[3.02–5.88]
n (%)		
3.0–3.5 years old	5 (3.0)	
3.5–4.0 years old	27 (16.4)	
4.0–5.0 years old	65 (39.4)	
5.0–6.0 years old	68 (41.2)	
Male, n (%)	122 (74)	
Ethnicity, n (%)		
White	104 (63)	
Black or African-American	29 (18)	
Hispanic or Latino	29 (18)	
Child assessment variables		
Differential Ability Scales IQ, mean (SD), [range]	97.93 (17.67)	[67–196]
Vineland Adaptive Behavior Composite, mean (SD), [range]	89.60 (14.63)	[61–128]
Clinical Global Impressions-Severity of Illness (CGI-S), mean (SD), [range]	4.71 (0.61)	[1–6]
Clinical Global Assessment Scale (CGAS), mean (SD), [range]	46.79 (4.26)	[35–60]
Comorbidity (clinical evaluation), n (%)[b]		
No comorbidity Subgroup (no co-morbid disorders)	47 (28.5)	
Low co-morbidity Subgroup (1 co-morbid disorder)	69 (41.8)	
Oppositional-defiant disorder	51 (74.0)	
Conduct disorder	2 (2.9)	
Communication disorder	6 (8.7)	
Elimination disorders (i.e., encopresis, enuresis)	5 (7.2)	
Anxiety disorder (i.e., separation, generalized, PTSD	2 (2.9)	
Specific phobia (i.e., animals, needles, social phobia)	2 (2.9)	
Pica	1 (1.4)	
Moderate co-morbidity subgroup (2 co-morbid disorders)	34 (20.6)	
Oppositional-defiant disorder	27 (79.4)	
Conduct disorder	1 (2.9)	
Communication disorder	13 (38.2)	
Anxiety disorder (i.e., separation, generalized, PTSD)	9 (26.5)	
Specific phobia (i.e., animals, needles, social phobia)	3 (8.8)	
Elimination disorders (i.e., encopresis, enuresis)	7 (20.6)	
Developmental coordination disorder	2 (5.9)	
Reactive attachment disorder	2 (5.9)	
Sleepwalking disorder	1 (2.9)	
Adjustment disorder	1 (2.9)	
Pica	1 (2.9)	
High co-morbidity subgroup (3 or 4 co-morbid disorders)	15 (9.0)	
Oppositional-defiant disorder	12 (80.0)	
Conduct disorder	2 (13.3)	
Communication disorder	13 (86.7)	
Anxiety disorder (i.e., separation, generalized, PTSD)	6 (40.0)	
Specific phobia (i.e., animals, needles, social phobia)	6 (40.0)	
Developmental coordination disorder	5 (33.3)	
Elimination disorders (i.e., encopresis, enuresis)	1 (6.7)	
Reactive attachment disorder	1 (6.7)	
Obsessive compulsive disorder	1 (6.7)	
Pica	1 (6.7)	
Conners' Parent Rating Scale, mean (SD), [range]		
Inattention	17.85 (5.40)	[2–27]
Hyperactivity	22.27 (3.48)	[15–27]
Total	40.16 (7.67)	[20–54]
Conners' Teacher Rating Scale, mean (SD), [range]		
Inattention	15.39 (5.84)	[2–27]
Hyperactivity	20.43 (4.62)	[2–27]
Total	35.91 (8.92)	[6–54]

(*continued*)

TABLE 1. CHARACTERISTICS OF THE CROSSOVER TITRATION SAMPLE (CONT'D)

Subject variables (n = 165)		
Number of DSM-IV ADHD symptoms, mean (SD), [range]		
Hyperactive	5.53 (0.70)	[3–6]
Impulsive	2.59 (0.59)	[1–3]
Inattentive	6.62 (1.75)	[1–9]
Total	14.74 (2.20)	[8–18]
ADHD subtype, *n* (%)		
Hyperactive-impulsive type	39 (24)	
Combined type	126 (76)	
Parent family variables		
High school graduate, *n* (%)		
Mother	154/161 (96)	
Father	130/133 (98)	
Employed, *n* (%)[c]		
Mother	120/160 (75)	
Father	112/158 (71)	
Welfare, *n* (%)	13/148 (9)	
Married, *n* (%)[d]	98/163 (60)	
Hollingshead Socio-Economic Status (SES), mean (SD), [range]	47.01 (9.58)	[13.50–63]
Family composition, *n* (%)		
2 parents	130 (79)	
1 parent	35 (21)	

[a]Age indicates age at screening.

[b]Percentage for the DSM-IV disorders in each co-morbid subgroup is relative to the total number of preschoolers in each co-morbid subgroup.

PTSD = Posttraumatic stress disorder; SD = standard deviation.

[c]Employed refers to the proportion of the sample whose parents held full- or part-time jobs, were unemployed and looking for work, or students full- or part-time.

[d]Married refers to those with intact two-parent families (married or common law).

parisons were made for the children living with both parents (married or common-law) versus living with a single parent. Employment status comparisons were made for parents who were employed full or part time versus unemployed parents. Mother's education level comparisons were made for mothers' self-reported education level of ≤ high school education and ≥ some college education. Number of caregivers in the home comparisons were made for the participant children living in a two-caregiver versus one-caregiver home. Referral source comparisons were made for clinical versus non-clinical source of referral.

Baseline child assessment variables were obtained from the screening assessments completed prior to randomization.

Intellectual and adaptive functioning level was assessed with the Differential Ability Scales (DAS; Elliott 1990) and the Vineland Adaptive Behavior Scales (VABS; Sparrow et al. 1984). Full-scale IQ equivalent scores on the

DAS and VABS composite scores were examined as continuous and categorical variables, and dose–response slope estimates were compared for children with IQ values between 70 and 85 (borderline IQ), 85 and 115 (average IQ), and above 115.

Severity of ADHD at study entry was determined using parent and teacher reports on the CRS-R (Conners 2001) clinician's endorsement of the number of ADHD symptoms on the clinical interview, clinician-rated C-GAS (Shaffer et al. 1983), and Clinical Global Impressions–Severity (CGI-S; Guy 1976) scores. Child's initial ADHD severity was examined as a continuous score for the parent and teacher CRS-R total scores and Hyperactive-Impulsive subscale scores separately and for the composite scores by averaging parent and teacher CRS-R total scores at study entry. Severity was also examined as a categorical variable by comparing participants with moderately high CRS-R scores, between 1.5 and 2 standard deviations

(SD) above age and gender expected mean, versus extremely high CRS-R scores (more than two SDs above age and gender expected mean) for the parent and teacher scores separately, as well as for the parent and teacher composite scores. Clinician's endorsement of the number of ADHD symptoms was examined both as continuous and categorical variables. Dose–response slope estimate comparisons were made between children with high (1 SD above the mean for the PATS sample), average, and low scores (1 SD below the mean for the PATS sample). CGI-S scores were examined both as continuous and categorical variables. Dose–response slope estimates comparisons were made between participants with "Moderately Ill," "Severely Ill," and "Extremely Ill" CGI-S ratings. C-GAS scores were examined as continuous and categorical variables. Dose–response slope estimates were compared for children with low, average, and high C-GAS scores.

ADHD Subtype was determined from the screening diagnosis based on clinical interview and confirmed by unanimous consensus by the PATS cross-site panel (Kollins et al. 2006). Comparisons were made between children with ADHD Hyperactive/Impulsive subtype versus children with ADHD Combined subtype.

Co-morbidity was assessed at study entry via the previously mentioned consensus diagnostic process. The number of co-morbid disorders was examined as a continuous variable, and comparisons were also made for children with no co-morbid disorders, one, two, or three or more co-morbid disorders.

Outcome measures

As mentioned previously, the primary outcome measure for the moderator analyses was the combined parent and teacher CLAM and SKAMP composite scores; we also conducted separate moderator analyses for the parent CLAM/SKAMP composite scores and the teacher CLAM/SKAMP composite scores.

Data analysis

The null hypothesis of no significant differences in treatment outcome based on the pos-

tulated moderators was tested. We assessed the fixed effects on the average slope in the regression of outcome on moderators, weight-adjusted dose, and the moderator-by-dose interaction using SAS PROC GENMOD. Omnibus tests for GENMOD were based on the Wald chi-square test. To evaluate the clinical significance of the impact of moderator on outcome, empirically-based effect sizes (Cohen's d, the standardized difference of the means) at the most effective dose, 7.5 mg three times/day, relative to placebo were calculated as $d =$ MC/SD placebo, where MC is the difference between the means for the primary outcome measure scores for the placebo and MPH 7.5 mg t.i.d. doses for the subjects with and without the moderator, and SD placebo is the standard deviation of the placebo group (Rosenthal et al. 2000).

Statistical significance (type 1 error rate) was set at 5% and all tests were two-tailed. Given the exploratory (hypothesis-generating) nature of these analyses and the small sample sizes for the moderator subgroups, no adjustments were made for multiple comparisons. The results obtained in this study will provide preliminary findings in need of further exploration and replication.

RESULTS

We tested for interactions of each of the moderator variables with weight-adjusted (mg/kg) dose effects on the trajectory of response for the parent and teacher CLAM/SKAMP composite scores (primary efficacy measure). Of all the variables examined as possible moderators of MPH response, a significant interaction effect was found only for the number of co-morbid disorders present at baseline ($p = 0.005$). None of the other variables examined moderated MPH dose response. There were no differences in the results from the separate moderator analyses for the parent CLAM/SKAMP composite scores and the teacher CLAM/SKAMP composite scores. Table 2 summarizes average slopes, dose effects, and effect sizes for moderator and weight-adjusted parent-teacher CLAM-SKAMP composite means.

As seen in Table 2, the participants with three

TABLE 2. Moderator and Weight-Adjusted (mg/kg) Methylphenidate Dose Effects, Slopes, and Effect Sizes at 7.5-mg Dose Relative to Placebo on the Primary Efficacy Measure (Parent–Teacher CLAM-SKAMP Composite) in Preschool Children with ADHD in the PATS Crossover Titration Sample

| | Moderator analysis | | | Parent-Teacher CLAM-SKAMP composite scores | | | | | | |
| | Moderator × dose interaction | | | MPH 7.5 mg t.i.d. | | | Placebo t.i.d. | | | |
Moderator variable	Chi square	p value**	Slope* (SE)	n	Mean	SD	n	Mean	SD	Effect size
Age at screen										
Continuous	$\chi^2_1 = 0.06$	p = 0.8058	−0.0183 (0.014)	133	0.923	(0.505)	152	1.254	(0.518)	0.64
Categorical	$\chi^2_2 = 2.05$	p = 0.3590								
Average			−0.0139 (0.002)	133	0.913	(0.505)	152	1.275	(0.518)	0.70
3–4 years			−0.0119 (0.004)	28	0.821	(0.491)	38	1.268	(0.610)	0.73
4–5 years			−0.0178 (0.003)	70	0.924	(0.529)	77	1.311	(0.432)	0.90
5–6 years			−0.0119 (0.004)	35	0.964	(0.471)	37	1.206	(0.586)	0.41
Gender	$\chi^2_1 = 0.06$	p = 0.6544								
Male			−0.0155 (0.002)	101	0.920	(0.504)	112	1.272	(0.478)	0.74
Female			−0.0133 (0.004)	32	0.891	(0.516)	40	1.284	(0.623)	0.63
Ethnicity	$\chi^2_2 = 4.62$	p = 0.0993								
Average			−0.0124 (0.002)	131	0.910	(0.510)	149	1.280	(0.520)	0.71
White			−0.0186 (0.003)	82	0.837	(0.467)	96	1.335	(0.516)	0.97
Black/African-American			−0.0112 (0.003)	26	0.965	(0.438)	27	1.200	(0.559)	0.42
Hispanic/Latino			−0.0076 (0.006)	23	1.115	(0.664)	26	1.164	(0.463)	0.11
Number of parents in the home	$\chi^2_1 = 0.42$	p = 0.5176								
2 parents			−0.0142 (0.002)	109	0.918	(0.509)	122	1.254	(0.488)	0.69
1 parent			−0.0180 (0.006)	24	0.892	(0.497)	30	1.359	(0.628)	0.74
Mother's education level	$\chi^2_1 = 2.21$	p = 0.1367								
At most high school Graduate/GED			−0.0082 (0.005)	20	1.114	(0.585)	23	1.257	(0.417)	0.34
Post high school			−0.0164 (0.002)	109	0.878	(0.484)	125	1.288	(0.534)	0.77
Referral source (categorical)	$\chi^2_1 = 0.05$	p = 0.8229								
Clinical			−0.0155 (0.003)	70	0.937	(0.558)	80	1.325	(0.512)	0.76
Nonclinical			−0.0145 (0.003)	59	0.897	(0.450)	66	1.247	(0.521)	0.67
Intelligence Quotient (IQ)										
Continuous	$\chi^2_1 = 3.22$	p = 0.0727	−0.0066 (0.013)	129	1.419	(0.484)	147	1.265	(0.514)	−0.30
Categorical	$\chi^2_2 = 1.87$	p = 0.3925								
Average			−0.0169 (0.002)	129	0.891	(0.484)	147	1.260	(0.510)	0.72
≤85			−0.0127 (0.004)	32	0.980	(0.495)	36	1.223	(0.477)	0.51
85–115			−0.0160 (0.003)	80	0.834	(0.455)	93	1.245	(0.531)	0.77
≥115			−0.0221 (0.005)	17	0.993	(0.581)	18	1.434	(0.485)	0.91

	χ^2	p	Slope (SE)	n	(SE)	n	(SE)	
Vineland Adaptive Behavior Scale (VABS)								
Composite score	$\chi^2_1 = 2.55$	$p = 0.1102$						
Slope at 74.97 (1 SD below mean)			−0.0105 (0.003)	115	1.016 (0.490)	132	1.251 (0.530)	0.44
Slope at 89.60 (mean VABS score)			−0.0140 (0.002)	115	0.907 (0.490)	132	1.223 (0.530)	0.60
Slope at 104.235 (1 SD above mean)			−0.0176 (0.003)	115	0.798 (0.490)	132	1.194 (0.530)	0.75
Conners' parent–teacher hyperactivity-impulsivity composite score	$\chi^2_1 = 0.25$	$p = 0.6189$						
Slope at 18.21 (1 SD below mean)			−0.0140 (0.003)	13	0.881 (0.505)	152	1.196 (0.518)	0.61
Slope at 21.35 (mean Conners' score)			−0.0150 (0.002)	133	0.904 (0.505)	152	1.241 (0.518)	0.65
Slope at 24.48 (1 SD above mean)			−0.0160 (0.003)	133	0.927 (0.505)	152	1.287 (0.518)	0.70
Conners' parent hyperactivity-impulsivity score	$\chi^2_1 = 0.02$	$p = 0.8861$						
Slope at 18.79 (1 SD below mean)			−0.0153 (0.003)	133	0.831 (0.505)	152	1.181 (0.518)	0.68
Slope at 22.27 (mean Conners' score)			−0.0150 (0.002)	133	0.928 (0.505)	152	1.262 (0.518)	0.65
Slope at 25.75 (1 SD above mean)			−0.0147 (0.003)	133	1.024 (0.505)	152	1.344 (0.518)	0.62
Conners' teacher hyperactivity-impulsivity composite score	$\chi^2_1 = 1.60$	$p = 0.2063$						
Slope at 15.81 (1 SD below mean)			−0.0126 (0.003)	126	0.918 (0.505)	145	1.201 (1.262)	0.22
Slope at 20.43 (mean Conners' score)			−0.0151 (0.002)	126	0.888 (0.505)	145	1.227 (1.262)	0.27
Slope at 25.05 (1 SD above mean)			−0.0176 (0.003)	126	0.858 (0.505)	145	1.254 (1.262)	0.31
Number of ADHD symptoms (continuous)	$\chi^2_1 = 0.70$	$p = 0.4040$						
Slope at 12.74 (1 SD below mean)			−0.0134 (0.003)	133	1.002 (0.505)	152	1.304 (0.518)	0.58
Slope at 14.74 (mean # symptoms for the group)			−0.0150 (0.002)	133	0.903 (0.505)	152	1.241 (0.518)	0.65
Slope at 16.74 (1 SD above mean)			−0.0166 (0.003)	133	0.804 (0.505)	152	1.177 (0.518)	0.72
ADHD subtype	$\chi^2_1 = 1.63$	$p = 0.2018$						
Hyperactive/Impulsive type			−0.0199 (0.005)	31	0.764 (0.471)	36	1.278 (0.509)	1.01
Combined type			−0.0135 (0.003)	102	0.958 (0.509)	116	1.274 (0.523)	0.60
Number of comorbid disorders								
Continuous	$\chi^2_1 = 9.21$	$p = 0.0024$	−0.0219 (0.003)	133	0.784 (0.505)	152	1.276 (0.518)	0.95
Categorical	$\chi^2_3 = 12.85$	$p = 0.0050$						
Average			−0.0104 (0.002)	133	0.913 (0.505)	152	1.275 (0.518)	0.70
None			−0.0182 (0.003)	43	0.889 (0.449)	45	1.280 (0.436)	0.90
One			−0.0185 (0.003)	54	0.826 (0.485)	61	1.314 (0.489)	1.00
Two			−0.0126 (0.005)	24	0.904 (0.438)	33	1.244 (0.610)	0.56
Three or Four			−0.0077 (0.007)	12	1.408 (0.670)	13	1.153 (0.685)	−0.37
CGI-S (continuous)	$\chi^2_1 = 0.33$	$p = 0.5646$						
Slope at 4.19 (1 SD below mean)			−0.0161 (0.003)	133	0.848 (0.505)	152	1.209 (0.518)	0.70
Slope at 4.79 (mean CGI-S for the group)			−0.0149 (0.002)	133	0.903 (0.505)	152	1.239 (0.518)	0.65
Slope at 5.39 (SD above mean)			−0.0139 (0.002)	133	0.958 (0.505)	152	1.268 (0.518)	0.60
CGAS score (continuous)	$\chi^2_1 = 0.49$	$p = 0.4865$						
Slope at 42.53 (1 SD below mean)			−0.0135 (0.003)	133	0.971 (0.505)	152	1.275 (0.518)	0.59

CLAM-SKAMP = Conners, Loney, and Milich–Swanson, Conners, Milich, and Pelham ratings; ADHD = attention-deficiect/hyperactivity; PATS = Preschoolers with ADHD Treatment Study; SE = standard error; t.i.d. = three times daily; SD = standard deviation; CGI-S = Clinical Global Impressions–Severity; C-GAS = Children's Global Assessment Scale.

or more co-morbid disorders displayed no dose response as evidenced by the positive slope of the primary outcome measure (0.008/mg MPH) compared to the negative and more steep slopes for the participants with no, one, or two co-morbid disorders (−0.018/mg MPH, −0.019/mg MPH, and −0.013/mg MPH, respectively). We examined the clinical significance of the variation in MPH outcome response in the different co-morbid groups by calculating effect sizes relative to placebo for the primary outcome measure at the most effective 7.5-mg dose. The estimated effect sizes (Cohen's d) for the MPH 7.5-mg t.i.d. dose relative to placebo were −0.37, 0.56, 1.00, and 0.89 for children with three or four co-morbid disorders (High co-morbidity subgroup), two co-morbid disorders (Moderate co-morbidity subgroup), one co-morbid disorder (Low comorbidity subgroup), and no co-morbid disorders (No co-morbidity subgroup), respectively. Table 3 shows the parent and teacher CLAM/SKAMP composite means and effect sizes for each randomized dose week for the comorbid subgroups.

Co-morbid subgroups

There were no differences in most of the demographic (age, gender, ethnicity, and type of preschool attended) and some of the family characteristics (parents' education and mothers' employment status) among children in the No, Low, Moderate, and High co-morbidity subgroups. The co-morbid subgroups differed based on fathers' employment status, families' welfare status, family composition (two-caregiver versus one-caregiver home), and parents' marital status. As seen in Table 4, the PATS sample showed a general linear upward trend in family adversity with increasing co-morbidity. Children in the High co-morbidity subgroup were found to have more family adversity compared to the children in the No, Low, and Moderate co-morbidity subgroups. In the High co-morbidity subgroup, comparatively fewer fathers were employed ($\chi^2_3 =$ 11.55, $p = 0.009$), more families were on welfare ($\chi^2_3 = 9.40, p = 0.024$), fewer children lived in two-caregiver homes ($\chi^2_3 = 11.41, p = 0.009$) or had parents who were married ($\chi^2_3 = 7.78$, $p = 0.05$).

There were no differences in most of the baseline assessment characteristics of the children (IQ, Autism Screener Questionnaire scores, parent and teacher CRS-R scores, ADHD subtype, and CGI-S) among the co-morbid subgroups, except for children's VABS and C-GAS scores, which were in the expected direction. The children in the High co-morbidity subgroup had lower VABS composite scores compared to the children in the No, Low, or Moderate co-morbidity subgroups ($F_{3,140} =$ 5.52, $p = 0.0013$). Children with co-morbid disorders (Low, Moderate, and High co-morbidity subgroups) had lower C-GAS scores compared to the children with no co-morbid disorders ($F_{3,161} = 4.45$, $p = 0.0049$).

There were no differences in the responder status determination by blinded ratings among

TABLE 3. PARENT–TEACHER CLAM-SKAMP MEANS AND SD VALUES FOR EACH CROSSOVER TITRATION RANDOMIZATION GROUP

Co-morbid Group	Crossover titration phase randomization										Effect size (Cohen's d) at 7.5 mg t.i.d. dose[a]
	Placebo		1.25 mg t.i.d.		2.5 mg t.i.d.		5 mg t.i.d.		7.5 mg t.i.d.		
	Mean	SD	Mean	SD	Mean	SD	Mean	SD	Mean	SD	
0	1.28	(0.4)	1.30	(0.7)	1.08	(0.6)	1.03	(0.5)	0.89	(0.4)	0.89
1	1.31	(0.5)	1.18	(0.6)	1.12	(0.5)	1.07	(0.7)	0.83	(0.5)	1.00
2	1.24	(0.6)	1.06	(0.4)	1.01	(0.5)	0.98	(0.6)	0.90	(0.4)	0.56
3 or 4	1.15	(0.7)	1.16	(0.6)	1.21	(0.5)	1.14	(0.7)	1.41	(0.7)	0.37

CLAM-SKAMP = Conners, Loney, and Milich–Swanson, Conners, Milich, and Pelham ratings; SD = standard deviation; t.i.d. = three times daily.

[a]Mean difference in parent–teacher CLAM-SKAMP composite score for placebo and 7.5 mg/standard deviation of the placebo group.

Table 4. Baseline Characteristics of the Co-morbid Groups for the Crossover Titration Sample[a] ($n = 166$)

Variable	No co-morbid disorders (n = 47)	1 Co-morbid disorder (n = 69)	2 Co-morbid disorders (n = 34)	3 or 4 co-morbid disorders (n = 15)	Comparison of groups[b]	
					Statistic	p Value
Subject variables						
Demographic variables						
Age, years, mean (SD)	4.52 (0.61)	4.31 (0.68)	4.35 (0.74)	4.58 (0.74)	$F_{3,161} = 1.28$	$p = 0.2843$
Male, n (%)	36 (76.60)	53 (76.81)	25 (73.53)	8 (53.33)	$\chi^2_3 = 3.78$	$p = 0.2867$
Ethnicity, n (%)						
White	30 (28.85)	47 (45.19)	21 (20.19)	6 (5.77)	$\chi^2_3 = 4.21$	$p = 0.2390$
Other	17 (27.87)	22 (36.07)	13 (21.31)	9 (14.75)		
Preschool/Daycare attendance, n (%)						
Nursery	40 (85.11)	51 (73.91)	25 (73.53)	9 (7.20)	$\chi^2_9 = 10.89$	$p = 0.2832$
Kindergarten	5 (10.64)	8 (11.59)	5 (14.71)	4 (26.67)		
Special school	2 (13.33)	9 (13.00)	2 (5.88)	2 (13.33)		
Not in school, play group, or daycare	0 (0.00)	1 (1.45)	2 (5.88)	0 (0.00)		
Child baseline assessment variables						
Conners' Teacher Rating Scale, mean (SD)						
Inattention	15.02 (6.27)	15.44 (6.12)	15.50 (5.04)	16.00 (5.20)	$F_{3,286} = 0.59$	$p = 0.6224$
Hyperactivity	20.57 (4.33)	20.62 (4.98)	20.25 (3.90)	19.50 (5.53)	$F_{3,287} = 0.35$	$p = 0.7864$
Total	35.55 (9.01)	36.24 (9.46)	35.91 (7.41)	35.50 (9.99)	$F_{3,287} = 0.19$	$p = 0.9045$
Conners' Parent Rating Scale, mean (SD)						
Inattention	17.36 (4.80)	17.86 (5.97)	17.71 (5.38)	19.67 (4.48)	$F_{3,316} = 0.98$	$p = 0.4034$
Hyperactivity	22.00 (3.72)	22.22 (3.30)	21.97 (3.41)	24.00 (3.46)	$F_{3,316} = 1.96$	$p = 0.1206$
Total	39.45 (7.37)	40.12 (8.06)	39.65 (7.09)	43.80 (7.73)	$F_{3,316} = 1.79$	$p = 0.1491$
Number of DSM-IV ADHD symptoms, mean (SD)						
Hyperactive	5.49 (0.75)	5.51 (0.70)	5.56 (0.70)	5.67 (0.62)	$F_{3,161} = 0.28$	$p = 0.8400$
Impulsive	2.55 (0.62)	2.58 (0.58)	2.56 (0.66)	2.80 (0.41)	$F_{3,161} = 0.72$	$p = 0.5429$
Inattentive	6.47 (1.90)	6.52 (1.71)	6.68 (1.80)	7.47 (1.19)	$F_{3,161} = 1.38$	$p = 0.2523$
Total	14.51 (2.41)	14.61 (2.07)	14.79 (2.31)	15.93 (1.53)	$F_{3,161} = 1.75$	$p = 0.1581$
ADHD subtype, n (%)						
Hyperactive-impulsive	12 (25.53)	17 (24.64)	9 (26.47)	1 (6.67)	$\chi^2_3 = 2.68$	$p = 0.4443$
Combined	35 (74.47)	52 (75.36)	25 (73.53)	14 (93.33)		
CGI-S, mean (SD)	4.66 (0.52)	4.87 (0.57)	4.85 (0.74)	4.67 (0.62)	$F_{3,161} = 1.48$	$p = 0.2221$
C-GAS Impairment Scale, mean (SD)	48.62 (3.26)	45.91 (3.87)	46.06 (5.58)	46.73 (3.94)	$F_{3,161} = 4.45^c$	$p = 0.0049$
					No co-morbidities > 1 co-morbidity, $p = 0.0007^c$	
					No co-morbidities > 2 co-morbidities, $p = 0.0067$	
Differential Ability Scales IQ, mean (SD)	100.74 (18.33)	95.38 (14.14)	99.41 (16.37)	97.54 (30.65)	$F_{3,148} = 0.88$	$p = 0.4508$
Vineland Adaptive Behavior Composite, mean (SD)	94.68 (12.86)	88.80 (14.50)	89.86 (14.63)	76.77 (13.40)	$F_{3,140} = 5.52$	$p = 0.0013$
					No co-morbidities > 1 co-morbidity, $p = 0.0391^c$	
					No co-morbidities > 3 or 4 co-morbidities, $p = 0.0001$	
					1 co-morbidity > 3 or 4 co-morbidities, $p = 0.0055$	
					2 co-morbidities > 3 or 4 co-morbidities, $p = 0.0057$	

(continued)

TABLE 4. Baseline Characteristics of the Co-morbid Groups for the Crossover Titration Sample[a] (n = 166) (Cont'd)

Variable	No co-morbid disorders (n = 47)	1 Co-morbid disorder (n = 69)	2 Co-morbid disorders (n = 34)	3 or 4 co-morbid disorders (n = 15)	Comparison of groups[b]	
					Statistic	p Value
Parent/family adversity variables						
High school graduate, n (%)						
Mother	44/45 (97.78)	65/67 (97.01)	32 (94.12)	13 (86.67)	$\chi^2_3 = 3.89$	p = 0.2733
Father	45/45 (100.00)	51/53 (96.23)	22/23 (95.65)	12/12 (100.00)	$\chi^2_3 = 2.33$	p = 0.5076
Employed, n (%)						
Mother	36 (76.60)	51/66 (77.27)	25/33 (75.76)	8/14 (57.14)	$\chi^2_3 = 2.64$	p = 0.4511
Father	40/46 (86.96)	46/65 (70.77)	19/33 (57.58)	7/14 (50.00)	$\chi^2_3 = 11.55$[c]	p = 0.0091
			No co-morbidities > 1 co-morbidity, p = 0.0443[c]			
			No co-morbidities > 2 co-morbidities, p = 0.0031			
			No co-morbidities > 3 or 4 co-morbidities, p = 0.0033			
Welfare, n (%)	1/43 (2.33)	6/60 (10.00)	2/29 (6.45)	4/14 (28.57)	$\chi^2_3 = 9.40$[c]	p = 0.0244
			No co-morbidities < 3 or 4 co-morbidities, p = 0.0026[c]			
			1 co-morbidity < 3 or 4 co-morbidities, p = 0.0672			
			2 co-morbidity < 3 or 4 co-morbidities, p = 0.0433			
Married, n (%)	33 (70.21)	43/68 (63.24)	17/33 (51.52)	5 (33.33)	$\chi^2_3 = 7.78$[c]	p = 0.0508
			No co-morbidities > 3 or 4 co-morbidities, p = 0.0107[c]			
			1 co-morbidity > 3 or 4 co-morbidities, p = 0.0338			
Family composition, n (%)						
2 parents	45 (95.74)	49 (71.01)	25 (73.53)	11 (73.33)	$\chi^2_3 = 11.41$	p = 0.0097
1 parent	2 (4.26)	20 (28.99)	9 (26.47)	4 (26.67)		
			No co-morbidities > 1 co-morbidity, p = 0.0009[c]			
			No co-morbidities > 2 co-morbidities, p = 0.0040			
			No co-morbidities > 3 or 4 co-morbidities, p = 0.0106			
Hollingshead SES, Mean (SD)	47.45 (8.47)	46.88 (10.12)	48.02 (9.10)	43.31 (11.98)	$F_{3,148} = 0.75$	p = 0.5232

SD = Standard deviation; DSM-IV = *Diagnostic and Statistical Manual of Mental Disorders*, 4th edition; ADHD = attention-deficit/hyperactivity disorder; CGI-S = Clinical Global Impressions-Severity; C-GAS = Children's Global Assessment Scale; IQ = intelligence quotient; SES = socioeconomic status.
[a]Employed refers to the proportion of the sample whose parents held full- or part-time jobs, were unemployed and looking for work, or students full-or part-time; married refers to those with intact two-parent families (married or common law).
[b]p value for Fisher's exact test.
[c]Posthoc analysis (p values unadjusted for multiple comparisons).

the co-morbid subgroups. As seen in Table 5, there were no differences in the percentage of children who were classified as responding best to placebo, 1.25 mg t.i.d., 2.5 mg t.i.d., 5 mg t.i.d., 7.5 mg t.i.d., or 10 mg t.i.d. among children in the No, Low, Moderate, or High co-morbidity subgroups.

DISCUSSION

The PATS crossover titration trial ($n = 165$) is the largest RCT of MPH treatment outcome in preschool children with ADHD. The efficacy data with four doses of MPH and placebo presented a unique opportunity to examine the possible impact of baseline moderator variables on MPH dose response in the PATS sample. As recommended by Kraemer et al. (2002, 2006), we planned the *post hoc* moderator analyses *a priori* by carefully selecting a comprehensive assessment battery to provide information about appropriate baseline moderator variables.

Of the 14 variables examined as potential moderators, only one (number of concurrent co-morbid disorders) served as a moderator of MPH dose response. Specifically, the High co-morbidity subgroup showed no improvement with the increasing MPH dose compared to significant improvement in the Moderate, Low, or No co-morbidity subgroups. The preschool children in the High co-morbidity subgroup had an effect size of -0.37 with a MPH dose of 7.5 mg t.i.d. relative to placebo compared to

high effect size (0.89 and 1.00) in children in the No and Low co-morbidity subgroups, respectively, and medium (0.56) in children in the Moderate co-morbidity subgroup (Cohen 1988). The effect sizes for children with no (0.89) or low co-morbidity (1.00) are slightly larger than the 0.72 effect size for our combined primary efficacy analysis sample (Greenhill et al. 2006), and are similar to school-aged children (MTA 1999a). The effect size for children with moderate co-morbidity (0.56) and the negative effect size for children with high co-morbidity (-0.37) are lower than the effect size for our combined primary efficacy analysis sample and school-aged children (MTA 1999a).

The association between poor treatment response and higher co-morbidity is consistent with the findings from the MTA study as previously mentioned (MTA 1999b) and the Treatment for Adolescents With Depression Study (TADS) of 439 depressed adolescents randomly assigned to acute intervention with fluoxetine, cognitive-behavioral therapy (CBT), both fluoxetine and CBT, or clinical management with pill placebo. The depressed adolescents with more than one concurrent co-morbid disorder diagnosis were reported to benefit less than the depressed adolescents with no or one co-morbid disorder diagnosis (Curry et al. 2006).

Even though the finding of poor response in preschool children in the High co-morbidity subgroup was not unexpected, it was surprising that a small number of preschool children in the High co-morbidity subgroup ($n = 15, 9\%$

TABLE 5. TREATMENT RESPONDER STATUS OF THE CO-MORBID SUBGROUPS FOR THE CROSSOVER TITRATION TRIAL COMPLETERS ($n = 147$)

Variable	No co-morbid disorders (n = 44)	1 Co-morbid disorder (n = 57)	2 Co-morbid disorders (n = 33)	3 or 4 Co-morbid disorders (n = 13)	Comparison of groups[b]	
					Statistic	p Value
Best dose determinations by blinded ratings						
Nonresponders	1 (2.27)	3 (5.26)	2 (6.06)	1 (7.69)		
Placebo	2 (4.55)	8 (14.04)	4 (12.12)	0 (0.00)		
1.25 mg t.i.d.	9 (20.45)	8 (14.04)	5 (15.15)	2 (15.38)		
2.5 mg t.i.d.	8 (18.18)	10 (17.54)	6 (18.18)	2 (15.38)	$\chi^2_{18} = 17.14$	$p = 0.5132$
5.0 mg t.i.d.	5 (11.36)	12 (21.05)	10 (30.30)	3 (23.08)		
7.5 mg t.i.d.	15 (34.09)	14 (24.56)	5 (15.15)	2 (15.38)		
10.0 mg t.i.d.	3 (6.82)	1 (1.75)	1 (3.03)	2 (15.38)		

[a]No best dose determination available for one child in this co-morbid subgroup.
[b]p value for Fisher's exact test.

of the crossover sample) had such an impact on the treatment outcome for the overall crossover sample. We wondered how the High co-morbidity subgroup was different from the Moderate, Low, and/or No co-morbidity subgroups. Did they have more severe ADHD symptoms? Were preschoolers in the high co-morbidity subgroup more developmentally immature? For example, were they younger? Did they have lower IQs? Were they more likely to have higher scores on the Autism Screener Questionnaire indicating some characteristics resembling pervasive developmental disorders? As previously mentioned, *post hoc* analysis showed that there were no differences in the proxy indicators of developmental immaturity (age, IQ, or Autism Screener Questionnaire scores), demographic, and ADHD severity among the High and No, Low, or Moderate co-morbidity subgroups.

Interestingly, even though some indicators of family adversity (family relationships and family financial status indicators) did not have a main effect on MPH dose response in the overall intent-to-treat crossover sample, children in the High co-morbidity subgroup were found to have more family adversity. As previously mentioned, comparatively fewer fathers were employed, more families were on welfare, fewer children lived in two-caregiver homes or had parents who were married in the high co-morbidity subgroup. These findings are consistent with previous reports of positive association of increased family adversity and increased risk for psychopathology in 6- to 17-year-old ADHD and normal control children (Biederman et al. 1995). The significance of the association between high co-morbidity and increased family adversity is unclear. Is it coincidental? Did the demands of caring for a child with multiple co-morbidities have an impact on family relationships and parents' ability to hold employment, thus resulting in an increased need for welfare help? Or was it the reverse that the impact of increased family adversity was reflected in increased number of co-morbid disorders in the preschool children? The PATS study design does not allow us to answer these questions. Further studies are needed to replicate these findings and to address the significance of the association of high co-morbidity and family adversity in preschool children with ADHD.

Contrary to our expectations and the currently prevalent belief among practitioners, age and IQ did not moderate MPH treatment response in the PATS sample of typically developing ADHD preschoolers with average intellectual functioning. Similarly, other moderator variables including demographic (gender, racial or ethnic status, SES), family characteristics, illness severity, and ADHD subtype also did not moderate MPH treatment response. Hence, it is reassuring to find that MPH was equally effective among younger and older preschool children, preschoolers with average and above average IQ, and preschoolers with a wide array of demographic, family, and illness characteristics. However, caution is needed in the generalization of the findings. Although the PATS included the largest sample of preschoolers with ADHD treated with MPH, sample sizes across different moderator categories/subgroups were relatively small. For example, there were only 32 (19%) children between 3.0 and 3.99 years of age. Furthermore, the distribution of IQ was truncated by the study exclusion criteria; the PATS sample excluded preschool children with mental retardation (IQ below 70). Therefore, we cannot address the suitability of MPH for ADHD preschoolers with mildly or moderately retarded intellectual functioning. Similarly, gender, ethnic status, and ADHD subtype and other illness characteristics-based subgroups had small sample sizes. Further studies with larger samples of preschoolers will serve to clarify whether there are any differences in the efficacy of MPH treatment among different ADHD subgroups among preschoolers.

Limitations

This study had several limitations. No adjustments were made for multiple comparisons. The findings should be considered preliminary and no firm conclusions can be drawn until results are replicated. The DISC-IV-P has not been validated in preschool children. However, there was general concordance across measures of ADHD symptoms at baseline (Posner et al., 2007). Additionally, the rigorous diagnostic procedures used in the PATS enhanced the validity of the diagnostic method. The High co-morbidity subgroup was relatively small in comparison to the other three co-morbid subgroups. Another limitation was missing data for medication compliance. Even though all parents were asked to complete daily medication diaries and return unused drug capsules at the time of each visit, parents were inconsistent in completing the medication diaries and/or returning unused drug capsules. Hence, we were unable to determine if the children in the High co-morbidity subgroup may have had lower medication compliance (and subsequently a lack of response) than children in the other co-morbid subgroups.

CONCLUSION

To summarize, in PATS, the preschoolers with ADHD and high co-morbidity did not respond to MPH and had more family adversity. Hence, it is important to assess an ADHD preschooler carefully for the presence of concurrent co-morbid disorders and the possible need for additional and/or more appropriate treatment strategies than MPH. Further studies are needed to confirm the association of co-morbidity to MPH response; and if confirmed in future studies, the ADHD preschoolers with high co-morbidity may not benefit from MPH.

In conclusion, diagnostic co-morbidity is an important moderator of MPH treatment response in preschool children with ADHD. Specifically, preschoolers with ADHD with no or one co-morbid disorder (primarily ODD) had very large treatment responses at the same level as found in school-aged children. In other words, the terrific responders either had no co-morbidity or had one co-morbid disorder, primarily ODD (74%). Preschoolers with two co-morbid disorders had moderate treatment response and preschoolers with three or more co-morbid disorders did not respond to MPH treatment.

DISCLOSURES

The following financial disclosures indicate potential conflicts of interest among the PATS investigators and industry sources for the period 2000–2007, inclusive. [1]Honoraria/consultant, [2]research support, [3]speaker's bureau, [4]significant equity (>$50,000). Dr. Ghuman: Bristol Myers-Squibb.[2] Dr. Murray: Eli Lilly,[2] Pfizer.[2] Dr. Kollins: McNeil,[1,2,3] Shire,[1,2] Eli Lilly,[1,2] Pfizer,[2] New River Pharmaceuticals,[2] Psychogenics,[2] Athenagen,[1,2] Cephalon.[1] Dr. Greenhill: Celltech,[1,2] Cephalon,[1,2] Eli Lilly,[1,2] Janssen,[1] McNeil,[1,2] Medeva,[2] Novartis Corporation,[1,2] Noven,[1,2] Otsuka,[1,2] Pfizer,[1] Sanofi,[1] Shire,[1,2] Solvay,[1,2] Somerset,[2] Thomson Advanced Therapeutics Communications.[1] Dr. Swanson: Alza,[1,2] Celgene,[1,2] Celltech,[1,2,3] Cephalon,[1,2,3] Eli Lilly,[1,2] Gliatech,[1,2] Janssen,[1,2,3] McNeil,[1,2,3] Organon,[1] Novartis,[1,2] UCB, Shire.[1,2] Dr. Sharon Wigal: Celltech,[1,2,3] McNeil,[1,2,3] Cephalon,[1,2,3] Novartis,[1,2,3] Shire,[1,2,3] New River Pharmaceuticals,[2] Janssen,[3] Eli Lilly.[2] Dr. Abikoff: Abbot Labs,[1] Cephalon,[1] McNeil,[1,2] Shire,[1,2] Eli Lilly,[1,2] Pfizer,[2] Celltech,[2] and Novartis.[2] Dr. McCracken: Abbott, UCB, Novartis, Johnson & Johnson, Eli Lilly,[1,2,3] Gliatech,[2] Shire,[1,2] Pfizer,[1,2] McNeil,[1,2] Noven,[1] Bristol Meyers Squibb,[1] Janssen,[1,3] Wyeth.[1] Dr. Riddle: Shire,[1] Janssen,[1] Glaxo-Smith-Kline,[1] Astra-Zeneca,[1] Pfizer.[2] Dr. McGough: Eli Lilly,[1,2,3] McNeil,[1,2,3] Novartis,[1,2,3] Shire,[1,2,3] Pfizer,[1,2,3] and New River Pharmaceuticals.[2] Dr. Posner: As part of an effort to help execute the FDA suicidality classification mandates, Dr. Posner has had research support[2] from GlaxoSmithKline, Forest Laboratories, Eisai Inc., Astra Zeneca Pharmaceuticals, Johnson and Johnson, Abbott Laboratories, Wyeth Research, Organon USA, Bristol Meyers Squibb, Sanofi-Aventis, Cephalon, Novartis, Shire Pharmaceuticals and UCB Pharma, Shire.[1,2] Dr. Tim Wigal: Celltech,[2] Cephalon,[2] Eli Lilly,[2,3] Janssen,[2] McNeil,[2,3] Novartis,[2] Shire.[2,3] Mr. Davies: Merck,[4] GlaxoSmithKline,[4] Amgen,[4] Bard,[4] Pfizer,[4] Amgen,[4] Johnson & Johnson,[4] Wyeth.[4] Drs. Cunningham, Kastelic, Scharko, and Vitiello, and Ms. Chuang and Skrobala have no conflicts of interest or financial ties to disclose.

REFERENCES

Aman MG, Buican B, Arnold LE: Methylphenidate treatment in children with borderline IQ and mental retardation: analysis of three aggregated studies. J Child Adolesc Psychopharmacol 13:29–40, 2003.

American Psychiatric Association. Diagnostic and Statistical Manual of Mental Disorders, 4th ed. (DSM-IV).

Washington, DC, American Psychiatric Association, 1994.

Barkley RA, Karlsson J, Strzelecki E, Murphy JV: Effects of age and Ritalin dosage on the mother-child interactions of hyperactive children. J Consult Clin Psychol 52:750–758, 1984.

Barkley RA, Karlsson J, Pollard S, Murphy JV: Developmental changes in the mother-child interactions of hyperactive boys: Effects of two dose levels of Ritalin. J Child Psychol Psychiatry 26:705–715, 1985.

Barkley RA, Fischer M, Newby RF, Breen MJ: Development of a multimethod clinical protocol for assessing stimulant drug response in children with attention deficit disorder. J Clin Child Psychol 17:14–24, 1988.

Baron RM, Kenny DA: The moderator-mediator variable distinction in social psychological research: conceptual, strategic, and statistical considerations. J Pers Soc Psychol 51:1173–1182, 1986.

Berument S, Rutter M, Lord C, Pickles A, Bailey A: Autism Screening Questionnaire: Diagnostic validity, Br J Psychiatry 175:444–451, 1999.

Biederman J, Milberger S, Faraone SV, Kiely K, Guite J, Mick E, Ablon S, Warburton R, Reed E: Family-environment risk factors for attention-deficit hyperactivity disorder. A test of Rutter's indicators of adversity. Arch Gen Psychiatry 52:464–470, 1995.

Campbell SB: Parent-referred problem three-year-olds: developmental changes in symptoms. J Child Psychol Psychiatry 28:835–845, 1987.

Campbell SB, Ewing LJ: Follow-up of hard-to-manage preschoolers: Adjustment at age 9 and predictors of continuing symptoms. J Child Psychol Psychiatry 31: 871–889, 1990.

Chacko A, Pelham WE, Gnagy EM, Greiner A, Vallano G, Bukstein O, Rancurello M: Stimulant medication effects in a summer treatment program among young children with attention-deficit/hyperactivity disorder. J Am Acad Child Adolesc Psychiatry 44:249–257, 2005.

Cohen J. Statistical Power Analysis for the Behavioral Sciences. Lawrence Erlbaum Associates; 1988.

Conners CK: Controlled trial of methylphenidate in preschool-children with minimal brain-dysfunction. Int J Mental Health 4:61–74, 1975.

Conners CK. Conners' Rating Scales–Revised (CRS-R): Technical Manual. Multi-Health Systems, 2001.

Cunningham CE, Siegel LS, Offord DR: A developmental dose-response analysis of the effects of methylphenidate on the peer interactions of attention deficit disordered boys. J Child Psychol Psychiatry 26:955–971, 1985.

Curry J, Rohde P, Simons A, Silva S, Vitiello B, Kratochvil C, Reinecke M, Feeny N, Wells K, Pathak S, Weller E, Rosenberg D, Kennard B, Robins M, Ginsburg G, March J: Predictors and moderators of acute outcome in the Treatment for Adolescents with Depression Study (TADS). J Am Acad Child Adolesc Psychiatry 45:1427–1439, 2006.

DuPaul GJ, McGoey KE, Eckert TL, VanBrakle J: Preschool children with attention-deficit/hyperactivity disorder: Impairments in behavioral, social, and school functioning. J Am Acad Child Adolesc Psychiatry 40:508–515, 2001.

Egger HL, Angold A: Common emotional and behavioral disorders in preschool children: Presentation, nosology, and epidemiology. J Child Psychol Psychiatry 47:313–337, 2006.

Elliott CD. Differential Ability Scales. The Psychological Corporation, Harcourt Brace Jovanovich, 1990.

Fischer M, Newby RF: Assessment of stimulant response in ADHD children using a refined multimethod clinical protocol. J Clin Child Psychol 20:232–244, 1991.

Greenhill L, Kollins S, Abikoff H, McCracken J, Riddle M, Swanson J, McGough J, Wigal S, Wigal T, Vitiello B, Skrobala A, Posner K, Ghuman J, Cunningham C, Davies M, Chuang S, Cooper T: Efficacy and safety of immediate-release methylphenidate treatment for preschoolers with ADHD. J Am Acad Child Adolesc Psychiatry 45:1284–1293, 2006.

Greenhill LL, Pliszka S, Dulcan MK, Bernet W, Arnold V, Beitchman J, Benson RS, Bukstein O, Kinlan J, McClellan J, Rue D, Shaw JA, Stock S: Practice parameter for the use of stimulant medications in the treatment of children, adolescents, and adults. J Am Acad Child Adolesc Psychiatry 41:26S–49S, 2002.

Guy W. ECDEU Assessment Manual for Psychopharmacology. U.S. Department of Health, Education, and Welfare, Public Health Service, Alcohol, Drug Abuse, and Mental Health Administration, National Institute of Mental Health, Psychopharmacology Research Branch, Division of Extramural Research Programs, 1976.

Handen BL, Feldman HM, Lurier A, Murray PJ: Efficacy of methylphenidate among preschool children with developmental disabilities and ADHD. J Am Acad Child Adolesc Psychiatry 38:805–812, 1999.

Kazdin AE, Mazurick JL: Dropping out of child psychotherapy: Distinguishing early and late dropouts over the course of treatment. J Consult Clin Psychol 62:1069–1074, 1994.

Kollins S, Greenhill L, Swanson J, Wigal S, Abikoff H, McCracken J, Riddle M, McGough J, Vitiello B, Wigal T, Skrobala A, Posner K, Ghuman J, Davies M, Cunningham C, Bauzo A: Rationale, design, and methods of the Preschool ADHD Treatment Study (PATS). J Am Acad Child Adolesc Psychiatry 45:1275–1283, 2006.

Kraemer HC, Wilson GT, Fairburn CG, Agras WS: Mediators and moderators of treatment effects in randomized clinical trials. Arch Gen Psychiatry 59:877–883, 2002.

Kraemer HC, Frank E, Kupfer DJ: Moderators of treatment outcomes: clinical, research, and policy importance. JAMA 296:1286–1289, 2006.

Lahey BB, Pelham WE, Stein MA, Loney J, Trapani C, Nugent K, Kipp H, Schmidt E, Lee S, Cale M, Gold E, Hartung CM, Willcutt E, Baumann B: Validity of DSM-IV attention-deficit/hyperactivity disorder for younger children. J Am Acad Child Adolesc Psychiatry 37: 695–702, 1998.

Lahey BB, Pelham WE, Loney J, Kipp H, Ehrhardt A, Lee SS, Willcutt EG, Hartung CM, Chronis A, Massetti G: Three-year predictive validity of DSM-IV attention deficit hyperactivity disorder in children diagnosed at 4–6 years of age. Am J Psychiatry 161:2014–2020, 2004.

Lavigne JV, Gibbons RD, Christoffel KK, Arend R, Rosenbaum D, Binns H, Dawson N, Sobel H, Isaacs C: Prevalence rates and correlates of psychiatric disorders among preschool children. J Am Acad Child Adolesc Psychiatry 35:204–214, 1996.

Martenyi F, Dossenbach M, Mraz K, Metcalfe S: Gender differences in the efficacy of fluoxetine and maprotiline in depressed patients: A double-blind trial of antidepressants with serotonergic or norepinhrinergic reuptake inhibition profile. Eur Neuropsychopharmacol 11:227–232, 2001.

Mayes SD, Crites DL, Bixler EO, Humphrey FJ, 2nd, Mattison RE: Methylphenidate and ADHD: influence of age, IQ and neurodevelopmental status. Dev Med Child Neurol 36:1099–1107, 1994.

McCracken JT, Smalley SL, McGough JJ, Crawford L, Del'Homme M, Cantor RM, Liu A, Nelson SF: Evidence for linkage of a tandem duplication polymorphism upstream of the dopamine D 4 receptor gene(DRD 4) with attention deficit hyperactivity disorder(ADHD). Molecular Psychiatry 5:531–536, 2000.

MTA: A 14-month randomized clinical trial of treatment strategies for attention-deficit/hyperactivity disorder. The MTA Cooperative Group. Multimodal Treatment Study of Children with ADHD. Arch Gen Psychiatry 56:1073–1086, 1999a.

MTA: Moderators and mediators of treatment response for children with attention-deficit/hyperactivity disorder: the Multimodal Treatment Study of children with Attention-deficit/hyperactivity disorder. Arch Gen Psychiatry 56:1088–1096, 1999b.

Musten LM, Firestone P, Pisterman S, Bennett S, Mercer J: Effects of methylphenidate on preschool children with ADHD: Cognitive and behavioral functions. J Am Acad Child Adolesc Psychiatry 36:1407–1415, 1997.

Owens EB, Hinshaw SP, Kraemer HC, Arnold LE, Abikoff HB, Cantwell DP, Conners CK, Elliott G, Greenhill LL, Hechtman L, Hoza B, Jensen PS, March JS, Newcorn JH, Pelham WE, Severe JB, Swanson JM, Vitiello B, Wells KC, Wigal T: Which treatment for whom for ADHD? Moderators of treatment response in the MTA. J Consult Clin Psychol 71:540–552, 2003.

Pierce EW, Ewing LJ, Campbell SB: Diagnostic status and symptomatic behavior of hard-to-manage preschool children in middle childhood and early adolescence. J Clin Child Psychol 28:44–57, 1999.

Posner K, Melvin GA, Murray DW, Gugga SS, Fisher P, Skrobala A, Cunningham C, Vitiello B, Abikoff HB, Ghuman JK, Kollins S, Wigal SB, Wigal T, McCracken JT, McGough JJ, Kastelic E, Boorady R, Davies M, Chuang SZ, Swanson JM, Riddle MA, Greenhill LL, Clinical Presentation of Moderate to Severe ADHD in Preschool Children: The Preschoolers with Attention-Deficit/Hyperactivity Disorder Treatment Study (PATS). J Child Adolesc Psychopharmacol, 17:547–562, 2007.

Rosenthal R, Rosnow RL, Rubin DB. Contrasts and Effect Sizes in Behavioral Research: A Correlational Approach. Cambridge University Press, 2000.

Ryan ND, Varma D: Child and adolescent mood disorders—experience with serotonin-based therapies. Biol Psychiatry 44:336–340, 1998.

Schachar R, Jadad AR, Gauld M, Boyle M, Booker L, Snider A, Kim M, Cunningham C: Attention-deficit hyperactivity disorder: Critical appraisal of extended treatment studies. Can J Psychiatry 47:337–348, 2002.

Shaffer D, Gould MS, Brasic J, Ambrosini P, Fisher P, Bird H, Aluwahlia S: A children's global assessment scale (CGAS). Arch Gen Psychiatry 40:1228–1231, 1983.

Shaffer D, Fisher P, Dulcan MK, Davies M, Piacentini J, Schwab-Stone ME, Lahey BB, Bourdon K, Jensen PS, Bird HR, Canino G, Regier DA: The NIMH Diagnostic Interview Schedule for Children Version 2.3 (DISC-2.3): Description, acceptability, prevalence rates, and performance in the MECA Study. Methods for the Epidemiology of Child and Adolescent Mental Disorders Study. J Am Acad Child Adolesc Psychiatry 35:865–877, 1996.

Short EJ, Manos MJ, Findling RL, Schubel EA: A prospective study of stimulant response in preschool children: insights from ROC analyses. J Am Acad Child Adolesc Psychiatry 43:251–259, 2004.

Sparrow SS, Balla DA, Cicchetti DV, Doll EA. Vineland Adaptive Behavior Scales: Interview Edition, Survey Form Manual. American Guidance Service, 1984.

Swanson JM. School-based Assessments and Interventions for ADD Students. KC Publishing, 1992.

Swanson JM, Kraemer HC, Hinshaw SP, Arnold LE, Conners CK, Abikoff HB, Clevenger W, Davies M, Elliott GR, Greenhill LL, Hechtman L, Hoza B, Jensen PS, March JS, Newcorn JH, Owens EB, Pelham WE, Schiller E, Severe JB, Simpson S, Vitiello B, Wells K, Wigal T, Wu M: Clinical relevance of the primary findings of the MTA: success rates based on severity of ADHD and ODD symptoms at the end of treatment. J Am Acad Child Adolesc Psychiatry 40:168–179, 2001.

Vitiello B, Jensen PS, Hoagwood K: Integrating science and ethics in child and adolescent psychiatry research. Biol Psychiatry 46:1044–1049, 1999.

Wigal SB, Gupta S, Guinta D, Swanson JM: Reliability and validity of the SKAMP rating scale in a laboratory school setting. Psychopharmacol Bull 34:47–53, 1998.

Wilens TE, Biederman J, Brown S, Tanguay S, Monuteaux MC, Blake C, Spencer TJ: Psychiatric comorbidity and functioning in clinically referred preschool children and school-age youths with ADHD. J Am Acad Child Adolesc Psychiatry 41:262–268, 2002a.

Wilens TE, Biederman J, Spencer TJ: Attention deficit/hyperactivity disorder across the lifespan. Annu Rev Med 53:113–131, 2002b.

Wood AJ: Ethnic differences in drug disposition and response. Ther Drug Monit 20:525–526, 1998.

ADVANCES IN PRESCHOOL PSYCHOPHARMACOLOGY
© 2009 Mary Ann Liebert, Inc.
140 Huguenot Street, 3rd Floor
New Rochelle, NY 10801-5215

Methylphenidate Effects on Functional Outcomes in the Preschoolers with Attention-Deficit/Hyperactivity Disorder Treatment Study (PATS)

Howard B. Abikoff, Ph.D.,[1] Benedetto Vitiello, M.D., M.S.,[2] Mark A. Riddle, M.D.,[3]
Charles Cunningham, Ph.D.,[4] Laurence L. Greenhill, M.D.,[5] James M. Swanson, Ph.D.,[6]
Shirley Z. Chuang, M.S.,[7] Mark Davies, M.P.H.,[5] Elizabeth Kastelic, M.D.,[3]
Sharon B. Wigal, Ph.D.,[6] Lori Evans, Ph.D.,[1] Jaswinder K. Ghuman, M.D.,[8] M.D.,
Scott H. Kollins, Ph.D.,[9] James T. McCracken, M.D.,[10] James J. McGough, M.D.,[10]
Desiree W. Murray, Ph.D.,[9] Kelly Posner, Ph.D.,[5] Anne M. Skrobala, M.A.,[5]
and Tim Wigal, Ph.D.[6]

ABSTRACT

Objective: **The purpose of this study was to examine the effects of methylphenidate (MPH) on functional outcomes, including children's social skills, classroom behavior, emotional status, and parenting stress, during the 4-week, double-blind placebo controlled phase of the Preschoolers with Attention Deficit/Hyperactivity Disorder (ADHD) Treatment Study (PATS).**

Methods: **A total of 114 preschoolers who had improved with acute MPH treatment, were randomized to their best MPH dose ($M = 14.22$ mg/day; $n = 63$) or placebo (PL; $n = 51$). Assessments included the Clinical Global Impression-Severity (CGI-S), parent and teacher ver-**

[1]New York University Child Study Center, New York, New York.
[2]National Institute of Mental Health,
[3]Johns Hopkins University, Baltimore, Maryland.
[4]McMaster University, Hamilton, Ontario.
[5]New York State Psychiatric Institute/Columbia University, New York, New York.
[6]University of California Irvine, Irvine, California.
[7]No current affiliation, formerly at New York State Psychiatric Institute/Columbia University.
[8]University of Arizona, Tucson, Arizona.
[9]Duke University Medical Center; Durham, North Carolina.
[10]University of California Los Angeles, Los Angeles, California.
Statistical consultants: Shirley Z. Chuang, M.S., Mark Davies, M.P.H. Ms. Chuang has no current affiliation; she was formerly at New York State Psychiatric Institute/Columbia University. Mr. Davies is affiliated with New York State Psychiatric Institute/Columbia University.

This research was supported by a cooperative agreement grants between the National Institute of Mental Health and the following institutions: Johns Hopkins University (U01 MH60642), NYSPI/Columbia University (U01 MH60903), University of California, Irvine (U01 MH60833), Duke University Medical Center (U01 MH60848), New York University Child Study Center (U01 MH60943), and University of California, Los Angeles (U01 MH60900); and by NIMH K23 MH01883-01A1 and Arizona Institute of Mental Health Research to J.K.G.

The opinions and assertions contained in this report are the private views of the authors and are not to be construed as official or as reflecting the views of the Department of Health and Human Services, the National Institutes of Health, or the National Institute of Mental Health.

sions of the Strengths and Weaknesses of ADHD-Symptoms and Normal Behaviors (SWAN), Social Competence Scale (SCS), Social Skills Rating System (SSRS), and Early Childhood Inventory (ECI), and Parenting Stress Index (PSI).

Results: Medication effects varied by informant and outcome measure. Parent measures and teacher SWAN scores did not differentially improve with MPH. Parent-rated depression ($p <$ 0.02) and dysthymia ($p < 0.001$) on the ECI worsened with MPH, but scores were not in the clinical range. Significant medication effects were found on clinician CGI-S ($p < 0.0001$) and teacher social competence ratings (SCS, $p < 0.03$).

Conclusions: Preschoolers with ADHD treated with MPH for 4 weeks improve in some aspects of functioning. Additional improvements might require longer treatment, higher doses, and/or intensive behavioral treatment in combination with medication.

INTRODUCTION

THE DIAGNOSIS OF attention-deficit/hyperactivity disorder (ADHD) is most commonly made in middle childhood, although onset during preschool years is typical. In contrast to an extensive treatment literature regarding the efficacy of psychostimulants in elementary school-aged children with ADHD, only a small number of such studies have been conducted with preschoolers. The efficacy of psychostimulants in reducing ADHD symptoms in preschoolers was first reported in the 1970s (Conners 1975; Schleifer et al. 1975). With few exceptions (Cohen 1981; Barkley et al. 1984), subsequent placebo-controlled studies, although varying in design, quality, and size, have confirmed medication effects on symptoms of ADHD. Monteiro-Musten et al. (1997) found that stimulants increased preschoolers' attention and decreased impulsiveness. Byrne et al. (1998) reported that stimulants improved behavior and significantly reduced errors of omission on visual and auditory vigilance tests. Short et al. (2004) found a clinically significant reduction in ADHD symptoms in 82% ($n = 28$) of preschoolers treated with stimulants. Findings from the National Institute of Mental Health (NIMH) multisite Preschoolers with ADHD Treatment Study (PATS) indicated that immediate release methylphenidate (MPH-IR), delivered in 2.5-, 5.0-, and 7.5-mg doses three times a day (t.i.d.), yielded significant reductions on ADHD symptom scales compared to placebo (Greenhill et al. 2006).

School-aged and preschool children with ADHD share not only a common symptom profile, but also a similar pattern of associated functional deficits and impairments (Sonuga-Barke et al. 2003). Both age groups have deficits in social skills, especially in social cooperation (Merrell and Wolfe 1998) and friendships (Lahey et al. 1998). They also experience problematic interactions with their parents and other relatives (DuPaul et al. 2001; Daley et al. 2003) that contribute to high levels of familial stress, which in turn exacerbate mental health problems among family members (DeWolfe et al. 2000).

Notably, functional impairments, especially in social functioning and parent–child interactions, as well as deficient regulation of emotions and problematic classroom behavior, typically result in clinic referrals in children with ADHD. Medication has been shown to improve these functional domains in elementary school-aged children with ADHD (MTA Cooperative Group 1999; Abikoff et al. 2004; Hechtman et al. 2004); however, information regarding medication effects on these aspects of functioning in preschoolers with ADHD is sparse and inconclusive. Acute MPH treatment has been reported to reduce the observed frequency of controlling and dominating peer interactions in 4–6 year olds with ADHD in a simulated classroom setting (Cunningham et al. 1985). Barkley (1988) reported that stimulants improved the quality of interactions between preschoolers and their mothers, whereas Monteiro-Musten et al. (1997) found that, although stimulants improved adjustment, they did not increase compliance with parental requests.

In recognition of the need to characterize the impact of stimulants on clinically relevant aspects of functioning in preschoolers with ADHD, the PATS trial evaluated the effects of MPH on children's social skills, classroom behavior, emotional status, and parenting stress. We hypothesized that medication effects in preschoolers with ADHD would parallel those found in school-aged children. Specifically, it was hypothesized that: (1) compared to children randomized to placebo (PL), preschoolers randomized to their "best dose" of MPH would show significant improvements in classroom behavior, social, and emotional functioning; and (2) parents of children receiving MPH would show significant reduction in parenting stress compared to parents of children on PL.

METHODS

Detailed descriptions of the PATS design and methods are provided elsewhere (Greenhill et al. 2006; Kollins et al. 2006); therefore, only key study features are presented here.

Subjects

Participants had to meet the following criteria: Stimulant-naive children of both sexes, ages 3–5.5 years with a *Diagnostic and Statistical Manual of Mental Disorders,* Fourth Edition (DSM-IV) consensus diagnosis of ADHD (American Psychiatric Association, 1994), combined or predominantly hyperactive subtype, based on the Diagnostic Interview Schedule for Children IV–Parent Version (DISC-IV-P) (Shaffer et al. 1996) and semistructured interview; an impairment scale score ≤ 55 on the Children's Global Assessment Scale (C-GAS) (Shaffer et al. 1983); hyperactive-impulsive subscale T score of 65 (1.5 SD above age- and sex-adjusted means) on both the Conners Revised Parent (CPRS) (Conners et al. 1998a) and Teacher (CTRS) (Conners et al. 1998b) Rating Scales; full scale intelligence quotient (IQ) > 70 on the Differential Ability Scales (DAS; Elliott 1990); participation in a preschool, day-care group setting or other school program at least 2 half-days per week with at least 8 same-age peers; and the same primary caretaker for at least 6 months prior to screening.

Exclusion criteria included current evidence of adjustment disorder, pervasive developmental disorders, psychosis, significant suicidality, or other psychiatric disorder that required treatment with additional medication; current stimulant or cocaine abuse in a relative living in the home; a confounding medical condition; inability of the parent to understand or follow study instructions; or history of bipolar disorder in both biological parents.

Study design

The PATS design consisted of several phases, detailed in Kollins et al. (2006). Briefly, 183 preschoolers who failed to improve significantly after parent participation in a 10-week parent training program, and whose parents consented to a medication trial for their youngsters, entered an open-label, lead-in phase to determine if they could tolerate doses of MPH used in the subsequent double-blind phases. Children ($n = 165$) who tolerated the lead-in doses entered the study's 5-week double-blind, within-subject, placebo-controlled, crossover-design, titration phase, and 147 children were randomized to, and completed, all five sequences of active MPH (1.25, 2.5, 5, 7.5 mg) and PL administered t.i.d.. At the end of each week, school and home behavior and side effects ratings were obtained from teachers and parents. At the conclusion of the 5-week trial, these weekly ratings were reviewed by two independent clinicians, blind to dosing information, who generated a consensus decision regarding each child's best dose. Following this crossover phase, children went on to participate in the between-subjects, randomized, 4-week, double-blind, parallel design study phase of the PATS trial, wherein they were randomized to either their best dose of MPH or PL. The parallel-design phase, unlike the preceding titration phase, included assessments of functional outcomes. Findings on these outcomes are reported here.

The study protocol and parental informed consent forms were approved by the institutional review boards at the six recruiting sites. The study was monitored by the Data and Safety Monitoring Board of the National Institute of Mental Health.

TABLE 1. DEMOGRAPHIC AND CLINICAL CHARACTERISTICS OF THE SAMPLE AT BASELINE

Variable	Best dose (n = 61)	Placebo (n = 53)
Age, years mean (SD)	4.39 (0.72)	4.45 (0.67)
Male, n (%)	49 (80.33)	36 (67.92)
Ethnicity, n (%)		
White	36 (59.02)	38 (71.70)
Black or African American	12 (19.67)	7 (13.21)
Hispanic or Latino	12 (19.67)	7 (13.21)
Other	1 (1.64)	1 (1.19)
High school graduate, n (%)		
Mother	58/60 (96.67)	49/51 (96.08)
Father	48/49 (97.96)	43/44 (97.73)
Employed, n (%)		
Mother	48/59 (81.36)	32/51 (62.75)
Father	44/58 (75.86)	36/51 (70.59)
Welfare, n (%)	5/53 (9.43)	2/45 (4.44)
Married, n (%)	35/60 (58.33)	33/52 (63.46)
Hollingshead SES, mean (SD)	46.65 (9.17)	48.75 (9.76)
Family Composition, n (%)		
2 Parents	50 (81.97)	42 (79.25)
1 Parent	11 (18.03)	11 (20.75)
CTRS, mean (SD)		
Inattention	15.00 (5.41)	14.65 (6.29)
Hyperactivity[a]	21.44 (4.12)	19.51 (5.12)
Total	36.56 (8.08)	34.24 (9.60)
CPRS, mean (SD)		
Inattention	16.95 (5.09)	18.34 (5.17)
Hyperactivity	22.00 (3.57)	22.62 (3.40)
Total	39.02 (7.31)	41.02 (7.62)
DAS IQ, mean (SD)	98.86 (16.84)	95.75 (15.17)
C-GAS Impairment Scale, mean (SD)	47.15 (4.42)	47.55 (3.93)
ADHD Subtype, n (%)		
Hyperactive-Impulsive	18 (29.51)	11 (20.75)
Combined	43 (70.49)	42 (70.25)

CTRS = Conners Teacher Rating Scale; CPRS = Conners Parent Rating Scale; DAS = Differential Ability Scale; C-GAS = Children's Global Assessment Scale; SD = standard deviation; IQ = intelligence quotient; SES = socio-economic status.

[a]$p < 0.04$, all other comparisons nonsignificant.

Participants

A total of 114 children participated in the parallel design study phase of the PATS: 61 were randomized to MPH and 53 to PL. Their characteristics are summarized in Table 1.

Domains and measures

ADHD behavior. Strengths and Weaknesses of ADHD-Symptoms and Normal Behaviors. The common occurrence of ADHD behaviors in preschoolers results in over-estimates of such behaviors with conventional ADHD rating scales. The SWAN's 7-point metric (from −3 "far above average" to +3 "far below average") of strengths and weaknesses of ADHD-Symptoms and Normal Behaviors (SWAN) was designed to protect against over-estimates

of ADHD behaviors, and yields ratings of preschool children's ADHD behaviors that are normally distributed, such that average, unaffected children would receive ratings of "0," which indicates no particular attentional or impulsive/motor problems compared to other children of the same age. Teacher and parent versions of the SWAN were used in the study (Swanson et al. 2001; Cornish et al. 2005).

Social behavior. Social Skills Rating System. The Social Skills Rating System (SSRS) is a standardized scale that assesses social functioning. Preschool and School-age parent (SSRS-P) and teacher (SSRS-T) versions are available (Gresham and Elliott 1990). The SSRS-P comprises 70 items, 60 of which assess prosocial skills and 10 assess problem behaviors. Fifty of the prosocial items overlap with the SSRS-T and the other 10 address social situations at home. The Total Social Skills score served as the study outcome measure, with higher scores indicating better functioning. Reliability and validity have been established (Gresham and Elliott, 1990).

Social Competence Scale. The 12-item parent (SCS-P) and teacher (SCS-T) versions of the Social Competence Scale Scale assess frustration tolerance, peer relationships, communication skills, and empathy (Conduct Problems Prevention Research Group 1992). The Total score served as the study outcome measure, with higher scores indicating more competence. The scale has demonstrated sensitivity to treatment effects in preschoolers (Webster-Stratton 1998).

Parental stress. Parenting Stress Index. The Parenting Stress Index (PSI) is a 101-item, 5-point Likert scale that measures stressful child, parental, relational, and situational characteristics (Abidin 1995). The Total score on the Parent Domain, which taps depression, attachment, restriction of role, sense of competence, social isolation, relation with spouse, and parent health, served as the outcome measure. Internal consistency and concurrent and discriminant validity have been documented. The scale has been shown to be sensitive to treatment effects in children with conduct disorders (Kazdin and Whitley, 2003).

Mood. Early Child Inventory. The Early Child Inventory (ECI) is a 108-item inventory that has been normed on preschool children, and the parent (ECI-P) and teacher (ECI-T) versions have acceptable reliability and validity data (Gadow and Sprafin, 1996; Sprafkin et al. 2002). The items assess behaviors and symptoms associated with a wide-range of childhood mental disorders. Scores on the two Mood Scales, Dysthymic Disorder and Major Depressive Disorder, served as outcome measures.

Severity of illness. Clinical Global Impressions–Severity. The Clinical Global Impressions–Severity (CGI-S) is a clinician completed 7-point rating scale (1 = not at all ill to 7 = among the most extremely ill) that assesses the child's current level of severity of illness (Guy 1976). The scale has adequate psychometric

properties (American Psychiatric Association, 2000) and is one of the most widely used outcome measures in psychopharmacology trials.

Data analyses

Measures were obtained at baseline at the beginning of the PATS trial (prior to initiation of medication) and at the end of the 4-week, double-blind, parallel design study phase. For participants who did not complete the 4-week phase, efforts were made to obtain outcome scores at the time of dropout. Data analysis was based on intent-to-treat, last observation carried forward (LOCF) procedures. Analyses of covariance of fixed effects, using baseline scores as the covariate, were conducted to evaluate medication effects on the study measures. Effect sizes (ES), using Cohen's d, were calculated for each outcome measure by dividing the difference between the post-treatment group means by the pooled SD.

The CGI-S, completed by the clinician at the end of each subject's participation in the parallel-design phase, was obtained on the full sample. Data on other measures were missing from some parents, and to a greater extent, from teachers. An *a priori* decision was made to analyze measures for which scores were available on at least half of the sample that entered the double-blind (DB) efficacy trial. Consequently, the teacher-completed ECI, which was unavailable on 60% of the sample (38 in the MPH group [62.6 %] and 30 in the PL group [56.6 %]) and the teacher-completed SSRS, missing for 51% of the sample (31 in the MPH group [50.8 %] and 27 in the PL group [50.1%]), were not analyzed. Descriptive statistics, analysis of covariance (ANCOVA) results and effect sizes are presented in Table 2.

RESULTS

Sample retention

Of the 114 children who entered the 4-week parallel-design phase, 36 (32%) dropped out. Of these, 33 had behavioral deterioration [24 were in the PL group (24/53, 45%), and 9 in the MPH group (9/61, 15%)], 2 declined study participation, and 1 had medication related ad-

TABLE 2. COMPARISON OF TREATMENT GROUPS ON STUDY OUTCOME MEASURES AT IMMEDIATE POSTTREATMENT

Outcome measure	N	Best dose ($n = 61$) Baseline mean (SD)	Best dose ($n = 61$) Posttreatment mean (SD)	n	Placebo ($n = 53$) Baseline mean (SD)	Placebo ($n = 53$) Posttreatment mean (SD)	ANCOVA treatment effect $F_{(NDF, DDF)}$	p <	Effect size
SWAN Parent[a]									
Total ADHD	48	1.66 (0.65)	1.09 (0.72)	38	1.83 (0.61)	1.41 (0.77)	2.09$_{(1, 78)}$	NS	0.43
Inattention	48	1.37 (0.82)	0.92 (0.81)	37	1.63 (0.72)	1.28 (0.86)	1.51$_{(1, 77)}$	NS	0.43
Hyp-Imp	47	1.92 (0.62)	1.26 (0.81)	38	2.04 (0.74)	1.52 (0.79)	1.41$_{(1, 77)}$	NS	0.32
SWAN Teacher[a]									
total ADHD	32	1.39 (0.58)	1.09 (0.80)	32	1.41 (0.79)	1.35 (0.77)	2.20$_{(1, 56)}$	NS	0.32
Inattention	31	1.10 (0.59)	0.85 (0.88)	32	1.31 (081)	1.14 (0.81)	0.86$_{(1, 55)}$	NS	0.34
Hyp-Imp	32	1.70 (0.71)	1.35 (0.87)	33	1.53 (0.95)	1.58 (0.89)	3.37$_{(1, 57)}$	0.08	0.27
Parent ECI[a]									
MDD	35	4.00 (2.36)	5.53 (2.85)	26	4.71 (2.86)	4.06 (2.46)	6.52$_{(1, 53)}$	0.02	0.55
Dysthymic	35	3.04 (1.85)	4.49 (2.56)	26	3.83 (2.49)	2.98 (1.74)	12.22$_{(1, 53)}$	0.001	0.67
CGI-S[a]	61	4.77 (0.59)	3.74 (1.09)	53	4.68 (0.51)	4.47 (0.89)	18.85$_{(1, 106)}$	0.001	0.73
PSI–Total Stress[a]	45	75.27 (27.36)	67.29 (32.84)	33	82.27 (23.77)	76.70 (24.76)	0.82$_{(1, 70)}$	NS	0.32
SCS–Parent[b]	50	1.16 (0.55)	1.43 (0.62)	37	1.23 (0.59)	1.36 (0.57)	1.44$_{(1, 79)}$	NS	0.13
SCS–Teacher[b]	31	1.14 (0.59)	1.56 (0.82)	31	1.31 (0.72)	1.27 (0.63)	5.17$_{(1, 54)}$	0.03	0.39
SSRS Parent[b]	44	84.48 (12.42)	89.41 (13.66)	31	81.52 (16.38)	87.39 (15.75)	0.00$_{(1, 67)}$	NS	0.14

[a]Lower scores indicate better outcome.

[b]Higher scores indicate better outcome.

SWAN = Strengths and Weaknesses of ADHD-Symptoms and Normal Behaviors; Hyp-Imp = Hyperactive/Impulsive scale; ECI = Early Child Inventory; MDD = major depressive disorder; CGI-S = Clinical Global Impressions-Severity; PSI = Parenting Stress Index; SCS = Social Compentence Scale; SSRS = Social Skills Rating System; ADHD = attention-deficit/hyperactivity disorder; SD = standard deviation; NS = not significant; ANCOVA = analysis of covariants.

verse effects. Nineteen children dropped out in week 1 (15 on PL, 4 on MPH), 13 in week 2 (PL = 8, MPH = 5) and one in week 3 (PL). Analyses comparing the baseline characteristics of completers and non-completers indicated no significant differences.

ADHD behavior

On the SWAN, the MPH and PL groups did not differ significantly in parent or teacher ratings of total ADHD or inattention, or parent ratings of hyperactivity/impulsivity, with scores improving in both groups from pre to post. However, teacher ratings of hyperactivity/impulsivity indicated a trend ($p = 0.08$; ES = 0.27) in favor of the MPH group.

Social behavior

Children's social competence and social skills, based on parent ratings on the SCS and SSRS, respectively, did not differ significantly between the groups. A significant treatment effect ($p < 0.03$; ES = 0.39) was found in teacher ratings on the SCS, with preschoolers treated with medication improving in their social competence scores, whereas those on placebo showing no change from pre to post.

Parental stress

There was no significant difference in the PSI ratings of parents of children in the MPH and PL groups, with the mean Total scores decreasing in both groups from pre to post.

Mood

Compared to preschoolers treated with PL, children in the MPH group had significantly higher mood scores on the parent rated ECI Major Depressive Disorder ($p < 0.02$) and Dysthymic scales ($p < 0.001$). The group difference reflected an increase in mood symptoms from pre- to posttreatment with MPH in contrast to a decrease over time with PL (see Table 2). Subsequent item analyses of the mood symptoms comprising these two ECI scales indicated that the item "Has become more sensitive or tearful than usual" was the only symptom that significantly differentiated MPH from PL ($p < 0.003$).

Severity of illness

Clinicians' global ratings of severity on the CGI-S at posttreatment were significantly lower for children in the MPH group compared to those on PL ($p < 0.0001$; ES = 0.73).

DISCUSSION

Contrary to expectations, the effects of MPH on functional outcomes in preschoolers did not parallel the functional improvements reported in elementary school-aged youngsters with ADHD treated with MPH. Rather, in the current study, medication effects varied as a function of informant and outcome measure. The absence of MPH effects was most evident on parent measures. Preschoolers' social skills and social competence, as well as their level of ADHD behaviors on the SWAN, did not improve differentially with medication on the basis of parent ratings. Similarly, self-ratings of parental stress were not significantly different in parents of children treated with MPH or PL. Moreover, parents' ratings of their children's mood symptoms indicated a worsening of symptoms with medication. In contrast, positive medication effects were detected in clinicians' global severity ratings and in teachers' ratings of improved social competence in children on MPH. However, like parents, teachers' ratings of ADHD behaviors on the SWAN were not differentially related to the children's medication status.

A variety of factors need to be considered in interpreting the study outcomes. Forty five percent of the children in the PL group dropped out before the end of the 4-week treatment phase because of behavioral deterioration, compared to 15% of children receiving MPH. At dropout, efforts to obtain outcome measures, which were intended to serve as LOCF data, were not always successful. Consequently, the power to detect treatment differences was decreased because of the reduced sample size available for analysis.

The lack of terminal data on all dropouts precludes an explication of the exact nature of the "behavioral deterioration" in these youngsters. In the PATS primary efficacy paper (Greenhill et al. 2006), we reported that attrition during the parallel group double-blind phase "was significantly correlated with elevated SNAP scores ($p < 0.009$)" (p. 1291), indicating that children withdrawn from the study had an increase in ADHD symptoms. It is unknown if these dropouts also showed an increase in functional impairment. To the extent that they did, the results reported here may be underestimates of MPH effects on functional outcomes. However, it is important to emphasize that the association between ADHD symptom severity and degree of functional impairment has been reported to be relatively small, with symptom severity predicting less than 25% of the variance in impairment in four separate studies (Gordon et al. 2006).

An underestimation of MPH effects could have also occurred if the completers were less functionally impaired on placebo than those who dropped out of the PL group. Here too, the absence of terminal ratings precludes a direct test of this possibility. However, as an indirect test of this notion, we examined if the completers and dropouts had a differential response to placebo during the preceding double-blind titration phase. Independent t-tests indicated no significant differences (p values ranged from 0.32 to 0.82) in the subgroups' scores on the parent and teacher Connors, Loney, and Milich (CLAM) and Swanson, Kotkin, Atkins, M-Flynn, and Pelhan (SKAMP) ADHD rating scales during the titration week when each child was on placebo.

The higher-than-expected rate of premature treatment discontinuation may be related to the multistage, sequential design of PATS. Children participating in the placebo-controlled trial reported here had previously completed a within-subject titration showing superiority of MPH over placebo at the individual patient level. Parents' experience during the titration phase presumably heightened their awareness of the behavioral differences associated with active and placebo medication. Such knowledge, in conjunction with study guidelines that allowed parents to forego or discontinue participation in the double-blind, parallel-group phase and have their child move directly to open maintenance treatment with MPH, likely contributed to dropout decisions for some parents.

We considered the possibility that the dropouts in the PL group showed more improvement with medication during titration than did the completers in the PL group, increasing the likelihood of dropout. To this end, we compared these two subgroups' parent and teacher scores on the CLAM and SKAMP ADHD rating scales when they were on their optimal dose of MPH during titration. The PL dropouts and completers did not differ significantly on any of these measures.

The MPH doses in the double-blind parallel group study phase were relatively low (M = 14.22 ± 8.1 mg/day), which may have limited functional improvements Findings from the PATS maintenance phase (Vitiello et al., this issue), provide some support for this notion. For example, the increase in children's MPH doses from the first to the tenth month of maintenance treatment (M = 19.98 ± 9.56 mg/day) was associated with improvements in children's social skills as rated by parents. These results must be tempered because of the absence of an untreated group as a temporal control. However, future studies might explore the possibility that children's social functioning is facilitated with higher doses.

Although MPH resulted in a significant increase in scores on the Major Depressive Disorder and Dysthymic Disorder scales on the ECI compared to PL, the scores were not in the clinical range. The higher score in the medication group on the item "Has become more sensitive or tearful than usual" likely reflects the significant increase in emotional outbursts/crying with MPH compared to PL reported in the initial titration phase of the study (Wigal et al. 2006). Notably, the frequency of emotional outbursts/crying decreased significantly during the 10-month maintenance period, even though the mean MPH total daily dose increased during this period (Wigal et al. 2006). A similar pattern of findings has been reported in 7- to 9-year-old children with ADHD, who showed initial increases in their Children's Depression Inventory scores after 5 weeks of MPH treatment, followed by a significant decrease in CDI scores after 6 months of treatment with MPH (Hechtman et al. 2004).

Teachers, unlike parents, reported gains in social competence with MPH. Poor concordance rates for parent and teacher ratings of ADHD symptoms in the PATS sample has been reported by Murray et al. (this issue). The lack of agreement between parent and teacher ratings of children's behavior is well established, and, in children with ADHD, it is considered to reflect the variability of children's behaviors across situations (McDermott et al. 2005). Relatedly, contextual factors could have facilitated teachers' ability to detect medication related changes in social competence, because they had more opportunities than parents to see children in social situations. These informant differences illustrate the importance of collecting and analyzing information from key individuals regarding preschool children's functioning to obtain a more complete picture of treatment outcome.

Stimulant medication in children with ADHD has been reported to have positive effects on some, but not all aspects of parenting. Improved parent–child interactions, decreased negative parenting practices, and improved ratings of parental effectiveness often occur with MPH treatment (Stein et al. 1996; Hechtman et al. 2004). In contrast, medication has not been shown to increase positive parenting practices (Hechtman et al. 2004) or positive changes in parent functioning, such as improved mood and ability to complete tasks (Chronis et al. 2003). In the current study, parental stress was not differentially reduced in parents whose children were treated with MPH relative to those on PL. The reasons for this are not clear. It is likely that children showed symptomatic improvement throughout much of the day. However, parental difficulties in managing their children in the morning, before medication effects were observable, or later in the day, when medication effects dissipated, conceivably continued to be salient, stressful events that influenced parents' judgments and self-ratings of stress levels.

Clinicians' global impressions of illness severity were significantly reduced in children treated with MPH compared to those on PL, yielding an ES of 0.73, the largest obtained on any outcome measure. CGI-S ratings, which take into account the youngster's overall functioning, have been reported to be influenced by a variety of factors, including severity of ADHD symptoms, peer relationship problems, oppositional defiant disorder (ODD), conduct disorder (CD), and internalizing symptoms (Coghill et al. 2006). Consequently, the degree to which clinicians' CGI-S ratings were influenced by functional improvements and/or reductions in children's ADHD symptoms is unknown. However, the absence of treatment effects in teacher and parent SWAN ratings of ADHD symptoms, with children in both groups improving over time, suggests that clinicians' judgments reflected, at least in part, improvements in non-ADHD-related areas of functioning.

Limitations

The present study has some limitations. First, as described above, the differential attrition rates in the two groups limited power to detect treatment differences and may have resulted in an underestimation of MPH effects on functional outcomes. Second, missing data, especially from teachers, precluded analyses of teacher ratings on the SSRS and ECI. As a result, it is unknown whether broader aspects of children's social skills, beyond those associated with social competence, improved in the school setting with MPH. Similarly, it is unknown whether the increase in sensitivity and tearfulness with MPH reported by parents occurred in school as well. Third, little is known about the psychometric properties of the CGI-S in preschool-aged children. The absence of reliability and validity information in this age group needs to be considered in interpreting the findings on the CGI-S. Fourth, in an effort to minimize treating preschoolers with medication unnecessarily, the PATS study design incorporated several features, including a 10-week parenting program, which preceded the study's medication phases, and a conservative set of diagnostic and inclusion criteria to minimize false positive diagnoses. These criteria included elevated scores on both the teacher and parent Conners Rating scales and an impairment score on the C-GAS $\leq$55. The resulting study sample had a mean C-GAS score of 47, which is considerably lower than the typical C-GAS score of 65 for children with ADHD seen in clinic settings. Consequently, the generalizability of the findings reported here to preschoolers with less severe levels of ADHD and impairment is uncertain.

Finally, although 4 weeks is typically sufficient to detect improvements in ADHD symptoms, a longer treatment period may be needed for functional changes to occur. However, because of design features of the PATS trial, it was not deemed ethical or clinically viable to keep children on placebo for more than 4 weeks. Specifically, the participants in the parallel-group phase had all participated in the previous within-subject titration phase and had demonstrated benefit with MPH treatment. In light of their prior experience with MPH, there was concern about the length of time individuals would tolerate treatment with PL, which led to the decision to limit the randomized, parallel-group phase to four weeks. Even with this design, the dropout rate was quite high in the PL group. It is likely that attrition in the PL group would have been even higher with an extended randomized, parallel-group phase. However, a parallel-group design that included randomization to MPH or PL for a longer treatment period, such as 8 weeks, might be viable in preschoolers without any prior exposure to MPH. Such an extended treatment period would provide greater opportunity for any functional improvements that occur to consolidate and be detected.

CONCLUSION

Preschoolers with ADHD treated with MPH for 4 weeks show some improvements in functioning, although not as extensive as those found in their elementary school-aged counterparts. We cannot rule out the possibility that these different outcome patterns are an artifact of the study design and uneven attrition rates in the MPH and PL groups. Nonetheless, it may be that additional functional improvements in preschoolers with ADHD require a longer treatment period, higher doses than those used in the current study, and/or the use of intensive behavioral treatment in combination with medication. Although there is a scarcity of evidence-based psychosocial interventions for preschool children with ADHD, the inclusion of "estab-

lished" parenting programs [e.g., New Forest Parenting Program (Sonuga-Barke et al. 2001); Parent-Child Interaction Therapy (Eyberg et al. 1995)], perhaps in conjunction with school-based behavioral approaches, might lead to additional improvements in children's social functioning and in parent stress levels beyond those reported here. Systematic, randomized controlled trials are needed to address this issue.

DISCLOSURES

The following financial disclosures indicate potential conflicts of interest among the PATS investigators and industry sources for the period 2000–2007. [1]Honoraria/consultant, [2]research support, [3]speaker's bureau, [4]significant equity (>$50,000). Dr. Abikoff: Abbott Laboratories,[1] Cephalon,[1] McNeil,[1,2] Shire,[1,2] Eli Lilly,[1,2] Pfizer,[2] Celltech,[2] Novartis.[2] Dr. Riddle: Shire,[1] Janssen,[1] Glaxo-Smith-Kline,[1] Astra-Zeneca,[1] Pfizer.[2] Dr. Swanson: Alza,[1,2] Celgene,[1,2] Celltech,[1,2,3] Cephalon,[1,2,3] Eli Lilly,[1,2] Gliatech,[1,2] Janssen,[1,2,3] McNeil,[1,2,3] Organon,[1] Novartis,[1,2] UCB, Shire.[1,2] Dr. Greenhill: Celltech,[1,2] Cephalon,[1,2] Eli Lilly,[1,2] Janssen,[1] McNeil,[1,2] Medeva,[2] Novartis Corporation,[1,2] Noven,[1,2] Otsuka,[1,2] Pfizer,[1] Sanofi,[1] Shire,[1,2] Solvay,[1,2] Somerset,[2] Thomson Advanced Therapeutics Communications.[1] Dr. Kollins: McNeil,[1,2,3] Shire,[1,2] Eli Lilly,[1,2] Pfizer,[2] New River Pharmaceuticals,[2] Psychogenics,[2] Athenagen,[1,2] Cephalon.[1] Dr. McCracken: Abbott, UCB, Novartis, Johnson & Johnson, Eli Lilly,[1,2,3] Gliatech,[2] Shire,[1,2] Pfizer,[1,2] McNeil,[1,2] Noven,[1] Bristol Meyers Squibb,[1] Janssen,[1,3] Wyeth.[1] Dr. McGough: Eli Lilly,[1,2,3] McNeil,[1,2,3] Novartis,[1,2,3] Shire,[1,2,3] Pfizer,[1,2,3] New River Pharmaceuticals.[2] Dr. Murray: Eli Lilly,[2] Pfizer,[2] Dr. Posner: As part of an effort to help execute the FDA suicidality classification mandates, Dr. Posner has had research support (2) from GlaxoSmithKline, Forest Laboratories, Eisai Inc., Astra Zeneca Pharmaceuticals, Johnson and Johnson, Abbott Laboratories, Wyeth Research, Organon USA, Bristol Meyers Squibb, Sanofi-Aventis, Cephalon, Novartis, Shire Pharmaceuticals and UCB Pharma; Shire.[1,2] Dr. Sharon Wigal: Celltech,[1,2,3] McNeil,[1,2,3] Cephalon,[1,2,3] Novartis,[1,2,3] Shire,[1,2,3] New

River Pharmaceuticals,[2] Janssen,[3] Eli Lilly.[2] Dr. Ghuman: Bristol Myers-Squibb.[2] Dr. Tim Wigal: Celltech,[2] Cephalon,[2] Eli Lilly,[2,3] Janssen,[2] McNeil,[2,3] Novartis,[2] Shire.[2,3] Drs. Vitiello, Cunningham, Kastelic, Evans, Ms. Chuang, and Ms. Skrobala have no conflict of interest as they have not received support from companies manufacturing medications.

REFERENCES

Abidin RR: Parenting Stress Index, 3rd ed. Lutz (Fl), Psychological Assessment Resource, 1995.

Abikoff H, Hechtman L, Klein R, Gallagher R, Fleiss K, Etcovitch J, Cousins L, Greenfield B, Martin D, Pollack S: Social functioning in children with ADHD treated with long-term methylphenidate and multimodal psychosocial treatment. J Am Acad Child Adolesc Psychiatry 43:812–819, 2004.

American Psychiatric Association. Diagnostic and Statistical Manual of Mental Disorders, 4th edition (DSM-IV). Washington (DC), American Psychiatric Association, 1994.

American Psychiatric Association: Handbook of Psychiatric Measures. Washington (DC), American Psychiatric Association, 2000.

Barkley RA: The effects of methylphenidate on the interactions of preschool ADHD children with their mothers. J Am Acad Child Adolesc Psychiatry 27:336–341, 1988.

Barkley RA, Karlsson J, Strzelecki E, Murphy JV: Effects of age and Ritalin dosage on the mother-child interactions of hyperactive children. J Consult Clin Psychol 52:750–758, 1984.

Byrne JM, Bawden HN, DeWolfe NA, Beattie TL: Clinical assessment of psychopharmacological treatment of preschoolers with ADHD. J Clin Exp Neuropsychol 20:613–627, 1998.

Chronis AM, Pelham WE Jr, Gnagy EM, Roberts JE, Aronoff HR: The impact of late-afternoon stimulant dosing for children with ADHD on parent and parent-child domains. J Clin Child Adolesc Psychol 32:118–126, 2003.

Coghill D, Spiel G, Baldursson G, Dopfner M, Lorenzo MJ, Ralston SJ, Rothenberger A, ADORE Study Group: Which factors impact on clinician-rated impairment in children with ADHD? Eur Child Adolesc Psychiatry 15 (Suppl 1):1/30–1/37, 2006.

Cohen NJ: Evaluation of the relative effectiveness of methylphenidate and cognitive behavior modification in the treatment of kindergarten-aged hyperactive children. J Abnorm Child Psychol 9:43–54, 1981.

Conduct Problems Prevention Research Group: A developmental and clinical model for the prevention of conduct disorders: The Fast Track program. Dev Psychopathol 4: 509–527, 1992.

Conners CK: Controlled trial of methylphenidate in preschool children with minimal brain dysfunction. Int J Ment Health 4:61-74, 1975.

Conners CK, Sitarenios G, Parker JD, Epstein JN: The revised Conners' Parent Rating Scale (CPRS-R): Factor structure, reliability, and criterion validity. J Abnorm Child Psychol 26 257–268, 1998a.

Conners CK, Sitarenios G, Parker JDA, Epstein JN: Revision and restandardization of the Conners' Teacher Rating Scale (CTRS-R): Factor structure, reliability, and criterion validity. J Abnorm Child Psychol 26:279–291, 1998b.

Cornish KM, Manly T, Savage R, Swanson J, Morisano D, Butler N, Grant C, Cross G, Bentley L, Hollis CP: Association of the dopamine transporter (DAT1) 10/10-repeat genotype with ADHD symptoms and response inhibition in a general population sample. Mol Psychiatry 10:686–698, 2005.

Cunningham CE, Siegel LS, Offord DR: A developmental dose response analysis of the effects of methylphenidate on the peer interactions of attention deficit disordered boys. J Child Psychol Psychiatry 26:955–971, 1985.

Daley D, Sonuga-Barke EJS, Thompson M: Assessing expressed emotion in mothers of preschool AD/HD children: Psychometric properties of a modified speech sample. Br J Clin Psychol 42:53–67, 2003.

DeWolfe N, Byrne JM, Bawden HN: ADHD in preschool children: Parent-rated psychosocial correlates. Dev Med Child Neurol 42:825–830, 2000.

DuPaul GJ, McGoey KE, Eckert TL, VanBrakle J: Preschool children with attention-deficit/hyperactivity disorder: Impairments in behavioral, social, and school functioning. J Am Acad Child Adolesc Psychiatry 40: 508–515, 2001.

Elliott CD: Differential Ability Scales. San Antonio (Texas), Harcourt Assessment Corporation, 1990.

Eyberg SM, Boggs SR, & Algina J: Parent-child interaction therapy: A psychosocial model for the treatment of young children with conduct problem behavior and their families. Psychopharmacol Bull 31:83–89, 1995.

Gadow KD, Sprafkin J: Child and Adolescent Symptom Inventories. Odessa (Florida), Psychological Assessment Resources, 1996.

Gordon M, Antshel K, Faraone S, Barkley R, Lewandowski L, Hudziak JJ, Biederman J, Cunningham C: Symptoms versus impairment: The case for respecting DSM-IV's Criterion D. J Attn Disorders 9:465–475, 2006.

Greenhill LL, Kollins SH, Abikoff H, McCracken J, Riddle M, Swanson J, McGough J, Wigal S, Wigal T, Vitiello B, Skrobala AM, Posner K, Ghuman J, Cunningham C, Davies M., Chuang S, Cooper T: Efficacy and safety of immediate-release methylphenidate treatment for preschoolers with ADHD. J Am Acad Child Adolesc Psychiatry 45:1284–1293, 2006.

Gresham FM, Elliott SN: Social Skills Rating System: Manual. Circle Pines (Minnesota), American Guidance Service, 1990.

Guy W: ECDEU Assessment Manual for Psychopharmacology: Revised. Washington (DC), U.S. Department of Health, Education and Welfare (DHEW), 1976.

Hechtman L, Abikoff H, Klein RG, Greenfield B, Etcovitch J, Cousins L, Fleiss K, Weiss M, Pollack S: Children with ADHD treated with long-term methylphenidate and multimodal psychosocial treatment: Impact on parental practices. J Am Acad Child Adolesc Psychiatry 43:830–838, 2004.

Kazdin AE, Whitley MK: Treatment of parental stress to enhance therapeutic change among children referred for aggressive and antisocial behavior. J Consult Clin Psychol 71:504–515, 2003.

Kollins SH, Greenhill LL, Swanson J, Wigal S, Abikoff H, McCracken JT, Riddle M, McGough JJ, Vitiello B, Wigal T, Skrobala AM, Posner K, Ghuman JK, Davies M, Cunningham C, Bauzo A: Rationale, design, and methods of the Preschool ADHD Treatment Study (PATS). J Am Acad Child Adolesc Psychol 45:1275–1283, 2006.

Lahey BB, Pelham WE, Stein MA, Loney J, Trapani C, Nugent K, Kipp H, Schmidt E, Lee S, Cale M, Gold E, Hartung CM, Willcutt E, Baumann B: Validity of DSM-IV attention-deficit/hyperactivity disorder for younger children. J Am Acad Child Adolesc Psychiatry 37:695–702, 1998.

McDermott PA, Steinberg CM, Angelo LE: Situational specificity makes the difference in assessment of youth behavior disorders. Psychol Sch 42:121–136, 2005.

Merrell KW, Wolfe TM: The relationship of teacher-rated social skills deficits and ADHD characteristics among kindergarten-age children. Psychol Sch 35:101–109, 1998.

Monteiro-Musten L, Firestone P, Pisterman S, Bennett S, Mercer J: Effects of methylphenidate on preschool children with ADHD: Cognitive and behavioral functions. J Am Acad Child Adolesc Psychiatry 36:1407–1415, 1997.

MTA Cooperative Group: A 14-month randomized clinical trial of treatment strategies for attention deficit/hyperactivity disorder. Arch Gen Psychiatry 56:1073–1086, 1999.

Murray DW, Kollins SH, Hardy KK, Abikoff HB, Swanson JM, Cunningham C, Vitiello B, Riddle MA, Davies M, Greenhill LL, McCracken JT, McGough JJ, Posner K, Skrobala AM, Wigal T, Wigal SB, Ghuman JK, Chuang SZ: Parent versus Teacher Ratings of Attention-Deficit/Hyperactivity Disorder Symptoms in the Preschoolers with Attention-Deficit/Hyperactivity Disorder Treatment Study (PATS). J Child Adolesc Psychopharmacol 17:605–619, 2007.

Schleifer M, Weiss G, Cohen NJ, Elman M, Cvejic H, Kruger E: Hyperactivity in preschoolers and the effect of methylphenidate. Am J Orthopsychiatry 45:38–50, 1975.

Shaffer D, Gould MS, Brasic J, Ambrosini P, Fisher P, Bird H, Aluwahlia S: A Children`s Global Assessment Scale (CGAS). Arch Gen Psychiatry 40:1228–1231, 1983.

Shaffer D, Fisher P, Dulcan MK, Davies M, Piacentini J, Schwab-Stone ME, Lahey BB, Bourdon K, Jensen PS, Bird HR, Canino G, Regier DA: The NIMH Diagnostic Interview Schedule for Children Version 2.3 (DISC–2.3): Description, acceptability, prevalence rates, and performance in the MECA study. J Am Acad Child Adolesc Psychiatry 35:865–877, 1996.

Short EJ, Manos MJ, Findling RL, and Schubel EA: A prospective study of stimulant response in preschool children: Insights from ROC analyses. J Am Acad Child Adolesc Psychiatry 43: 251–259, 2004.

Sonuga-Barke EJS, Daley D, Thompson M, Laver-Bradbury C, and Weeks B: A Parent-based therapies for preschool attention-deficit/hyperactivity disorder: A randomized, controlled trial with a community sample. J Am Acad Child Adolesc Psychiatry 40:402–408, 2001.

Sonuga-Barke EJS, Daley D, Thompson M, Swanson J: The management of preschool AD/HD: Addressing uncertainties about syndrome validity, diagnostic validity and utility, and treatment efficacy and safety. Expert Rev Neurother 3:465–476, 2003.

Sprafkin J, Volpe RJ, Gadow KD, Nolan EE, Kelly K : A DSM-IV-referenced screening instrument for preschool children: The Early Childhood Inventory-4. J Am Acad Child Adolesc Psychiatry 41:604–612, 2002.

Stein MA, Blondis TA, Schnitzler ER, O'Brien T, Fishkin J, Blackwell B, Szumowski E, Roizen NJ: Methylphenidate dosing: Twice daily versus three times daily. Pediatrics 98:748–56, 1996.

Swanson JM, McStephen M, Hay D, Levy F: The potential of the SWAN rating scale in the genetic analysis of ADHD. Vancouver (BC), Presentation at the 10th Meeting of the International Society for Research in Child and Adolescent Psychiatry, 2001.

Vitiello B, Abikoff HB, Chuang SZ, Kollins SH, McCracken JT, Riddle MA, Swanson JM, Wigal T, McGough JJ, Ghuman JH, Wigal SB, Skrobala AM, Davies M, Posner K, Cunningham C, Greenhill LL: Effectiveness of methylphenidate in the 10-month continuation phase of the Preschoolers with Attention-Deficit/Hyperactivity Disorder Treatment Study (PATS). J Child Adolesc Psychopharmacol 17:593–603, 2007.

Webster-Stratton C: Preventing conduct problems in Head Start children: Strengthening parenting competencies. J Consult Clin Psychol 66:715–730, 1998.

Wigal T, Greenhill L, Chuang S, McGough J, Vitiello B, Skrobala A, Swanson J, Wigal S, Abikoff H, Kollins S, McCracken J, Riddle M, Posner K, Ghuman J, Davies M, Thorp B, Stehli A: Safety and tolerability of methylphenidate in preschool children with ADHD. J Am Acad Child Adolesc Psychiatry 45: 1294–1303, 2006.

ADVANCES IN PRESCHOOL PSYCHOPHARMACOLOGY
© 2009 Mary Ann Liebert, Inc.
140 Huguenot Street, 3rd Floor
New Rochelle, NY 10801-5215

Effectiveness of Methylphenidate in the 10-Month Continuation Phase of the Preschoolers with Attention-Deficit/Hyperactivity Disorder Treatment Study (PATS)

Benedetto Vitiello, M.D.,[1] Howard B. Abikoff, Ph.D.,[2] Shirley Z. Chuang, M.S.,[3]
Scott H. Kollins, Ph.D.,[4] James T. McCracken, M.D.,[5] Mark A. Riddle, M.D.,[6]
James M. Swanson, Ph.D.,[7] Tim Wigal, Ph.D.,[7] James J. McGough, M.D.,[5]
Jaswinder K. Ghuman, M.D.,[8] Sharon B. Wigal, Ph.D.,[7] Anne M. Skrobala, M.A.,[3]
Mark Davies, M.P.H.,[3] Kelly Posner, Ph.D.,[3] Charles Cunningham, Ph.D.,[9]
and Laurence L. Greenhill, M.D.[3]

ABSTRACT

Objective: The aim of this study was to examine immediate-release methylphenidate effectiveness during the 10-month open-label continuation phase of the Preschoolers with attention-deficit/hyperactivity disorder (ADHD) Treatment Study (PATS).

Methods: One hundred and forty preschoolers with ADHD, who had improved with acute immediate-release methylphenidate (IR-MPH) treatment, entered a 10-month, open-label medication maintenance at six sites. Assessments included the Clinical Global Impression-Severity (CGI-S), CGI-Improvement (CGI-I), Children's Global Assessment Scale (C-GAS), Swanson, Nolan, and Pelham Questionnaire (SNAP), Scale Strengths and Weaknesses of ADHD-Symptoms and Normal Behaviors (SWAN), Social Competence Scale, Social Skills Rating System (SSRS), and Parenting Stress Index–Short Form (PSI-SF).

---

[1]Child and Adolescent Treatment and Preventive Intervention Research Branch, National Institute of Mental Health, Bethesda, Maryland.
[2]Child Study Center, New York University School of Medicine, New York, New York.
[3]New York State Psychiatric Institute, Columbia University, New York, New York.
[4]Duke University Medical Center, Durham, North Carolina.
[5]University of California Los Angeles, Los Angeles, California.
[6]Johns Hopkins Medical Institutions, Baltimore, Maryland.
[7]University of California Irvine, Irvine, California.
[8]University of Arizona, Tucson, Arizona.
[9]McMaster University, Hamilton, Ontario, Canada.

This research was supported by cooperative agreement grants between the National Institute of Mental Health and the following institutions: University of California, Irvine (U01 MH60833), Duke University Medical Center (U01 MH60848), NYSPI/Columbia University (U01 MH60903), New York University Child Study Center (U01 MH60943), University of California, Los Angeles (U01 MH60900), and Johns Hopkins University (U01 MH60642).

The opinion and assertions contained in this report are the private views of the authors and are not to be construed as official or as reflecting the views of the National Institute of Mental Health, the National Institutes of Health, or the U.S. Department of Health and Human Services.

Results: For the 95 children who completed the 10-month treatment, improvement occurred on the CGI-S ($p = 0.02$), CGI-I ($p < 0.01$), C-GAS ($p = 0.001$), and SSRS ($p = 0.01$). SNAP and SWAN scores remained stable. Forty five children discontinued: 7 for adverse effects, 7 for behavior worsening, 7 for switching to long-acting stimulants, 3 for inadequate benefit, and 21 for other reasons. The mean MPH dose increased from 14.04 mg/day ± SD 7.57 ($0.71 ± 0.38$ mg/kg per day) at month 1 to 19.98 mg/day ± 9.56 ($0.92 ± 0.40$ mg/kg per day) at month 10.

Conclusions: With careful monitoring and gradual medication dose increase, most preschoolers with ADHD maintained improvement during long-term IR-MPH treatment. There was substantial variability in effective and tolerated dosing.

INTRODUCTION

ATTENTION-DEFICIT/HYPERACTIVITY DISORDER (ADHD) is characterized by developmentally abnormal and functionally impairing levels of hyperactivity, impulsivity, and inattention with onset prior to 7 years of age (American Psychiatric Association 2000). Although ADHD is typically first diagnosed in elementary school years, onset is often in preschool years (Lahey et al. 1998; Connor 2002). Methylphenidate (MPH) is not approved by the Food and Drug Administration (FDA) for use under age 6 years, but several reports have documented its community off-label use in preschoolers (Zito et al. 2000; DeBar et al. 2003; Zuvekas et al. 2006).

The recently completed Preschoolers with ADHD Treatment Study (PATS) documented the acute efficacy of immediate-release (IR)-MPH at doses between 2.5 and 7.5 mg three times a day (Greenhill et al. 2006). In PATS, 165 children age 3–5.5 years participated in a 5-week, placebo-controlled, crossover trial. Of them, 75% best responded to MPH as compared to 8% responding to placebo. IR-MPH was well tolerated by most preschoolers, but 11% discontinued treatment due to adverse effects (Wigal et al. 2006).

ADHD is a chronic condition that often requires long-term treatment (Lahey et al. 2004). A number of studies of the long-term treatment of ADHD in school-age children have been conducted and the continuous effectiveness of stimulant medication over time has been documented for at least 14 months (MTA Cooperative Group 1999; McGough et al. 2005). In the Multimodal Treatment of ADHD study (MTA), to maintain optimal control of ADHD symptoms, the dose of IR-MPH was gradually increased from an average of 30.5 mg/day at the beginning of maintenance treatment to a final average dose of 34.4 mg/day 14 months later (Vitiello et al. 2001).

Little information is available on the extended use of MPH in preschoolers. The PATS 10-month open-label treatment phase offers an opportunity to investigate long-term effectiveness of IR-MPH in preschoolers. The primary aim of this phase was to examine whether preschoolers who had acutely responded to IR-MPH during the placebo-controlled phase of PATS would continue to show adequate control of ADHD symptoms and whether dose was adjusted to meet the individual child's clinical needs. On the basis of similar studies in school-aged children, it was anticipated that preschoolers continuing IR-MPH treatment would maintain the improvement in ADHD symptoms observed during acute treatment and that the medication dose would be gradually increased.

METHODS

Design

This was a 10-month, open-label, uncontrolled, outpatient, follow-on IR-MPH treatment phase for preschoolers with ADHD who had shown clinically significant improvement in ADHD symptoms and acceptable drug tolerability during the previous controlled phases of PATS. The rationale, design, and methods of PATS have been reported (Kollins et al. 2006), as well as the results of the placebo-controlled trial (Greenhill et al. 2006) and the safety outcomes, also including effects of stimulany treatment on growth (Swanson et al. 2006; Wigal et al. 2006).

Subjects

The characteristics of the PATS sample have been described in detail in previous publications (Greenhill et al. 2006; Kollins et al. 2006). Briefly, preschoolers of both genders, age 3.0–5.5 years, with a diagnosis of ADHD combined or hyperactive subtype (American Psychiatric Association 2000) and a hyperactive-impulsive subscale T-score of 65 or above on both the revised Conners Parent Rating Scale (CPRS) and the revised Conners Teacher Rating Scale (CTRS) (Conners et al. 1998a; Conners et al. 1998b) were eligible for PATS. The parents of all children meeting entry criteria were first trained in child behavior management and asked to implement it to avoid unnecessary exposure to medications (Kollins et al. 2006). Nonresponders to behavior therapy entered the medication phase of PATS, which included: (1) an open-label titration; (2) a 5-week crossover, double-blind, placebo-controlled trial of MPH at doses ranging from 1.25 to 7.5 mg three times a day; (3) a 4-week double-blind, placebo-controlled, parallel-group trial; and (4) the 10-month maintenance treatment, which is the focus of this report.

Of the 165 children who entered the crossover trial, 140 entered the long-term maintenance. Their characteristics are summarized in Table 1 (below).

The study protocol and parental informed consent forms were approved by the institutional review boards at the six recruiting sites. The study was monitored by the Data and Safety Monitoring Board of the National Institute of Mental Health.

Treatment

Short-acting IR-MPH was administered orally on a three times a day schedule (in the morning at breakfast, around noon after lunch, and at about 3:30 pm) 7 days a week. Each child started maintenance at the dose of MPH that was found to control best the ADHD symptoms without unacceptable adverse effects during the preceding placebo-controlled double-blind trial (Greenhill et al. 2006). Children were seen for monthly visits during which clinical status was reviewed by the study psychopharmacologist, and the dosage was modified if there were clinically significant adverse effects or re-sidual symptoms, as indicated by a score of 3 (mildly ill) or above on the Clinical Global Impression–Severity Scale (CGI-S; Guy 1976).

Measures

For each child, the study clinician completed the CGI-S and CGI–Improvement (CGI-I) scales and recorded adverse effects after reviewing the side-effect checklist completed by parent and teacher at each monthly visit (Wigal et al. 2006). The CGI-I scored improvement as compared with the PATS premedication status. At month 1 and at the end of the 10-month maintenance, the clinician also completed the Children's Global Assessment Scale (C-GAS) (Shaffer et al. 1983).

At month 1 and at the end of the 10-month maintenance, the parent completed the following ratings:

- The Swanson Nolan and Pelham questionnaire (SNAP), which included the 18 symptom items for ADHD of the Diagnostic and Statistical Manual of Mental Disorders, Forth Edition (DSM-IV; American Psychiatric Association 2000), each scored on a four-point scale (from 0 = not at all to 3 = very much) (Swanson 1992).
- The Strengths and Weaknesses of ADHD Symptoms and Normal Behavior Scale (SWAN), which, like the SNAP, is based on the 18 ADHD symptoms listed in the DSM-IV, but reworded to reflect normal behavior and scored along a seven-point scale (from far above average = −3 to far below average = 3) (Swanson et al. 2001b; Cornish et al. 2005).
- The parent version of the Social Skills Rating Scale (SSRS), a 70-item standardized scale to assess social functioning in preschool children (Gresham and Elliot 1990).
- The Parenting Stress Index–Short Form (PSI–SF), which is a 36-item five-point scale measuring the level of parental stress with respect to the parent-child relationship and other situational interactions (Reitman et al. 2002).
- The Social Competence Scale–Parent version, a 12-item measure of the child's

positive social behaviors, communication skills, and frustration tolerance, which was created for the Fast Track Project (Conduct Problems Prevention Research Group 1992).

At the same time points, the teacher completed the SNAP, SWAN, SSRS, and the Social Competence Scale–Teacher version.

Data analyses

Descriptive statistics were applied. Analyses included the outcome variables for which data were available on at least 50% of the children entering the maintenance study (i.e., on at least 70 children). Pre-post, within subject Cohen's d

effect sizes [i.e., $mean_{pre} - mean_{post}$/pooled standard deviation (SD)] were computed for the outcome variables as a way of quantifying differences. Thus, for symptom scores, small effect sizes between month 1 and end of maintenance indicate little clinical change and consequently maintenance of improvement. The significance of pre-post differences was tested with paired t-tests at a two-tail $\alpha < 0.05$.

RESULTS

Sample retention

Of the 140 children who entered maintenance, 95 (67.8%) completed the 10 months of

TABLE 1. DEMOGRAPHICS AND CLINICAL CHARACTERISTICS[a]

	Entered maintenance	Completed maintenance	Discontinued maintenance	Completers vs. noncompleters[b] (p)
n	140	95	45	
Age, years, mean (SD)	4.4 (0.7)	4.4 (0.7)	4.4 (0.7)	0.91
Males, n (%)	104 (74.3)	72 (75.8)	32 (71.1)	0.55
Race/ethnicity, n (%)				0.79
White	91 (65.0)	61 (64.2)	30 (66.7)	
African American	24 (17.1)	17 (17.9)	7 (15.6)	
Hispanic	22 (15.7)	14 (14.7)	8 (17.8)	
Asian	2 (1.4)	2 (2.1)	0 (0.0)	
American Indian	1 (0.7)	1 (1.1)	0 (0.0)	
ADHD type, n (%)				0.80
Hyperactive-impulsive	33 (23.6)	23 (24.2)	10 (22.2)	
Combined	107 (76.4)	72 (76.0)	35 (77.8)	
Co-morbidity,[c] n (%)				
Oppositional-defiant disorder	74 (52.9)	52 (54.7)	22 (48.9)	0.59
Communication disorder	27 (19.3)	20 (21.0)	7 (15.6)	0.44
Anxiety disorder	16 (11.4)	12 (12.6)	4 (8.9)	0.58
Hollingshead socio-economic status, mean (SD)	47.2 (9.5)	47.1 (9.6)	47.7 (9.2)	0.74
Family on welfare, n (%)	10 (8.1)	9 (10.6)	1 (2.6)	0.17
Family composition, n (%)				0.15
2 parents	92 (81.4)	71 (84.5)	21 (72.4)	
1 parent	21 (18.6)	13 (15.5)	8 (27.6)	
Conners' Parent Rating Scale				
Total, mean (SD)	39.96 (7.52)	40.32 (7.42)	39.22 (7.76)	0.42
Inattention, mean (SD)	17.70 (5.32)	17.95 (5.05)	17.18 (5.87)	0.43
Hyperactive, mean (SD)	22.21 (3.44)	22.33 (3.52)	21.98 (3.29)	0.56
Conners' Teacher Rating Scale				
Total, mean (SD)	35.36 (8.71)	36.09 (8.11)	33.71 (9.84)	0.15
Inattention, mean (SD)	14.90 (5.70)	15.26 (5.58)	14.10 (5.95)	0.43
Hyperactive, mean (SD)	20.35 (4.60)	20.70 (4.15)	19.56 (5.47)	0.24
Children's Global Assessment Scale, mean (SD)	47.20 (4.09)	47.38 (3.97)	46.82 (4.36)	0.45

SD = Standard deviation; ADHD = attention-deficit hyperactivity disorder; PATS = Preschoolers with ADHD Treatment Study.

[a]At baseline, before starting medication treatment in PATS.

[b]t-test for continuous variables and χ^2 for categorical variables.

[c]Common comorbidities with prevalence of 10% or greater.

treatment, while 45 (32.1%) left the study prematurely. A comparison between the subgroup that completed maintenance and the subgroup that discontinued it showed that there were no statistically significant differences in demographics or clinical characteristics between the two subgroups (Table 1).

Reasons for discontinuation are provided in Table 2. Among these, 7 children (5.0% of 140) discontinued because of adverse effects, 7 (5.0%) for behavioral deterioration, 6 (4.3%) for switching to a long-acting formulations of stimulant, and 3 (2.1%) for inadequate benefit.

Clinician-, parent-, and teacher-rated outcome measures are summarized in Tables 3 and 4. The completion rate of these assessments was above 90% for clinician-rated instruments, between 59% and 89% for parent-rated instruments, and about 60% for teacher-rated instruments.

Overall severity of illness and level of improvement

For children who remained in treatment until the end of maintenance, a statistically significant decline in the CGI-S ($p = 0.02$) and CGI-I ($p < 0.01$) occurred between month 1 and end of maintenance, denoting a decrease in severity of illness and an increase in level of improvement, with small pre-post effect sizes (Tables 3 and 4). At the end of maintenance, the mean CGI-S score was 3.07 ± SD 1.11 (corresponding to "mildly ill") and the mean CGI-I score was 2.73.07 ± SD 1.06 (corresponding to "much improved").

ADHD symptoms

The parent- and teacher-rated SNAP and SWAN scores showed minimal, nonstatistically significant variation during maintenance treatment, with pre-post effect size ranging from −0.29 to 0.13 for the SNAP and from 0.08 to 0.22 for the SWAN (Tables 3 and 4). At the end of maintenance, the parent and teacher ADHD composite score was 1.26 ± SD 0.59, unchanged from the month 1 assessment, and significantly lower than the 2.02 ± 0.42 score obtained before the children entered the acute treatment phase of PATS ($p < 0.0001$).

In school-aged children, a SNAP ADHD score of 1 or below is considered an index of normalization and therefore of "excellent response" (Swanson et al. 2001a). In the PATS maintenance phase, 42% of the children had a parent SNAP ADHD score of 1 or below at month 1, and 34% at month 10 ($p = 0.23$).

TABLE 2. REASONS FOR PREMATURE DISCONTINUATION FROM METHYLPHENIDATE MAINTENANCE

	n (%)
Entered maintenance	140 (100)
Completed maintenance	95 (67.9)
Discontinued prematurely	45 (32.1)
Reasons for discontinuation	
Adverse effects	7
Irritability	3
Emotionality	1
Motor tics	2
Weight loss	1
Behavior worsening	7
Inadequate benefit	3
Switched to long-acting stimulant medication	6
Switched to atomoxetine	1
Emergence of other psychopathology	3
Anxiety	1
Unspecified	2
Parents did not want to use medication any more	3
Parents did not feel child needed medication any more	1
Parents withdrew consent/no reason provided	3
Moved out of the area	1
Did not return to the clinic/no reason provided	10

Table 3. Symptom and Functioning Scores during the 10-Month Maintenance Treatment[a]

Rating scale[b]	Measure of	Rater	End of month 1			End of maintenance			End of month 1 vs. end of maintenance Cohen's effect size
			n	Mean	SD	n	Mean	SD	
CGI–S[c]	Severity of illness	Clinician	136	3.38	1.08	127	3.07	1.11	0.28
CGI–I[d]	Improvement	Clinician	133	3.24	1.31	128	2.73	1.06	0.42
SNAP[e]	Inattention	Parent	123	1.20	0.61	91	1.12	0.57	0.13
	Hyperactivity impulsivity	Parent	122	1.43	0.75	91	1.40	0.69	0.04
	ADHD symptoms	Parent	124	1.31	0.63	91	1.26	0.58	0.08
	Inattention	Teacher	86	1.03	0.58	68	1.22	0.74	−0.29
	Hyperactivity impulsivity	Teacher	86	1.27	0.73	68	1.33	0.85	−0.08
	ADHD symptoms	Teacher	86	1.15	0.60	68	1.23	0.76	−0.12
	ADHD symptoms composite	Parent and/or teacher	128	1.26	0.56	96	1.26	0.59	0.00
SWAN[f]	Inattention	Parent	123	0.77	0.81	90	0.62	0.85	0.18
	Hyperactivity impulsivity	Parent	125	1.14	0.88	90	0.94	0.92	0.22
	ADHD symptoms	Parent	125	0.95	0.77	90	0.78	0.83	0.21
	Inattention	Teacher	85	0.54	0.88	66	0.34	1.15	0.20
	Hyperactivity impulsivity	Teacher	86	0.93	0.86	67	0.85	1.17	0.08
	ADHD symptoms	Teacher	86	0.74	0.80	67	0.60	1.10	0.15
C–GAS[g]	Functioning	Clinician	127	59.18	11.03	106	65.76	12.82	−0.55
Social Competence Scale	Social competence	Parent	93	1.49	0.61	92	1.74	0.76	−0.36
	Social competence	Teacher	83	1.71	0.69	53	1.93	0.92	−0.28
Social Skills Rating System	Social Skills	Parent	113	90.70	16.04	87	94.66	16.35	−0.24
Parenting Stress Index-Short Form	Difficult child	Parent	73	76.47	26.58	83	70.72	28.59	0.21
	Defensive responding	Parent	73	58.62	35.67	83	55.71	36.83	0.08
	Dysfunctional interaction	Parent	73	57.57	30.42	83	54.39	27.57	0.11
	Parental distress	Parent	73	42.88	33.58	83	45.18	33.88	−0.07
	Total stress	Parent	73	68.18	29.81	83	64.18	31.32	0.13

SD = standard deviation; ADHD = attention-deficit hyperactivity disorder.

[a]For all the children entered into maintenance for whom assessments were available.

[b]Table includes measures for which there were data from at least 50% (n = 70) of the total sample that entered into treatment maintenance (n = 140).

[c]CGI-S = Clinical Global Impressions-Severity Scale (Guy 1976).

[d]CGI-I = Clinical Global Impressions-Improvement Scale (Guy 1976).

[e]SNAP = Swanson Nolan and Pelham questionnaire (Swanson 1992).

[f]SWAN = Strengths and Weaknesses of ADHD Symptoms and Normal Behavior Scale (Swanson et al. 2001b; Cornish et al. 2005).

[g]C-GAS = Children's Global Assessment Scale (Shaffer et al. 1983).

Level of functioning

Clinician-rated C-GAS scores increased ($p < 0.001$) during the 10 months, with a moderate pre-post effect size, denoting improved functioning (Tables 3 and 4). End-of-maintenance C-GAS was 65.76 ± 12.82. Effect sizes of −0.36 and −0.28 were found on the parent and teacher Social Competence Scale, denoting increased level of social competence (Table 3). Parent-rated SSRS significantly improved ($p = 0.01$) (Table 4).

Parental stress

Parental Stress Index scores showed little change during maintenance as indicated by pre-post absolute effects sizes between 0.07 and 0.21 (Table 3). On this index, the mean Total Stress Score was 68.18 ± SD 29.81 at month 1 and 64.18 ± 31.32 at end of the maintenance, both scores being within 1 SD above the normal population mean (Reitman et al. 2002).

TABLE 4. OUTCOME MEASURES FOR CHILDREN WITH BOTH MONTH-1 AND MONTH-10 ASSESSMENTS[a]

| Rating scale[b] | Measure of | Rater | End of month 1 | | | End of maintenance | | | End of month 1 vs. end of maintenance | |
			n	Mean	SD	n	Mean	SD	Cohen's effect size	Paired t-test (p)
CGI	Severity of illness	Clinician	127	3.31	1.04	127	3.07	1.11	0.22	0.02
	Improvement		127	3.17	1.27	127	2.73	1.07	0.37	<0.01
SNAP	ADHD	Parent	85	1.23	0.62	85	1.26	0.58	−0.05	0.68
	Inattention	Parent	85	1.14	0.59	85	1.12	0.58	0.02	0.84
	Hyperactivity-impulsivity	Parent	84	1.34	0.74	84	1.41	0.70	−0.10	0.41
	ADHD symptom composite	Parent and/or teacher	92	1.20	0.57	92	1.25	0.58	−0.08	0.49
SWAN	ADHD symptoms	Parent	85	0.85	0.75	85	0.77	0.84	0.10	0.37
	Inattention	Parent	83	0.68	0.79	83	0.61	0.87	0.08	0.44
	Hyperactivity-impulsivity	Parent	85	1.03	0.87	85	0.93	0.93	0.10	0.38
C-GAS	Functioning	Clinician	99	60.01	10.59	99	64.56	12.24	−0.40	<0.001
SSRS	Social Skills	Parent	77	91.19	16.05	77	95.08	17.00	−0.23	0.01

SD = standard deviation; CGI = Clinical Global Impression; SNAP = Swanson Nolan and Pelham Questionnaire; SWAN = Strengths and Weaknesses of ADHD Symptoms and Normal Behavior Scale; C-GAS = Children's Global Assessment Scale; SSRS = Social Skills Rating Scale.

[a]For the children for whom both month 1 and end of maintenance assessments were available.

[b]Table includes measures for which there were data from at least 50% ($n = 70$) of the total sample that entered into treatment maintenance ($n = 140$).

Medication dose

The mean average dose of MPH increased from 14.4 ± SD 7.57 mg/day (0.71 ± 0.38 mg/kg per day) at month 1 to 19.94 ± 8.6 mg/day (0.92 ± 0.40 mg/kg per day) at the end of 10-month maintenance ($p < 0.0001$) (Table 5, Fig. 1). The mean dose for completers only was 13.64 ± 7.19 mg/day (0.69 ± 0.38 mg/kg per day) at month 1 and 19.61 ± 8.70 mg/day (0.92 ± 0.40 mg/kg per day) at month 10. Noncompleters started with a somewhat higher mean dose (15.01 ± 8.42 mg/day, or 0.75 ± 0.40 mg/kg/day) than noncompleters. In repeated measures random regression analyses, however, there were no differences in dose trend between completers and noncompleters, so that no statistically significant main effects of completion/non-completion status on dose increase emerged.

DISCUSSION

In this study, preschoolers with ADHD, who had improved after short-term administration of MPH, entered a 10-month maintenance treatment. The open-label and uncontrolled nature of the study prevents disentangling treatment effects from the natural course of illness or possible influence of contextual factors. With these limitations in mind, the data indicate that symptomatic improvement was maintained during long-term treatment.

Children who remained in treatment for the entire maintenance phase continued to improve as documented by statistically significantly better CGI and C-GAS scores (Table 4). The exact source of this modest improvement cannot be determined, but it may reflect continuous medication monitoring with dose adjustment. The mean Parent- and Teacher-rated rating scales showed that ADHD symptoms remained stable during treatment. Thus, while symptomatic improvement was maintained, global functioning continued to improve during long-term treatment. This finding suggests that the maximum effect of treatment on symptoms emerges early, followed by slower improvement in functioning.

The end-of-treatment ADHD symptom SNAP mean scores of 1.26, based on parent rat-

A

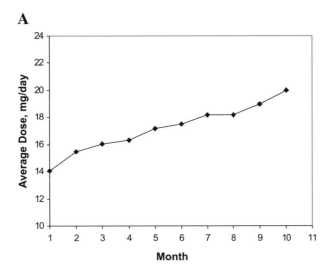

B

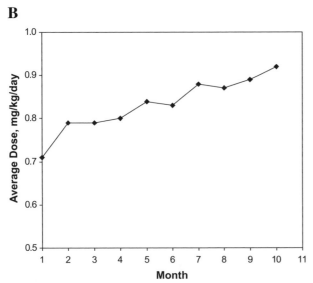

FIG. 1. Methylphenidate dose during maintenance (mean). (**A**) Absolute dose (mg/day). Dose increased an average of 0.57 mg/day per month ($p < 0.0001$). (**B**) Weight-adjusted dose (mg/kg per day). Dose increased an average of 0.022 mg/kg per day per month ($p < 0.0007$).

ing, and 1.23, based on teacher rating, indicate persistence of mild symptoms. In fact, full "normalization," defined according the criterion of SNAP scores of 1 or below (Swanson et al. 2001a), was not achieved for most children, in spite of careful pharmacological treatment. Likewise, the mean CGAS at end of maintenance was 65.76 (± SD 12.82), which is substantially better than the 47.33 (± 4.07) registered at the entry into PATS (Greenhill et al. 2006), but still short of normal functioning (i.e., CGAS score >70).

The end-of-maintenance mean score of 95 on the SSRS, which is below the normative mean, suggests that social functioning was not optimized in preschoolers, as similarly reported in elementary school-aged children with ADHD after 2 years of MPH treatment (Abikoff et al. 2004). These data indicate that there is room for further improvement in the treatment of ADHD.

About one-third of the children who had entered maintenance in PATS left the study prematurely (Table 2). The reasons for premature discontinuation were diverse and reflect the range of situations likely to happen in routine clinical practice. Because MPH is widely available in the community, discontinuation from the study does not necessarily mean the MPH treatment was discontinued. For instance, 6 children switched to long-acting stimulant formulations, which were not provided in PATS. The fact that about 5% of the children discontinued treatment due to adverse effects suggests that tolerability to acute MPH administration predicts tolerability to long-term treatment for most, though not all cases. Likewise, the finding that about 7% of the children discontinued due to behavioral deterioration or inadequate benefit suggests that response to acute treatment is predictive of continuous benefit with long-term treatment in more than 90% of the cases.

In this study, treatment was monitored through monthly visits, and the IR-MPH dose was gradually increased from an average of

TABLE 5. METHYLPHENIDATE DOSE DURING MAINTENANCE

	Mg/day			Mg/kg per day		
Month	n	Mean	SD	n	Mean	SD
1	135	14.04	7.57	126	0.71	0.38
2	126	15.49	6.88	118	0.79	0.34
3	118	16.08	6.84	113	0.80	0.34
4	115	16.27	7.42	111	0.80	0.36
5	111	17.21	7.88	103	0.84	0.40
6	106	17.53	7.69	100	0.83	0.38
7	106	18.43	9.38	99	0.89	0.46
8	97	18.46	8.40	87	0.89	0.42
9	94	18.98	8.20	90	0.89	0.39
10	94	19.94	8.66	89	0.92	0.40

SD = standard deviation.
[a]n is based on all data available at each time point, including both completers and noncompleters.

0.71 mg/kg per day at month 1 to 0.92 mg/kg per day at month 10 (Table 5). Nevertheless, the final average dose remained lower than that reported in several previous short-term studies of MPH in preschoolers (Firestone et al. 1998; Handen et al. 1999). The need for upward dose adjustments during maintenance treatment is consistent with the findings of the MTA in 7- to 9-year-old children. During the 13-month MTA maintenance treatment, the IR-MPH dose increased from a mean 0.97 ± 0.50 mg/kg per day to 1.09 ± 0.48 mg/kg per day (Vitiello et al. 2001). Compared with the MTA, the steeper increase observed in PATS reflects a lower mean dose at entry, thus suggesting that the rather conservative dose escalation in the acute titration phase resulted in underdosing.

As already pointed out, the main limitation of this study consists in the lack of experimental control as all the children received MPH during the 10-month treatment. This design allows only for pre-post, within-subject comparisons to be made, but not for between group analyses. Due to this design limitation, it is not possible to partial out treatment effects from changes due to passage of time. Still, this long-term study, although uncontrolled, offers an opportunity to assess prospectively preschoolers with ADHD under treatment conditions close to usual community practice. Another limitation is the relatively high rate of premature discontinuation, which, however, likely reflects the clinical reality. In fact, the course of treatment is subject to change due to evolving symptom presentation, parental preferences, or other contextual factors. A third limitation pertains to the use of an immediate release formulation of MPH. PATS was designed in the late 1990s, before long-lasting formulations became widely available.

In conclusion, consistent with similar studies in school-aged children with ADHD, long-term pharmacological treatment with IR-MPH of preschoolers with ADHD was accompanied by maintenance of the symptomatic improvement seen during the acute treatment phases and by further improvement in overall level of functioning. Variability seen in optimal doses over long-term treatment was substantial. Even if carefully determined at the initial, acute titra-

tion, the optimal dose of medication had to be adjusted on the basis of parent and teacher reports, and was gradually increased during the long-term maintenance treatment.

DISCLOSURE

The authors' relationships with for-profit organizations, including research support, consultant fees, honoraria, and significant equity, for the period 2000–2007 are as follows: Dr. Abikoff—McNeil, Shire, Eli Lilly, Pfizer, Celltech, and Novartis; Mr. Davies—Pfizer, Amgen, Johnson & Johnson, Wyeth; Dr. Greenhill—Wyeth Ayerst, Glaxo Wellcome, Eli Lilly, Alza, Shire, Medeva, Cephalon, Noven, Somerset, McNeil, Celltech, Novartis Corporation, Solvay, Sanofi Aventis, Otsuka, Janssen, Thomson Advanced Therapeutics Communications; Dr. Ghuman—Bristol-Myers Squibb; Dr. Kollins—Athenagen, Pfizer, Shire, Eli Lilly, New River Pharmaceuticals, McNeil, Novartis, Cephalon, Celltech, Janssen/Cilag, Psychogenics; Dr. McCracken—McNeil, Eli Lilly, Abbott, Wyeth, Shire, Pfizer, Celltech, Cephalon, Novartis, Bristol-Myers Squibb, Janssen; Dr. McGough—Eli Lilly, McNeil, Novartis, Shire, Pfizer, New River Pharmaceuticals; Dr. Posner—Glaxo-SmithKline, Forest, Eisai, AstraZeneca, Johnson&Johnson, Abbott, Wyeth, Organon, Bristol-Myers Squibb, Sanofi-Aventis, Cephalon, Novartis, and UCB; Dr. Riddle—Shire, Janssen, Glaxo-Smith-Kline, AstraZeneca, Pfizer; Dr. Swanson—Alza, Celgene, Celltech, Cephalon, Eli Lilly, Janssen, McNeil, Novartis, Shire, Targacept; Dr. Tim Wigal—Celltech, Cephalon, Eli Lilly, Janssen, McNeil, Novartis, Shire; Dr. Sharon Wigal—Celltech, McNeil, Cephalon, Novartis, Shire, Janssen, Eli Lilly; Drs. Cunningham and Vitiello, Ms. Chuang and Ms. Skrobala, have no conflicts of interest or financial ties to disclose.

REFERENCES

Abikoff H, Hechtman L, Klein RG, Gallagher R, Fleiss K, Etcovitch J, Cousins L, Greenfield B, Martin D, Pollack S: Social functioning in children with ADHD treated with long-term methylphenidate and multimodal psychosocial treatment. J Am Acad Child Adolesc Psychiatry 43:812–819, 2004.

American Psychiatric Association: Diagnostic and Statistical Manual of Mental Disorders, 4th ed. Text Revision (DSM-IV-TR). Washington (DC), American Psychiatric Association, 2000.

Conduct Problems Prevention Research Group: A developmental and clinical model for the prevention of conduct disorder: The Fast Track Program. Dev Psychopathol 4:509–527, 1992.

Connor DF: Preschool attention deficit hyperactivity disorder: A review of prevalence, diagnosis, neurobiology, and stimulant treatment. Dev Behav Pediatrics 23:S1–S9, 2002.

Conners CK, Sitarenios G, Parker J, Epstein J: The revised Conners' Parent Rating Scale (CPRS-R): Factor structure, reliability, and criterion validity. J Abnorm Child Psychology 26, 257–268, 1998a.

Conners CK, Sitarenios G, Parker J, Epstein J: Revision and restandardization of the Conners' Teacher Rating Scale (CTRS-R): Factor structure, reliability and criterion validity. J Abnorm Child Psychology 26: 279–293, 1998b.

Cornish KM, Manly T, Savage R, Swanson J, Morisano D, Butler N, Grant C, Cross G, Bentley L, Hollis CP: Association of the dopamine transporter (DAT1) 10/10-repeat genotype with ADHD symptoms and response inhibition in a general population sample. Mol Psychiatry 10:686–698, 2005.

Debar LL, Lynch F, Powell J, Gale J: Use of psychotropic agents in preschool children: Associated symptoms, diagnoses, and health care services in a health maintenance organization. Arch Pediatr Adolesc Med 157:150–157, 2003.

Firestone P, Musten LM, Pisterman S, Mercer K, Bennet S: Short-term side effects of stimulant medication are increased in preschool children with attention-deficit/hyperactivity disorder: A double-blind placebo-controlled study. J Child Adolesc Psychopharmacol 8:13–25, 1998.

Greenhill LL, Abikoff H, Chuang S, Cooper T, Cunningham C, Davies M, Ghuman J, Kollins S, McCracken JT, McGough J, Posner K, Riddle MA, Skrobala A, Swanson A, Vitiello B, Wigal S, Wigal T: Efficacy and safety of immediate-release methylphenidate treatment for preschoolers with ADHD. J Am Acad Child Adolesc Psychiatry 45:1284–1293, 2006.

Gresham FM, Elliott SN: Social Skills Rating System: Manual. Circle Pines (Minnesota), American Guidance Service, 1990.

Guy W: ECDEU Assessment Manual for Psychopharmacology. 2nd ed. DHEW Publication 76-388. Washington (DC), U.S. Government Printing Office, 1976.

Handen BL, Feldman HM, Lurier A, Murray PJ: Efficacy of methylphenidate among preschool children with developmental disabilities and ADHD. J Am Acad Child Adolesc Psychiatry 38:805–812, 1999.

Kollins SH, Greenhill LL, Swanson S, Wigal S, Abikoff H, McCracken JT, Riddle M, McGough JJ, Vitiello B, Wigal T, Skrobala AM, Posner K, Ghuman JK, Davies M,

Cunningham C, Bauzo A: Rationale, design, and methods of the Preschool ADHD Treatment Study (PATS). J Am Acad Child Adolesc Psychiatry 45:1275–1283, 2006.

Lahey BB, Pelham WE, Syein MA, Loney J, Trapani C, Nugent K, Kipp H, Schmidt E, Lee S, Cale M, Gold E, Hartung CM, Willincutt E, Baumann B: Validity of DSM-IV attention-deficit/hyperactivity disorder for younger children. J Am Acad Child Adolesc Psychiatry 37:695–702, 1998.

Lahey BB, Pelham WE, Loney J, Kipp H, Erhardt A, Lee SS, Willcull EG, Hartung CM, Chronis A., Massetti G: Three-year predictive validity of DSM-IV attention-deficit/hyperactivity disorder in children diagnosed at 4–6 years of age. Am J Psychiatry 161:2014–2020, 2004.

McGough JJ, Biederman J, Wigal SB, Lopez FA, McCracken JT, Spencer T, Zhang Y, Tulloch SJ: Long-term tolerability and effectiveness of once-daily mixed amphetamine salts (Adderall XR) in children with ADHD. J Am Acad Child Adolesc Psychiatry 44:530–538, 2005.

MTA Cooperative Group: A 14-Month randomized clinical trial of treatment strategies for attention-deficit/hyperactivity disorder (ADHD). Arch Gen Psychiatry 56:1073–1086, 1999.

Reitman D, Currier RO, Stickle TR: A critical evaluation of the Parenting Stress Index-Short Form (PSI-SF) in a head start population. J Clin Child Adolesc Psychol 31:384–392, 2002.

Shaffer D, Gould MS, Brasic J, Ambrosini P, Fisher P, Bird H, Aluwahlia S: A children's global assessment scale (CGAS). Arch Gen Psychiatry 40:1228–1231, 1983.

Sparrow S, Balla D, Cicchetti D: Vineland Adaptive Behavior Scales–Survey Edition. Circle Pines (Minnesota), American Guidance Service, 1984.

Swanson JM: School-based Assessments and Interventions for ADD Students. Irvine (California), K.C. Publications, 1992.

Swanson JM, Kraemer HC, Hinshaw SP, Arnold LE, Conners CK, Abikoff HB, Clevenger W, Davies M, Elliott GR, Greenhill LL, Hechtman L, Hoza, B, Jensen PS, March JS, Newcorn JH, Owens EB, Pelham WE, Schiller E, Severe JB, Simpson S, Vitiello B, Wells K, Wigal T, Wu M: Clinical relevance of the primary findings of the MTA: Success rate based on severity of ADHD and ODD symptoms at the end of treatment. J Am Acad Child Adolesc Psychiatry 40:168–179, 2001a.

Swanson JM, McStephen M, Hay D, Levy F: The potential of the SWAN rating scale in the genetic analysis of ADHD. Presentation at the 10th Meeting of the International Society for Research in Child and Adolescent Psychiatry, Vancouver (BC), 2001b.

Swanson JM, Greenhill LL, Wigal T, Kollins SH, Stehli-Nguyen A, Davies M, Chuang S, Vitiello B, Skrobala AM, Abikoff HB, Oatis M, McCracken JT, McGough JJ, Riddle M, Ghuman J, Cunningham C, Wigal SB: Stimulant-related reductions of growth rates in the PATS. J Am Acad Child Adolesc Psychiatry 45:1304–1313, 2006.

Vitiello B, Severe JB, Greenhill LL, Arnold LE, Abikoff HB, Bukstein O, Elliott GR, Hechtman L, Jensen PS,

Hinshaw SP, March JS, Newcorn JH, Swanson JM, Cantwell DP: Methylphenidate dosage for children with ADHD over time under controlled conditions: Lessons from the MTA. J Am Acad Child Adolesc Psychiatry 40:188–196, 2001.

Wigal T, Greenhill LL, Chuang S, McGough JJ, Vitiello B, Skrobala AM, Swanson J, Wigal S, Abikoff H, Kollins SH, McCracken JT, Riddle M, Posner K, Ghuman JK, Davies M, Thorp B, Stehli A: Safety and tolerability of methylphenidate in preschool children with ADHD. J Am Acad Child Adolesc Psychiatry 45:1294–1303, 2006.

Zito JM, Safer DJ, DosReis S, Gardner JF, Boles M, Lynch F: Trends in the prescribing of psychotropic medications to preschoolers. JAMA 283:1025–1030, 2000.

Zuvekas SH, Vitiello B, Norquist NS: Recent trends in stimulant medication use among U.S. children. Am J Psychiatry 163:579–585, 2006.

ADVANCES IN PRESCHOOL PSYCHOPHARMACOLOGY
© 2009 Mary Ann Liebert, Inc.
140 Huguenot Street, 3rd Floor
New Rochelle, NY 10801-5215

Parent versus Teacher Ratings of Attention-Deficit/Hyperactivity Disorder Symptoms in the Preschoolers with Attention-Deficit/Hyperactivity Disorder Treatment Study (PATS)

Desiree W. Murray, Ph.D.,[1] Scott H. Kollins, Ph.D.,[1,2] Kristina K. Hardy, Ph.D.,[1]
Howard B. Abikoff, Ph.D.,[3] James M. Swanson, Ph.D.,[4] Charles Cunningham, Ph.D.,[5]
Benedetto Vitiello, M.D.,[6] Mark A. Riddle, M.D.,[7] Mark Davies, M.P.H.,[8]
Laurence L. Greenhill, M.D.,[8] James T. McCracken, M.D.,[2] James J. McGough, M.D.,[2]
Kelly Posner, Ph.D.,[8] Anne M. Skrobala, M.A.,[8] Tim Wigal, Ph.D.,[6] Sharon B. Wigal, Ph.D.,[6]
Jaswinder K. Ghuman, M.D.,[9] and Shirley Z. Chuang, M.S.[10]

ABSTRACT

Objective. To assess parent-teacher concordance on ratings of DSM-IV symptoms of attention-deficit/hyperactivity disorder (ADHD) in a sample of preschool children referred for an ADHD treatment study.

Methods. Parent and teacher symptom ratings were compared for 452 children aged 3–5 years. Agreement was calculated using Pearson correlations, Cohen's kappa, and conditional probabilities.

Results. The correlations between parent and teacher ratings were low for both Inattentive (r = .24) and Hyperactive-Impulsive (r = .26) symptom domains, with individual symptoms ranging from .01–.28. Kappa values for specific symptoms were even lower. Conditional probabilities suggest that teachers are only moderately likely to agree with parents on the presence or abscence of symptoms. Parents were quite likely to agree with teachers' endorsement of symptoms, but much less likely to agree when teachers indicated that a symptom was not present.

Conclusions. Results provide important data regarding base rates and concordance rates in this age group and support the hypothesis that preschool-aged children at risk for ADHD exhibit significant differences in behavior patterns across settings. Obtaining ratings from multiple informants is therefore considered critical for obtaining a full picture of young children's functioning.

---

[1]Duke University Medical Center, Durham, North Carolina.
[2]University of California, Los Angeles, Los Angeles, California.
[3]New York University Child Study Center, New York, New York.
[4]University of California, Irvine, Irvine, California.
[5]McMaster University, Hamilton, Ontario, Canada.
[6]National Institute of Mental Health, Bethesda, Maryland.
[7]Johns Hopkins University, Baltimore, Maryland.
[8]New York State Psychiatric Institute/Columbia University, New York, New York.
[9]University of Arizona, Tucson, Arizona.
[10]Formerly at New York State Psychiatric Institute/Columbia University.

INTRODUCTION

$\mathbf{T}$HE *DIAGNOSTIC AND STATISTICAL MANUAL of Mental Disorders*, 4th edition (DSM-IV) (American Psychiatric Association 1994) criteria for attention-deficit/hyperactivity disorder (ADHD) require that symptoms and impairment occur in multiple settings. To evaluate this criterion, practice guidelines recommend collecting information from both parents and teachers about the behavior of the child in different settings (American Psychiatric Association 1994; AACAP 1997; AAP 2000; McDermott et al. 2005). However, the utility of this pervasiveness criterion has been questioned (e.g., Biederman et al. 1990), especially with respect to the benefits of multiple informants for diagnostic validity relative to the burden of collecting such data. This concern is especially salient in preschool-aged children, because the kinds of settings from which teacher ratings may be gathered are more variable than settings for school-aged children, and many 3 and 4 year olds do not attend preschool. Furthermore, integrating discrepant data from parents and teachers is challenging because there are not empirically supported guidelines to support the reliability and validity of different approaches. Understanding the patterns of parent–teacher agreement for ADHD symptoms is important not only for clinical decision making but also for a more valid characterization of the disorder, especially in young children.

Parent–teacher agreement for behavior ratings has been found to be low to moderate across a range of ages and types of behaviors. An early yet influential meta-analysis demonstrated an average correlation of $r = 0.27$ across 26 studies, with externalizing behaviors such as hyperactivity generally having higher agreement than internalizing behaviors (Achenbach et al. 1987). More recent large-scale studies have found similar results across different samples, with correlations in the range of $r = 0.13–0.54$ across behaviors (Kumpulainen et al. 1999; Frigerio et al. 2004). Concordance rates for ADHD behaviors fall in this range, although they may be lower than for oppositional and conduct disordered behaviors (Loeber et al. 1991; Biederman et al. 1993).

Two recent studies examining clinical sam-

ples of ADHD youth also demonstrate a lack of association between parent and teacher identification of disorder subtypes and ratings. One study assessed agreement on DSM-IV symptoms of ADHD using structured diagnostic interviews with 74 7–11 year olds. They found significant correlations between the total number of symptoms reported by parents and teachers ($r = 0.42$), the number of hyperactive-impulsive symptoms ($r = 0.39$), and the number of inattentive symptoms ($r = 0.30$). However, agreement with regard to diagnostic subtype based on parents and teachers each endorsing a threshold number of symptoms was poor (i.e., 17 of 55 cases; 31%). The authors attributed some of this discrepancy to the categorical cutpoint of six symptoms required for diagnosis as well as to cross-situational differences in children's behavior (Mitsis et al. 2000).

In a sample of 6–12 year olds diagnosed with ADHD, correlations on DSM-IV ADHD symptom scales rated on a 0–3 Likert scale were very low ($r = 0.13$ and 0.09 for inattention and hyperactivity-impulsivity, respectively) although ratings of oppositional and conduct disordered behavior were moderate ($r = 0.56$ and 0.36, respectively). Agreement at the item level ranged from $r = 0.20$ to 0.52 for inattentive items and from $r = 0.06$ to 0.32 for hyperactive-impulsive items. Significant Spearman correlation coefficients were found for only 5 of 18 symptoms: forgetful, not listening, difficulty following instructions or completing tasks, difficulty engaging in activities quietly, and leaving seat (Antrop et al. 2002). In addition to reflecting the situational specificity of ADHD children's behaviors, the authors suggest that lower agreement on ADHD behaviors may be due to the nature of ADHD symptoms being less concrete than aggression and defiance.

Additional explanations for low correlations between raters in clinical samples, often assessed by Pearson's r, are the effects of restricted-range, nonnormally distributed data, and the fact that rating scales data are ordinal rather than continuous. However, evidence that agreement in ADHD clinical samples is comparable to that found for ADHD-related behaviors in large community samples suggests that range restriction may have limited impact. In any case, examining agreement in clinical samples from a variety of approaches can be potentially informative from a clinical perspective, provided the caveat of restricted range is observed.

Although a sizable body of literature has addressed parent–teacher agreement in school-aged children, few published studies address the association of parent and teacher ratings in preschool children. Concordance rates at this age may be negatively affected by the wide range of day-care and preschool settings with varying levels of structure and demands as compared to elementary school, or by different developmental manifestations of disorders. Indeed, lower agreement for younger children was identified in a community-based study directly comparing agreement in 4–5 year olds and 6–12 year olds, where the number of significant correlations at the item level on the Achenbach Child Behavior Checklist and Teacher Report Form (CBCL, TRF) was over three times as large for the older group as compared to the younger group (Verhulst and Akkerhuis 1989). However, this may be partly attributable to the difference in sample sizes (271 younger vs. 890 older).

Two additional studies of nonclinical preschool samples provide further indications that concordance rates for preschoolers are no better than, if not lower than, rates cited for older children. In a small sample of 3–6 year olds identified as either "at-risk" or comparison, one study found that parent–teacher ratings of externalizing behavior on the Achenbach were modestly associated ($r = 0.32$), although ratings of internalizing behaviors were not ($r = 0.13$) (Hinshaw et al. 1992). Second, parent–teacher agreement at the item level on the Achenbach in a large sample of predominantly African-American children attending Head Start averaged 0.06, with only 18 of 82 common items achieving statistically significant correlation values (Cai et al. 2004).

The presentation of ADHD symptoms in younger children may also contribute to lower concordance rates than in older samples. ADHD behaviors have been reported by parents of 2–6 year olds at relatively high base rates (Gimpel and Kuhn 2000), with over 20% of 253 mothers with children in day care endorsing fidgeting, being on the go, talking excessively, difficulty waiting, and interrupting as occurring often or very often and almost 1 in 10 preschool children being identified as having some ADHD behaviors. In addition, there is indication that inattentive symptoms and subtypes of ADHD may be unstable at this age (Gadow et al. 2001; Lahey et al. 2005), which may contribute to variable symptom presentation across settings as well as time. More specifically, young children who meet criteria for the Hyperactive-Impulsive subtype are more likely to shift to another subtype (most typically Combined Type) and/or desist over time, although almost 80% of preschoolers with ADHD continued to meet criteria for diagnosis 7 years later. Consistent with this finding, the mean number of hyperactive-impulsive symptoms appears to decrease over time whereas the number of inattentive symptoms remains constant. Thus, in preschool children, the common occurrence of ADHD behaviors in the population as well as the individual variability of symptoms over time may make it more difficult for parents and teachers to agree on what specific symptoms are problematic.

In sum, previous work has provided useful information on parent–teacher agreement in clinical samples of school-aged children with ADHD and in community samples of preschoolers. However, parent–teacher agreement for clinically referred preschoolers with ADHD has not been examined previously. Moreover, varying methodological approaches to assessing agreement across studies complicate the conclusions that can be drawn. Given additional factors that may lower concordance rates in preschoolers with ADHD (e.g., high base rates and instability of symptom presentation) and recent concerns related to increasing rates of diagnosis and treatment, this gap in the literature is significant. Advancing understanding of the nature and extent of parent–teacher agreement for ADHD symptoms will also assist clinicians in making diagnostic decisions and may inform future revisions to diagnostic classification criteria for this age group. Therefore, the present study examined patterns of parent and teacher agreement on ADHD symptoms in children referred to the Preschool ADHD Treatment Study (PATS) from a variety of statistical approaches. This study was the largest treatment study to date for preschool children with ADHD (Kollins et al. 2006) and allowed for extensive data collection of both parent and teacher ratings of the behavior of children in the home and preschool settings.

METHODS

Participants

Participants were children aged 3–5.5 years referred for participation in the PATS study at six academic sites (Columbia University, Duke University, Johns Hopkins, New York University, University of California Irvine, and University of California Los Angeles). As will be described further, not all participants in the present analyses met criteria for inclusion in the PATS study. At each site, paid advertisements and public service announcements were placed in newspapers and radio broadcasts for a treatment study for preschoolers with ADHD symptoms. The primary incentives for participation were a 10-week course of parent training and the possibility of a carefully monitored trial of methylphenidate (MPH) free of charge. Notices were distributed to primary-care physicians, nursery schools, day-care centers, and kindergartens. There were no restrictions on the basis of sex, race, or ethnicity. A total of 553 participants signed consent forms for the study during the period between February, 2001, and April, 2003, and 452 provided both parent and teacher ratings as part of the screening process.

Sixty five percent (295/452) of the sample met all of the criteria for entry into the PATS study, including being stimulant naïve, meeting consensus diagnosis for ADHD (American Psychiatric Association 1994) based on the Diagnostic Interview Schedule for Children IV–Parent Version (DISC-IV-P; Shaffer et al. 1996) and semistructured interview; combined or predominately hyperactive subtype; an impairment scale score ≤55 on the Children's Global Assessment Scale (C-GAS; Shaffer et al. 1983); full-scale IQ of greater than 70 on the Differential Ability Scales (DAS; Elliott 1990); participation in a preschool, day-care group setting or other school program for at least 2

TABLE 1. SAMPLE CHARACTERISTICS ($n = 452$)

Variable	Mean (SD)	n (%)
Age	4.39 (.70)	
Male		339 (75)
Ethnicity		
White		276 (61.1)
Black or		
African-American		74 (16.4)
Asian American		6 (1.3)
American Indian or		
Alaskan Native		2 (0.4)

SD = Standard deviation.

half-days per week with at least 8 same-age peers; and the same primary caretaker for at least 6 months prior to screening. These subjects also had ratings on both the Conners' Revised Parent (CPRS) and Teacher (CTRS) Rating Scales (Conners 1997) that were at or above a T score of 65, 1.5 standard deviations (SD) above the age- and sex-adjusted means, on the DSM-IV Hyperactive-Impulsive subscale T score. Children were excluded from the treatment study if there was current evidence of adjustment disorder, pervasive developmental disorders, psychosis, significant suicidality, or other psychiatric disorder in addition to ADHD that required treatment with additional medication; current stimulant or cocaine abuse in a relative living in the home; a confounding medical condition; inability of the parent to understand or follow study instructions; or history of bipolar disorder in both biological parents. For the purpose of the present study, 8 enrolled subjects were excluded due to the absence of teacher rating data.

The additional 157 participants with data analyzed were also referred to the PATS study by parents or teachers due to ADHD symptoms, but did not meet full criteria for inclusion. Although we are unable to report on the specific reasons these participants were excluded given the data collection procedures used, parents and teachers of nonenrolled participants reported fewer inattentive [t (teachers) = 5.59, t (parents) = 2.95, $p < 0.001$] and hyperactive-impulsive symptoms [t (teachers) = 13.10, (parents) = 6.55, $p < 0.001$]. Thus, our sample was designed to consider limitations created by restriction of range typically found in clinical samples, and is considered more generalizable than a sample based only upon participants who met strict criteria for a specific treatment study. There were no significant differences in age or ethnicity of enrolled versus nonenrolled children, although there was a trend for fewer females to be enrolled than males ($\chi^2 = 3.34$, $p = 0.07$). As can be seen in Table 1, the total sample analyzed was demographically diverse, with 61% Caucasian and 75% male participants.

Dependent measures

As indicated, subscales of the parent and teacher versions of the Conners' Rating Scales, Revised (Conners 1997) collected at screening were used as the primary dependent measures. These scales are widely used to assess disruptive behavior disorders in clinical and research settings, have well-established psychometric properties, and have normative data available for the age range used in this study (Conners et al. 1998a; Conners et al. 1998b). Both parent and teacher versions of the rating scales include questions corresponding to each of the 18 DSM-IV symptoms of ADHD. These items are rated on a scale from 0 to 3, with the following descriptors as anchors: 0 = Not at all, Never; 1 = Just a little, Once in a while; 2 = Pretty much, Often; 3 = Very Much, Very frequently. The average (or sum) of items for the two ADHD domains (DSM-IV Inattentive and Hyperactive-Impulsive subscales) was the primary outcome measure for this report.

Data analysis

To determine the extent of absent items and to identify any nonrandom sources of missing data, we conducted a missing values analysis for the 18 DSM-IV ADHD items on both the CPRS-R and the CTRS-R. With regard to the CPRS-R, the analysis indicated that less than 1% of data ($n = 57/8136$) was missing across all responses. An examination of each participant's data revealed only 38 participants with any missing items; of these, there were just 2 participants who were missing ratings on 4 or more of the 18 DSM-IV symptoms. Furthermore, an item analysis indicated that missing values were randomly distributed across the 18 symptoms. On the CTRS-R, 2.6% ($n = 213/8136$) of responses were missing. There were 15 cases with 4 or more responses missing. In addition, 11.5% ($n = 52/452$) of teachers failed to provide a response for one item ("Loses things necessary for tasks or activities"). All other missing values appeared to be randomly occurring, and, as such, mean-substitution was employed to replace missing values for the purpose summary statistics. However, no substitutions were made for four participants with four or more missing values or for the CTRS-R item "Loses things necessary for tasks or activities," as this did not appear to be missing randomly, nor for analyses at the item level.

Parent–teacher agreement was assessed in several ways. First, overall concordance was evaluated for the severity ratings of each individual symptom (range = 0–3), as well as the total scores from the Inattention and Hyperactive-Impulsive subscales (range = 0–27 each) using Pearson's correlations. Although we considered nonparametric analysis such as Spearman's correlation, we report Pearson's so our results will be comparable with other studies in this area. Next, ratings for each symptom

TABLE 2. DESCRIPTIVE CHARACTERISTICS OF THE DSM-IV SYMPTOM INDICES

Scale	Number of symptoms		Index total		Internal Consistency
	M	SD	M	SD	α
CPRS-R:L					
DSM-IV Inattentive	5.64	2.37	16.17	5.66	0.85
DSM-IV Hyperactive-Impulsive	7.41	1.62	20.68	4.21	0.72
CTRS-R:L					
DSM-IV Inattentive	4.31	2.78	13.20	6.69	0.89
DSM-IV Hyperactive-Impulsive	5.84	2.92	17.11	7.31	0.90

DSM-IV = *Diagnostic and Statistical Manual of Mental Disorders*, 4th edition; SD = standard deviation; CPRS-R:L = Connors' Parent Rating Scale-Revised: Long Version; CTRS-R:L = Connors' Teacher Rating Scale-Revised: Long Version.

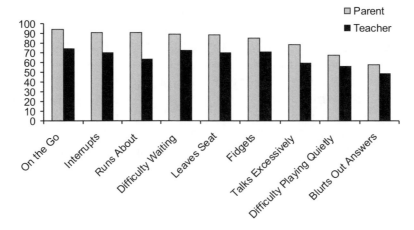

FIG. 1. Percentage of parents and teachers reporting hyperactive-impulsive symptoms.

were dichotomized as "absent" (rated as a 0 or 1) or "present" (rated as a 2 or 3). This approach for determining symptom presence or absence has been used previously (Pelham et al. 1992; Lahey et al. 2005). We compared the total number of Inattentive and Hyperactive-Impulsive symptoms reported by parents to the number reported by teachers using paired *t*-tests. Agreement for individual symptoms was then evaluated using Cohen's kappa statistic based upon the presence or absence of symptoms as described above. Because calculation of the kappa statistic is heavily influenced by base rates of symptoms (Spitznagel and Helzer 1985; Feinstein and Cicchetti 1990; Byrt et al. 1993), and because overall base rates of symptom reporting in this at-risk sample was high, we conducted an additional analysis of agreement to assess the conditional probabilities of parent and teacher en-

dorsement of symptoms, based on what the other informant reported (Cicchetti and Feinstein 1990). This approach for calculating concordance has been used previously in studies of rater agreement in ADHD samples (Faraone et al. 2005). Of note, kappas and conditional probabilities were calculated using original raw scores with no mean substitution of missing values.

RESULTS

Reliability of dependent measure

Reliability of the parent and teacher ratings was first assessed to ensure that results from our agreement analyses were interpretable. To assess the reliability of parent and teacher ratings of DSM-IV ADHD symptoms, internal consistency for each symptom domain was cal-

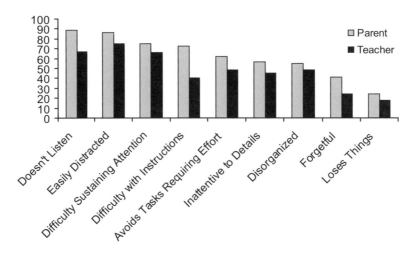

FIG. 2. Percentage of parents and teachers reporting inattentive symptoms.

TABLE 3.   RANK ORDER OF DSM-IV ADHD SYMPTOMS BY PARENT AND TEACHER REPORT

	Parent rank	Percentage reporting	Teacher rank	Percentage reporting
DSM-IV Inattentive symptoms				
Does not listen	1	89.2	2	67.7
Easily distracted	2	85.6	1	74.1
Difficulty sustaining attention	3	75.2	3	66.8
Does not follow instructions	4	73.5	7	38.9
Avoids tasks requiring effort	5	61.7	4	47.3
Fails to give close attention to details	6	56.0	6	44.0
Difficulty organizing	7	55.3	4	47.3
Forgetful	8	41.4	8	23.9
Loses things	9	25.0	9	15.5
DSM-IV Hyperactive-Impulsive symptoms				
Always "on the go"	1	93.8	1	73.7
Interrupts others	2	90.9	5	69.5
Runs about	3	90.7	6	63.1
Difficulty waiting	4	89.4	2	72.8
Leaves seat	5	88.2	4	69.7
Fidgets	6	85.4	3	71.0
Talks excessively	7	78.1	7	59.1
Difficulty playing quietly	8	67.9	8	55.8
Blurts out answers	9	57.3	9	47.6

DSM-IV = *Diagnostic and Statistical Manual of Mental Disorders*, 4th edition; ADHD = attention-deficit/hyperactivity disorder.

culated. Cronbach's alpha was found to be adequate or better ($\alpha \geq 0.70$) for both informants across both domains (see Table 2). Teacher reliability was somewhat higher than parent reliability, particularly for the Hyperactive-Impulsive domain (CTRS HI $\alpha = 0.90$, CPRS HI $\alpha = 0.72$). Overall, however, reliability results suggest that both parents and teachers are relatively consistent in their own reports of ADHD symptoms. In addition, both parent and teacher ratings of the ADHD symptom domains (hyperactivity-impulsivity and inattention) were significantly related (teachers $r = 0.50$, $p < 0.001$; parents $r = 0.37$, $p < 0.001$).

Descriptive analyses and main effects

Prior to the assessment of rater concordance, the frequency of individual symptoms by parent and teacher report across domains was examined and global differences between responses of parents and teachers were evaluated. As can be seen in Fig. 1, parents and teachers reported that individual hyperactive-impulsive symptoms (defined as a 2 or 3 on the Conners' rating scales) were present in 57–94% of the sample. This finding is not surprising given that two-thirds of the sample met the in-clusion criteria of elevated ratings on these symptoms. What is also apparent is that parents consistently reported symptoms in more children than did teachers, a pattern that is also seen for inattentive symptoms in Fig. 2. Given that parents initiated referrals to the PATS study in most cases, this is also not surprising. Figure 2 also demonstrates that overall base rates of individual inattentive symptoms in the sample are lower than the rates of hyperactive-impulsive symptoms, as might be expected for this age range. There also appeared to be a wider range in the percentage of children exhibiting different inattentive symptoms as compared to those exhibiting hyperactive-impulsive symptoms.

Regarding global differences between informants, parents reported significantly more Inattentive [$t(397) = 8.24$, $p < 0.001$] and Hyperactive-Impulsive [$t(444) = 11.04$, $p < 0.001$] symptoms than did teachers (see Table 2). In addition, the total raw scores for the DSM-IV Inattentive and Hyperactive-Impulsive subscales were significantly higher for parents compared to teachers [$t(287) = 4.40$, $p < 0.001$, $d = 0.48$ and $t(290) = 4.76$, $p < 0.001$, respectively, $d = 0.60$]. We next examined a rank ordering of the frequency with which individual

TABLE 4.   AGREEMENT BETWEEN PARENT AND TEACHER RATINGS OF DSM-IV
INATTENTIVE AND HYPERACTIVE-IMPULSIVE SYMPTOMS

	r	κ
DSM-IV Inattentive symptoms	0.24**	
Forgetful	0.14**	0.09
Fails to give close attention to details	0.26**	0.20
Avoids tasks requiring effort	0.27**	0.15
Does not listen	0.13	0.12
Difficulty organizing	0.14**	0.13
Difficulty sustaining attention	0.21**	0.04
Loses things	0.01	0.12
Does not follow instructions	0.16**	0.12
Easily distracted	0.10*	0.07
DSM-IV Hyperactive-Impulsive symptoms	0.26**	
Always "on the go"	0.15**	0.09
Leaves seat	0.28**	0.18
Difficulty waiting	0.13*	0.10
Talks excessively	0.27**	0.19
Runs about	0.11*	0.08
Difficulty playing quietly	0.12*	0.08
Fidgets	0.21**	0.12
Blurts out answers	0.27**	0.20
Interrupts others	0.11*	0.07

r = Pearson's; κ = Cohen's kappa; DSM-IV = *Diagnostic and Statistical Manual of Mental Disorders*, 4th edition.
*$p < 0.05$; **$p < 0.01$.

DSM-IV Inattentive and Hyperactive-Impulsive symptoms were reported across groups. As may be seen in Table 3, teachers and parents were quite similar in terms of which symptoms were endorsed most often.

Analysis of rater concordance

Correlations between parent and teacher ratings of individual Inattentive and Hyperactive-Impulsive symptoms were generally low, ranging from 0.01 to 0.28 (see Table 4). Pearson's correlations for the total DSM-IV Inattentive Symptom subscale ($r = 0.24$, $p < 0.01$) and total DSM-IV Hyperactive-Impulsive subscale ($r = 0.26$, $p < 0.01$) also indicated low concordance. Correlations were of similar magnitude across domains. To examine agreement regarding the presence of clinical significant symptoms, we also calculated kappas based upon categorizing participants by T scores above and below 70 on each subscale. Results were similarly low for both domains ($\kappa = 0.11$ for the Hyperactive-Impulsive domain, and 0.16 for Inattention). Given these low values, we calculated correlations on the four non-ADHD scales common to both the CPRS-R and

the CTRS-R. Correlations were similar to those obtained for the ADHD scales on the Oppositional subscale ($r = 0.29$, $p < 0.01$) and Social Problems subscale ($r = 0.25$, $p < 0.01$), although associations were somewhat lower on the Perfectionism ($r = 0.15$, $p < 0.01$) and Anxious-Shy ($r = 0.16$, $p < 0.01$) subscales.

Within the Inattentive domain, the greatest concordance for individual symptoms was achieved for "avoids tasks requiring sustained mental effort" ($r = 0.27$, $p < 0.01$) and "fails to give close attention to details" ($r = 0.26$, $p < 0.01$). With regard to Hyperactive-Impulsive symptoms, three items describing impulsivity achieved modest correlation: "talks excessively" ($r = 0.27$, $p < 0.01$), "blurts out" ($r = 0.27$, $p < 0.01$), and "leaves seat" ($r = 0.28$, $p < 0.01$). It should be noted that Spearman correlations and Intra-Class Correlations (ICC), which are sometimes used in reliability analyses, were almost identical to Pearson r values.

To provide direct comparison to Mitsis et al. (2000), we also calculated correlations between the number of symptoms reported by parents and teachers for each domain. Again, we found low, albeit significant, correlations for both the number of hyperactive-impulsive symptoms

TABLE 5. CONDITIONAL PROBABILITIES FOR DSM-IV INATTENTIVE AND HYPERACTIVE SYMPTOMS

	Sensitivity	Specificity	+PP	−PP
DSM-IV Inattentive symptoms				
Forgetful	54/184 (**29.3**)	208/262 (**79.4**)	54/108 (**50.0**)	208/338 (**61.5**)
Fails to give close attention	133/247 (**53.8**)	128/193 (**66.3**)	133/247 (**67.2**)	128/242 (**52.9**)
Avoids tasks requiring effort	150/276 (**54.3**)	103/167 (**61.7**)	150/214 (**70.1**)	103/229 (**45.0**)
Does not listen	280/402 (**69.7**)	26/49 (**53.1**)	280/303 (**92.4**)	26/148 (**17.6**)
Difficulty organizing	131/243 (**53.9**)	114/197 (**57.9**)	131/214 (**61.2**)	114/197 (**50.4**)
Difficulty sustaining attention	237/338 (**70.1**)	50/112 (**44.6**)	237/299 (**79.3**)	50/151 (**33.1**)
Loses things	20/98 (**20.4**)	253/303 (**83.5**)	20/70 (**28.6**)	253/331 (**83.5**)
Does not follow instructions	142/317 (**44.8**)	85/119 (**71.4**)	142/176 (**80.7**)	85/260 (**32.7**)
Easily distracted	293/385 (**76.1**)	21/63 (**33.3**)	293/335 (**87.5**)	21/113 (**18.6**)
Mean (SD)	**52.5 (18.70)**	**61.2 (16.16)**	**68.6 (19.97)**	**43.9 (21.14)**
DSM-IV Hyperactive–Impulsive symptoms				
Always "on the go"	318/423 (**75.2**)	13/28 (**46.4**)	318/333 (**95.5**)	13/118 (**11.0**)
Leaves seat	291/396 (**73.5**)	30/53 (**56.6**)	291/314 (**92.7**)	30/135 (**22.2**)
Difficulty waiting	301/404 (**74.5**)	20/48 (**41.7**)	301/329 (**91.5**)	20/123 (**16.3**)
Talks excessively	228/352 (**64.8**)	60/99 (**60.6**)	228/267 (**85.4**)	60/184 (**32.6**)
Runs about	266/410 (**64.9**)	23/42 (**54.8**)	266/285 (**93.3**)	23/167 (**13.8**)
Difficulty playing quietly	179/305 (**58.7**)	73/146 (**50.0**)	179/305 (**71.0**)	73/199 (**36.7**)
Fidgets	284/386 (**73.6**)	29/66 (**43.9**)	284/321 (**88.5**)	29/131 (**22.1**)
Blurts out answers	146/256 (**57.0**)	120/189 (**63.5**)	146/215 (**67.9**)	120/230 (**52.2**)
Interrupts others	291/410 (**71.0**)	18/41 (**43.9**)	291/314 (**92.7**)	18/137 (**13.1**)
Mean (SD)	**68.1 (7.00)**	**51.3 (7.93)**	**86.5 (10.13)**	**24.4 (13.63)**

DSM-IV = *Diagnostic and Statistical Manual of Mental Disorders*, 4th edition.
Note: See text for explanations of column headings. Values in column represent frequencies (reported/total number respondents). Bold values represent percentages.

($r = 0.23$, $p < 0.001$) and the number of inattentive symptoms ($r = 0.21$, $p < 0.001$). Rater agreement was further examined at the individual symptom level using Cohen's κ to correct for chance agreement. Across individual Inattentive and Hyperactive-Impulsive symptoms, kappa values were poor, ranging from 0.04 to 0.20 (see Table 4). We did not observe any consistent pattern between kappa values and base rates of individual symptoms. However, kappa values were likely restricted by overall relatively high base rates of symptoms in this sample. We saw this effect when we examined kappa values for only those participants who met inclusion criteria for the PATS study ($\kappa = 0.13$ for Inattentive and 0.07 for hyperactive-impulsive, much lower than for the full sample).

To ascertain whether rater agreement differed according to child demographic variables, kappa values were calculated separately for gender, age group (3–4 vs. 5-year-olds), and race (white vs. non-white). For Inattentive symptoms, there were no differences in rater agreement by age or gender, but for Hyperactive-Impulsive symptoms, there was a trend for

rater agreement to be better for children of ethnic minority groups ($r = 0.35$) than for white children ($r = 0.17$, $z = 1.91$, $p = 0.06$).

As can be seen in Table 5, conditional probabilities were calculated for individual symptoms to determine the diagnostic efficiency of parent reports as predictors of teacher reports, and vice versa using guidelines previously reported (Faraone et al. 2005). Sensitivity, defined as the probability that a teacher reported a symptom given that a parent had done so, was variable across symptoms (range = 20.4–76.1%) and somewhat better for Hyperactive-Impulsive ($M = 68.1$, SD = 7.00) than Inattentive ($M = 52.5$, SD = 18.70) symptoms. Specificity, the probability that a teacher did not report a symptom given that a parent had not, fell in a similar range (33.3–83.5%), although was slightly higher for inattentive ($M = 61.2$, SD = 16.16) than hyperactive-impulsive symptoms ($M = 51.3$, SD = 7.93). Positive predictive power was defined as the probability that symptoms were rated by parents as present given that teachers had endorsed them. These probabilities were the most robust of all the conditional probabilities across both Hyperactive-Impulsive symptoms ($M = 86.5$, SD = 10.13) and Inattentive symptoms ($M = 68.6$, SD = 19.97). Finally, negative predictive power was the probability that a parent did not endorse a symptom that had not been reported by a teacher. These probabilities were considerably lower, ranging from 11% to 83.5%, with most symptoms below 50% and with lower probability of agreement for hyperactive-impulsive symptoms ($M = 24.4$, SD = 13.63) than inattentive symptoms ($M = 43.9$, SD = 21.14).

DISCUSSION

The major aim of this study was to describe the concordance between parent and teacher ratings of ADHD symptoms in preschool-aged children referred for participation in an ADHD medication treatment study. Given that this likely represents the population that presents most often to clinicians for evaluation, we believe our sample is ideal for evaluating this important, yet unexamined topic. Therefore, we examined concordance rates through a variety of statistical methods, and interpreted them in relation to base rates and relative rankings of symptoms in this age group as well as to concordance rates reported in school-aged clinical samples.

As predicted, overall parent–teacher agreement was poor, as demonstrated by low correlations for individual items, subscale scores, total number of symptoms, and kappa values. Compared to a small clinical sample of school-aged children with ADHD, the magnitude of association in our sample at the subscale level ($r = 0.26$ and 0.24) is actually higher (Antrop et al. 2002), although this may be due to the increased range of our sample. On the other hand, our agreement for the number of ADHD symptoms endorsed (0.23 and 0.21 for Hyperactive-Impulsive and Inattentive, respectively) was lower than that reported by Mitsis et al. (2000), $r = 0.39$ and 0.30. What is perhaps more interesting is that the range of agreement we found was much more similar to Antrop et al. (2002) for hyperactive-impulsive items (0.11–0.28 in our sample vs. 0.06–0.32 for Antrop) than for inattentive items (0.01–0.27 vs. 0.2–0.52). We also found differences across the age

groups in the specific items that occurred most frequently. For example, Antrop et al. (2002) identified leaving seat, difficulty playing quietly, forgetful, difficulty listening, and difficulty following directions as having the highest parent–teacher agreement rates, whereas the highest agreement rates in our sample were for leaving seat, talking excessively, blurting out, difficulty attending to details, and avoiding tasks. In the present sample, demographic characteristics of the participants (i.e., gender, age) did not appear to influence concordance rates as has been found in some studies of older children (Achenbach et al. 1987; Verhulst and Akkerhuis 1989; Kumpulainen et al. 1999; Frigerio et al. 2004). Overall, the pattern of our results varies somewhat from that reported previously for school-aged samples, although this may be due more to differences in analytic approaches and sample characteristics than to any developmental differences. Present results cannot empirically evaluate whether parent–teacher concordance differs as a function of developmental level, but our data do not provide as much support for this as we had expected.

Consistent with poor parent–teacher concordance rates, diagnostic efficiency statistics reflect only moderate probability that teachers will agree with parents on the presence or absence of individual ADHD symptoms, for most inattentive and hyperactive-impulsive symptoms. This is particularly relevant for clinicians evaluating young children who present to the clinic with their parents, and for whom obtaining teacher ratings may be difficult. Although less clinically informative given that diagnostic information is usually obtained from parents first, we also found that predictive power for the presence of symptoms was higher than for the absence of symptoms, suggesting that there is a reasonable likelihood that parents will agree with teachers that specific symptoms are present, but if teachers do not endorse a given symptom, parents may or may not endorse it. These results are understandable in that parents of preschool-aged children may receive information about their child's behavior in the school setting that could increase their agreement with teacher reports, although teachers are less likely to be familiar with the child's home behavior. Our conditional probability rates are actually somewhat higher than those assessed in older ADHD clinical samples (Biederman et al. 1990; Faraone et al. 2005), which may be a function of our lower and more variable base rates. That is, if almost all the cases exhibit symptoms such as expected in a purely clinical sample, it will be more likely that parents and teachers will agree with each other than if there is more of a range in the prevalence rates of symptoms. However, conditional probabilities based on such clinical samples are less likely to be useful to clinicians presented with possible cases.

In interpreting the meaning of poor parent–teacher concordance rates, it is important to recognize some of the differences in the settings in which parents and teachers observe young children. In contrast to homes, where a child may have no or few siblings and the expectations and structure may be variable, preschools typically require children to interact with groups of peers, may place greater or at least different demands for attention and impulse control upon children, and expose them to a range of activities that generally follow a consistent schedule. In particular for first-born children, parents may lack knowledge of what is developmentally appropriate. On the other hand, parents certainly have a greater sample of behavior upon which to rate their child, not just across time historically but also at different times of day than when teachers are making observations. Young children in particular may be more likely to demonstrate emotional and behavioral difficulties with parents with whom they feel comfortable. Thus, there are many setting differences that may contribute to low concordance rates.

Support for the hypothesis that parent–teacher discrepancies reflect the variability of children's behaviors across situations is provided by data verifying behavioral differences across settings when rater variability is controlled (McDermott et al. 2005). Moreover, both parent and teacher reports were reliable in the present sample as evidenced by adequate internal consistency. Previous studies also support the validity of teacher ratings, which have been found to relate to observations of preschoolers' externalizing behaviors and to predict long-term impairment (Hinshaw et al.

1992; Mannuzza et al. 2002). Thus, parents and teachers appear to be reporting on important but distinct aspects of child functioning, and the lack of agreement on symptom ratings suggests that cross-situational informants are needed to provide a full picture of a child's functioning and to make diagnostic decisions.

Overall, six of nine hyperactive-impulsive symptoms were endorsed by more than 80% of parents and 60% of teachers, whereas only two of nine inattentive symptoms were reported at these rates. Again, this is not surprising given that two thirds of our sample met criteria for elevated hyperactivity-impulsivity ratings and were diagnosed with ADHD, Combined or Hyperactive-Impulsive subtype. There was also considerably more variability in the rates of inattentive symptoms, with several identified in less than 50% of the sample, particularly by teacher report. One implication of this finding is that the distribution of symptoms across domains in this age group may not be consistent. As was seen, however, parent–teacher agreement was low across both domains, and across symptoms with high base rates as well as those with much lower base rates. Also of note, more than 1 in 10 teachers failed to respond to the CTRS-R:L item assessing "loses things," which appeared nonrandom, and may reflect the lack of relevance of that behavior at this age.

Although parents identified more symptoms occurring more frequently than did teachers, as has been found in other clinic-referred samples (Mitsis et al. 2000; Antrop et al. 2002), there was overlap in the specific symptoms identified as occurring most often by rank order. The most commonly reported inattentive symptoms, reported by >65% of parents and teachers in this sample were not listening, distractibility, and difficulty sustaining attention. In addition, parents reported that many of their children often demonstrated difficulty following instructions (72%). Several hyperactive-impulsive symptoms were reported at a similar rate: being on the go, leaving seat, fidgeting, difficulty waiting, and interrupting. Talking excessively, running about, and difficulty playing quietly were also endorsed frequently by parents. Interestingly, however, these symptoms mirror those reported by parents most often in a nonclinical sample of preschoolers aged 2–6 years recruited from day-care centers (Gimpel et al. 2000), albeit at a much higher rate (15–92% across symptoms vs. 4–28% in the nonclinical sample). In both samples, hyperactive–impulsive behaviors were considerably more common than inattentive behaviors by parent and teacher report. This may reflect the developmental nature of the symptoms at this age, and is consistent with the more frequent diagnosis of Hyperactive-Impulsive subtype in this age than at other ages (Lahey et al. 2005).

Despite poor parent–teacher concordance for specific ADHD symptoms, the careful clinical integration of symptoms across informants identified a subset of young children qualifying for the PATS study that demonstrated considerable impairment and clinical correlates resembling that of older children (Posner et al., this issue). Epidemiological work also suggests that current DSM-IV symptom criteria are identifying a group of preschoolers with nonnormative hyperactivity, impulsivity, and inattention (Egger and Angold 2006) who have a disorder similar to that seen at other stages of life. As is carefully detailed in Posner et al. (this issue), ADHD can be validly diagnosed in preschool-aged children despite developmental features such as increased base rates of symptoms and variation in the presentation of symptoms.

CLINICAL IMPLICATIONS

Information on the base rates of ADHD symptoms and poor parent–teacher agreement in an at-risk preschool sample may be useful to clinicians when making diagnostic decisions. For example, if a preschooler presents with a few relatively low base-rate symptoms reported by either parents or teachers (e.g., loses things, forgetful, blurts out answers, inattentive to details), this may increase confidence in the developmental inappropriateness of such behaviors. On the other hand, if the only behaviors reported are those that occur commonly in high-risk children this age (e.g., distractibility, being "on the go," interrupting, and fidgeting), then the clinician may wish to obtain additional information to ascertain symptom presence. Given that parents are the primary referral source for children with disruptive behavior at

this age, and that they tend to report much higher rates of symptoms than teachers, one implication is that clinician confidence in symptom presence may increase when endorsed by teachers.

These data also have direct implications for diagnostic algorithms that could be developed for clinicians in the future. For example, preschool-aged children might need to demonstrate fewer low base-rate symptoms for valid diagnosis, whereas more symptoms might be necessary to diagnose ADHD in a preschooler presenting with only high base-rate symptoms. Alternately, as suggested by Hardy et al. (this issue), some symptoms may be more diagnostic than others, given how unique they are in terms of the different dimensions of inattention, hyperactivity, and impulsivity.

Although study results emphasize lack of agreement between parents and teachers on the presence of specific symptoms, it is important to note that agreement at the level of diagnosis was likely much higher given that two thirds of the sample had elevations on both parent and teacher ratings of hyperactivity-impulsivity. Indeed, this emphasizes that behavior ratings are best used in aggregate rather than in isolation and suggests that the expectation that all symptoms are reported across settings is unreasonable. This point is one that could be addressed further in future DSM revisions, providing some guidance for clinicians faced with symptom-level disagreements. Clinically, we propose that disagreements be opportunities for further investigation to understand and explain discrepancies, and to determine how situational factors or informant bias may be contributing to any differences. Finally, lack of agreement on any symptom should not be cause for dismissing the possibility that a symptom exists. This is consistent with the DSM-IV field trial approach that counted symptoms as present if endorsed by either parents or teachers.

The lack of agreement reported here does not suggest that either parent or teacher ratings are necessarily invalid, but rather highlight the variability in presentation of ADHD symptoms across settings. In fact, despite the low levels of agreement between raters, the reliability of reports within rating source were adequate.

From a clinical perspective, this means that only collecting data from parents or teachers in assessment will provide an incomplete view of preschool child functioning. In particular, the low conditional probabilities for absence of symptoms raise some concern of under diagnosis if cases are ruled out on the basis of only one reporter. Another implication of these results is that when developing treatment plans, data from both parents and teachers should be used to obtain an accurate view of how children respond to certain interventions.

LIMITATIONS

Although approximately one third of our sample did not meet inclusion criteria for the PATS study and likely had subclinical levels of ADHD symptoms across settings, the majority met very strict inclusion criteria, including obtaining elevated scores on the Hyperactive-Impulsive subscale of the CPRS-R:L and CTRS-R:L. There are clearly some unique characteristics of this sample that may not generalize to all samples presenting for clinical evaluation, primarily that this was a moderately to markedly severe group of young children whose parents were willing to consider medication as a treatment option. Moreover, part of our sample was defined by a high level of hyperactive-impulsive ratings by both parents and teachers, which restricted our range on our dependent variables and may have decreased concordance rates while some of our sample was characterized by lower teacher ratings that contributed to a wider range of scores. Nonetheless, evidence that poor agreement on the hyperactive-impulsive symptoms was not due to restriction of range was provided by the similarly low agreement rates for inattentive symptoms and for subscales assessing other behaviors. In addition, the range for the primary dependent measure used in this study was comparable to or greater than that reported in other clinical studies of rater agreement for ADHD (e.g., Mitsis et al. 2000; Antrop et al. 2002). Thus, we believe that our sample is generalizable to a population of preschool-aged children with ADHD symptoms presenting for clinical evaluation. Finally, as noted previously, examining the data in a number of different ways increases our confidence in the interpretation of the findings.

CONCLUSION AND FUTURE DIRECTIONS

This study has a number of strengths, the most salient of which is a large and well-characterized sample of young children with ADHD. It is also the first study to address parent–teacher agreement specifically for DSM-IV ADHD symptoms in a clinical sample of preschoolers. This study also contributes important information about parent and teacher ratings in this age group, which may be useful in increasing the diagnostic accuracy of ADHD assessment in preschoolers. It also provides data related to base rates and concordance rates that may be relevant for future DSM revisions.

Future research identifying which symptoms may be more validly identified by parents versus teachers given varying situational demands would also be an important contribution in informing DSM revisions. Further understanding of the developmental nature of ADHD may be provided by directly comparing parent–teacher agreement between diagnosed preschool and school-aged children. In addition, future research should evaluate the agreement of parents and teachers on ratings of improvement following treatment. Although this kind of agreement is not as germane to the diagnostic validity of ADHD in preschoolers, parent and teacher agreement for ratings of behavior change following treatment is very important and will be the focus of a separate paper based on the follow-up data from the PATS dataset. This follow-up analysis will be particularly important in light of recent data on how parent teacher agreement may be associated with response to medication. This was documented in the school-aged children in the MTA study, in which only 25% of the children who met the DSM-IV criteria for a diagnosis of ADHD-Combined Type also met the ICD-10 criteria for a diagnosis of Hyperkinetic Disorder, and this subset showed better response to stimulant medication and worse response to behavioral intervention (Santosh et al. 2005).

DISCLOSURES

The following financial disclosures indicate potential conflicts of interest among the PATS investigators and industry sources for the period 2000–2007. [1]Honoraria/consultant, [2]research support, [3]speaker's bureau, [4]significant equity (>$50,000). Dr. Murray: Eli Lilly,[2] Pfizer.[2] Dr. Kollins: Athenagen,[1,2] Cephalon,[1] Eli Lilly,[1,2] McNeil, New River Pharmaceuticals,[2] Pfizer,[2] Psychogenics,[2] Shire.[1,2] Dr. Greenhill: Alza,[2] Aventis,[1] Celltech,[2] Cephalon,[2] Eli Lilly,[1,2] Glaxo Wellcome,[2] Janssen,[1] McNeil,[2] Medeva,[2] Novartis Corporation,[2] Noven,[2] Otsuka,[1] Sanofi, Shire,[1,2] Solvay,[1] Somerset,[2] Thomson Advanced Therapeutics Communications,[1] Wyeth Ayerst.[2] Dr. Swanson: Alza,[1,2] Celgene,[1,2] Celltech,[1,2,3] Cephalon,[1,2,3] Eli Lilly,[1,2] Gliatech,[1,2] Janssen,[1,2,3] McNeil,[1,2,3] Novartis,[1,2] Shire,[1,2] UCB. Dr. Sharon Wigal: Celltech,[1,2,3] Cephalon,[1,2,3] Eli Lilly,[2] Janssen,[3] McNeil,[1,2,3] New River Pharmaceuticals,[2] Novartis,[1,2,3] Shire.[1,2,3] Dr. Abikoff: Abbot Labs,[1] Celltech,[2] Cephalon,[1] Eli Lilly,[1,2] McNeil,[1,2] Novartis,[2] Pfizer,[2] Shire.[1,2] Dr. McCracken: Abbott, Bristol Meyers Squibb,[1] Eli Lilly,[1,2,3] Gliatech,[2] Janssen,[1,3] Johnson & Johnson, McNeil,[1,2] Novartis, Noven,[1] Pfizer,[1,2] Shire,[1,2] UCB, Wyeth. Dr. Riddle: AstraZeneca,[1] Glaxo-Smith-Kline,[1] Janssen,[1] Pfizer,[2] Shire.[1] Dr. McGough: Eli Lilly,[1,2,3] McNeil,[1,2,3] New River Pharmaceuticals,[2] Novartis,[1,2,3] Pfizer,[1,2,3] Shire.[1,2,3] Dr. Posner: Abbott Laboratories, AstraZeneca Pharmaceuticals, Aventis, Bristol-Meyers Squibb, Cephalon, Eisai, Forest Laboratories, GlaxoSmithKline, Johnson & Johnson, Novartis, Organon USA, Sanofi-Shire,[1,2] Wyeth Research, UCB. Dr. Tim Wigal: Celltech,[2] Cephalon,[2] Eli Lilly,[2,3] Janssen,[2] McNeil,[2,3] Novartis,[2] Shire.[2,3] Mr. Davies: Amgen,[4] Bard, GlaxoSmithKline,[4] Johnson & Johnson,[4] Merck,[4] Pfizer,[4] Wyeth.[4] Dr. Ghuman: Bristol Myers-Squibb,[2] Drs. Vitiello and Cunningham and Ms. Chuang, and Ms. Skrobala have no conflicts of interest as they have not received support from companies manufacturing medications.

ACKNOWLEDGMENTS

The authors wish to acknowledge Rachel Baden, previously as Duke University Medical Center and currently at the University of Alabama, for her assistance with an earlier draft of this manuscript.

REFERENCES

Achenbach T, McConaughy S, Howell C: Child/adolescent behavioral and emotional problems: Implications of cross-informant correlations for situational specificity. Psycholog Bull 101:213–231, 1987.

American Academy of Child and Adolescent Psychiatry (AACAP): Practice parameters for the assessment and treatment of children, adolescents, and adults with attention-deficit/hyperactivity disorder. J Am Acad Child Adolesc Psychiatry 36:85S–121S, 1997.

American Academy of Pediatrics (AAP): Clinical practice guideline: Diagnosis and evaluation of the child with attention-deficit/hyperactivity disorder. Pediatrics 105:1158–1170, 2000.

American Psychiatric Association: Diagnostic and statistical manual of mental disorders, 4th edition. Washington (DC), American Psychiatric Association, 1994.

Antrop I, Roeyers H, Oosterlaan J, Van Oost P: Agreement between parent and teacher ratings of disruptive behavior disorders in children with clinically diagnosed ADHD. J Psychopathol Behav Assess 24:67–73, 2002.

Biederman J, Keenan K, Faraone SV: Parent-based diagnosis of attention deficit disorder predicts a diagnosis based on teacher report. J Am Acad Child Adolesc Psychiatry 29:698–701, 1990.

Biederman J, Faraone SV, Milberger S, Doyle A: Diagnoses of attention-deficit hyperactivity disorder from parent reports predict diagnoses based on teacher reports. J Am Acad Child Adolesc Psychiatry 32:315–317, 1993.

Byrt T, Bishop J, Carlin JB: Bias, prevalence and kappa. J Clin Epidemiol 46:423–429, 1993.

Cai X, Kaiser AP, Hancock TB: Parent and teacher agreement on child behavior checklist items in a sample of preschoolers from low-income and predominantly African American families. J Clin Child Adolesc Psychol 33:303–312, 2004.

Cicchetti DV, Feinstein AR: High agreement but low kappa: II Resolving the paradoxes. J Clin Epidemiol 43:551–558, 1990.

Conners CK: Conners' Rating Scales–Revised: Technical Manual. North Tonawanda (New York), Multi-Health Systems, 1997.

Conners CK, Sitarenios G, Parker, JA, Epstein JN: The Revised Conners' Parent Rating Scale (CPRS-R): Factor structure, reliability, and criterion validity. J Abnorm Child Psychol 26:257–268, 1998a.

Conners CK, Sitarenios G, Parker JA, Epstein JN: Revision and restandardization of the Conners' Teacher Rating Scale (CTRS-R): Factor structure, reliability, and criterion validity. J Abnorm Child Psychol 26:279–291, 1998b.

Egger HL, Angold A: Common emotional and behavioral disorders in preschool children: Presentation, nosology, and epidemiology. J Child Psychol Psychiatry 47:313–337, 2006.

Elliott CD: Differential Abilities Scale. San Antonio (Texas), The Psychological Corporation, 1990.

Faraone SV, Biederman J, Zimmerman B: Correspondence of parent and teacher reports in medication trials. Eur Child Adolesc Psychiatry 14:20–27, 2005.

Feinstein AR, Cicchetti DV: High agreement but low kappa: I. The problems of two paradoxes. J Clin Epidemiol 43:543–549, 1990.

Frigerio A, Cattaneo C, Cataldo M, Achiatti A, Molteni M, Battaglia M: Behavioral and emotional problems among Italian children and adolescents aged 4 to 18 years as reported by parents and teachers. Eur J Psycholog Assess 20:124–133, 2004.

Gadow KD, Sprafkin J, Nolan EE: DSM-IV Symptoms in community and clinic preschool children. J Am Acad Child Adolesc Psychiatry 40:1383–1392, 2001.

Gimpel GA, Kuhn BR: Maternal report of attention deficit hyperactivity disorder symptoms in preschool children. Child Care Health Dev 26:163–179, 2000.

Hardy KK, Kollins SH, Murray DW, Riddle MA, Greenhill LL, Cunningham C, Abikoff HB, McCracken JT, Vitiello B, Davies M, McGough JJ, Posner K, Skrobala AM, Swanson JM, Wigal T, Wigal SK, Ghuman JK, Chuang SZ: Factor structure of parent- and teacher-rated attention-deficit/hyperactivity disorder symptoms in the Preschoolers with Attention-Deficit/Hyperactivity Disorder Treatment Study (PATS). J Child Adolesc Psychopharmacol 17:621–633, 2007.

Hinshaw SP, Han SS, Erhardt D, Huber A: Internalizing and externalizing behavior problems in preschool children: Correspondence among parent and teacher ratings and behavior observations. J Clin Child Psychol 21:143–150, 1992.

Kollins SH, Greenhill LL, Swanson JM, Wigal S, Abikoff H, McCracken JT, Riddle M, McGough JJ, Vitiello B, Wigal T, Skrobala AM, Posner K, Ghuman JK, Davies M, Cunningham C, Bauzo A: Rationale, design, and methods of the Preschool ADHD Treatment Study (PATS). J Am Acad Child Adolesc Psychiatry 45: 1275–1283, 2006.

Kumpulainen K, Rasanen E, Henttonen I, Moilanen I, Piha J, Puura K, Tamminen T, Almqvist F: Children's behavioural/emotional problems: a comparison of parents' and teachers' reports for elementary school-aged children. Eur Child Adolesc Psychiatry 8(Suppl 4): 41–47, 1999.

Lahey BB, Pelham WE, Loney J, Lee SS, Willcutt E: Instability of the DSM-IV Subtypes of ADHD from preschool through elementary school. Arch Gen Psychiatry 62:896–902, 2005.

Loeber R, Green SM, Lahey BB, Stouthamer-Loeber M: Differences and similarities between children, mothers, and teachers as informants on disruptive child behavior. J Abnorm Child Psychol 19:75–95, 1991.

Mannuzza S, Klein RG, Moulton JL 3rd: Young adult outcome of children with "situational" hyperactivity: A prospective, controlled follow-up study. J Abnorm Child Psychol 30:191–198, 2002.

McDermott PA, Steinberg CM, Angelo LE: Situational specificity makes the difference in assessment of youth behavior disorders. Psychology in the Schools 42: 121–136, 2005.

Mitsis EM, McKay KE, Schulz KP, Newcorn JH, Halperin JM: Parent-teacher concordance for DSM-IV attention-deficit/hyperactivity disorder in a clinic-referred sample. J Am Acad Child Adolesc Psychiatry 39:308–313, 2000.

Pelham WE Jr, Gnagy EM, Greenslade KE, Milich R: Teacher ratings of DSM-III-R symptoms for the disruptive behavior disorders. J Am Acad Child Adolesc Psychiatry 31:210–218, 1992.

Posner K, Melvin GA, Murray DW, Gugga SS, Fisher P, Skrobala AM, Cunningham C, Vitiello B, Abikoff HB, Ghuman JK, Kollins SH, Wigal SB, Wigal T, McCracken JT, McGough JJ, Kastelic E, Boorady R, Davies M, Chuang SZ, Swanson JM, Riddle MA, Greenhill LL: Clinical presentation of attention-deficit/hyperactivity disorder in preschool children: The Preschoolers with Attention-Deficit/Hyperactivity Disorder Treatment Study (PATS). J Child Adolesc Psychopharmaccol 17:547–562, 2007.

Santosh PJ, Taylor E, Swanson J, Wigal T, Chuang S, Davies M, Greenhill L, Newcorn J, Arnold LE, Jensen PS, Vitiello B, Elliott G, Hinshaw S, Hechtman L, Abikoff H, Pelham W, Hoza B, Molina BS, Wells K, Epstein J, Posner M: Refining the diagnoses of inattention and overactivity syndromes: A reanalysis of the Multimodal Treatment study of attention deficit hyperactivity disorder (ADHD) based on ICD-10 criteria for hyperkinetic disorder. Clin Neurosci Res 5:307–314, 2005.

Shaffer D, Gould MS, Brasic J, Ambrosini P, Fisher P, Bird H, Aluwahlia S: A children's global assessment scale (CGAS). Arch Gen Psychiatry 40:1228–1231, 1983.

Shaffer D, Fisher P, Dulcan MK, Davies M, Piacentini J, Schwab-Stone ME, Lahey BB, Bourdon K, Jensen PS, Bird HR, Canino G, Regier D: The NIMH Diagnostic Interview Schedule for Children Version 2.3 (DISC-2.3): Description, acceptability, prevalence rates, and performance in the MECA Study. Methods for the Epidemiology of Child and Adolescent Mental Disorders Study. J Am Acad Child Adolesc Psychiatry 35:865–877, 1996.

Spitznagel EL, Helzer JE: A proposed solution to the base rate problem in the kappa statistic. Arch Gen Psychiatry 42:725–728, 1985.

Verhulst FC, Akkerhuis GW: Agreement between parents' and teachers' ratings of behavioral/emotional problems of children aged 4–12. J Child Psychol Psychiatry 30:123–136, 1989.

ADVANCES IN PRESCHOOL PSYCHOPHARMACOLOGY
© 2009 Mary Ann Liebert, Inc.
140 Huguenot Street, 3rd Floor
New Rochelle, NY 10801-5215

Factor Structure of Parent- and Teacher-Rated Attention-Deficit/Hyperactivity Disorder Symptoms in the Preschoolers with Attention-Deficit/Hyperactivity Disorder Treatment Study (PATS)

Kristina K. Hardy, Ph.D.,[1] Scott H. Kollins, Ph.D.,[1] Desiree W. Murray, Ph.D.,[1]
Mark A. Riddle, M.D.,[6] Laurence Greenhill, M.D.,[7] Charles Cunningham, Ph.D,[4]
Howard B. Abikoff, Ph.D.,[2] James T. McCracken, M.D.,[8] Benedetto Vitiello, M.D.,[5]
Mark Davies, M.Ph.,[7] James J. McGough, M.D.,[8] Kelly Posner, Ph.D.,[7]
Anne M. Skrobala, M.A.,[7] James M. Swanson, Ph.D.,[3] Tim Wigal, Ph.D.,[3]
Sharon B. Wigal, Ph.D.,[3] Jaswinder K. Ghuman, M.D.,[9] and Shirley Z. Chuang[7]

ABSTRACT

Objective: This study examines one-, two-, and three-factor models of attention-deficit/hyperactivity disorder (ADHD) using the existing 18 *Diagnostic and Statistical Manual of Mental Disorder,* 4th edition (DSM-IV) symptoms in a sample of symptomatic preschoolers.

Methods: Parent and/or teacher ratings of DSM-IV symptoms were obtained for 532 children (aged 3–5.5) who were screened for the Preschool ADHD Treatment Study (PATS). Confirmatory factor analysis (CFA) using symptoms identified on the Conners' Parent and Teacher Rating Scales was conducted to assess a two-factor model representing the DSM-IV dimensions of inattention (IN) and hyperactivity/impulsivity (H/I), a three-factor model reflecting inattention, hyperactivity, and impulsivity, and a single-factor model of all ADHD symptoms. Exploratory factor analysis (EFA) was subsequently used to examine the latent structure of the data.

Results: For parent ratings, the two-factor and three-factor models were marginally acceptable according to several widely used fit indices, whereas the one-factor model failed to meet minimum thresholds for goodness-of-fit. For teachers, none of the models was a solid fit for the data. Maximum likelihood EFAs resulted in satisfactory two- and three-factor models for

[1]Duke University Medical Center, Durham, North Carolina.
[2] New York University Child Study Center, New York, New York.
[3] University of California Irvine, Irvine, California.
[4] McMaster Universtity, Toronto, Ontario, Canada
[5] National Institute of Mental Health, Bethesda, Maryland.
[6]Johns Hopkins University, Baltimore, Maryland.
[7] New York State Psychiatric Institute/Columbia University, New York, New York.
[8]University of California Los Angeles, Los Angeles, California.
[9]University of Arizona, Tucson, Arizona.
This work was supported by NIMH U01MH60848.

both parents and teachers, although all models contained several moderate cross loadings. Factor loadings were generally concordant with those published for older children and community-based samples.

Conclusion: ADHD subtypes according to current DSM-IV specifications may not be the best descriptors of the disorder in the preschool age group.

INTRODUCTION

DESPITE GROWING DATA supporting the validity of the attention-deficit/hyperactivty disorder (ADHD) diagnosis in preschool-aged children (DuPaul et al. 2001; Wilens et al. 2002; Lahey et al. 2004; Lahey et al. 2005), to our knowledge the factorial structure of *Diagnostic and Statistical Manual of Mental Disorders,* 4th edition (DSM-IV) (American Psychiatric Association 1994) symptoms in the 3- to 5-year-old age range has not been evaluated. Children under the age of 6 have been included in larger cross-age studies, but not in numbers sufficient for separate factor analytic techniques (DuPaul et al. 1997; Conners et al. 1998a; DuPaul et al. 1998). Moreover, we are not aware of any studies that have examined the factor structure of teacher ratings of DSM-IV items for children who are not yet in kindergarten. Given age-related differences in symptom presentation with younger children being rated as more symptomatic by parents and teachers (DuPaul et al. 1997; Conners et al. 1998a), it is reasonable to question whether differences may be found in the latent structure of the 18 DSM-IV symptoms for preschool-aged children.

Another reason to examine the dimensional structure of ADHD symptomatology in this age group is that DSM-IV subtypes, which are inherently related to differential symptom presentation across the Hyperactive-Impulsive (H/I) and Inattentive (IN) domains, do not appear to be stable across time for 4 to 6 year olds. Lahey et al. (2005) reported that, although a clinical sample of young children demonstrated consistent differences in mean levels of H/I symptoms by subtype, the majority met criteria for a different subtype at least twice over an 8-year follow up. Children who initially met criteria for the H/I type were most likely to change subtypes, with almost all of the 23 subjects either shifting or remitting by year 8. This may be related, in part, to a decline in H/I symptoms across subtypes and an increase in inattention in the H/I type with age, resulting in a later diagnosis of Combined Type (CT) for the majority of those initially classified as H/I. Consistent with this finding, the base rates of inattentive symptoms in clinically referred preschoolers have been found to be lower and more variable (25–89%) than H/I symptoms (57–94%; Murray et al., this issue). These data raise questions about whether a two-dimensional model of DSM-IV ADHD symptoms for younger children is conceptually and structurally valid.

For school-aged children, a two-factor model of ADHD symptoms has generally been supported by factor analyses demonstrating better fit indices for a two-factor than a one-factor model (DuPaul et al. 1998; Gomez et al. 1999; Collett et al. 2000; Molina et al. 2001). However, factor loadings have not been consistently high, and some items have loaded onto both factors. Correlations between the two factors tend to be high, with relatively small gains in variance explained by the two-factor solution (DuPaul et al. 1997; DuPaul et al. 1998). Nonetheless, because the two factors of H/I and IN represent the current theoretical conceptualization of ADHD, and because children may be high on one dimension without being high on the other (Lahey et al. 1994), a two-factor interpretation has been preferred.

The purpose of this study was to evaluate the factor structure of the DSM-IV ADHD symptoms as reported by parents and teachers in a large, clinical sample of preschoolers referred to the Preschool ADHD Treatment Study (PATS). We were first interested in confirming the current two-factor model from DSM-IV and then determining whether exploratory analyses yielded factors that better represented the reported symptoms.

TABLE 1. SAMPLE CHARACTERISTICS

Variable	Total sample (n = 532)		Enrolled (n = 303)		Nonenrolled (n = 229)	
	Mean (SD)	n (%)	Mean (SD)	n (%)	Mean (SD)	n (%)
Age	4.4 (0.694)		4.4 (0.685)		4.4 (0.710)	
Male		389 (73.1)		228 (75.2)		161 (70.3)
Ethnicity						
White		305 (57.3)		190 (62.7)		115 (50.2)
African-American		92 (17.3)		58 (19.1)		34 (14.8)
Latino/Hispanic		87 (16.4)		46 (15.2)		41 (17.9)
Asian American		13 (2.4)		6 (2.0)		7 (3.1)
American Indian/ Alaskan Native		3 (0.6)		2 (0.7)		1 (0.4)
Missing/not reported		32 (6.0)		1 (0.0)		31 (13.5)
DSM-IV IN[a]						
Parent[b]	15.8 (5.85)		16.8 (5.53)		14.6 (6.03)	
Teacher[c]	13.4 (6.94)		15.2 (5.87)		10.0 (7.47)	
DSM-IV H/I[a]						
Parent[d]	20.3 (4.62)		21.7 (3.65)		18.3 (5.07)	
Teacher[e]	17.0 (7.40)		20.2 (4.63)		11.3 (8.05)	

SD = Standard deviation; DSM-IV = *Diagnostic and Statistical Manual of Mental Disorders*, 4th edition; IN = inattentive; H/I = hyperactive/impulsive.

[a]Scores from DSM-IV: Inattentive and DSM-IV: Hyperactive scales from the Conners' Rating Scales (Conners 1997); Range, 0 to 27.

[b]$t = 4.41, p < 0.001$.

[c]$t = 6.34, p < 0.001$.

[d]$t = 8.49, p < 0.001$.

[e]$t = 12.25, p < 0.001$.

METHODS

Participants

Table 1 describes demographic characteristics for the participants used in this analysis. Participants were children aged 3–5.5 years (M = 4.4, SD = 0.70) referred to the PATS study between 2001 and 2003 at six academic sites across the country, whose parents provided written consent for study participation. Data for the present analyses were collected from teachers and/or parents of 532 preschool children initially screened for the PATS study. Of those, 303 (57.0%) met all study criteria and were enrolled into the PATS study, including being rated 1.5 SD above the mean on the H/I scale of both the Conners' Parent and Teacher Rating Scales. Further details on inclusion criteria have been reported elsewhere (Greenhill et al. 2006; Kollins et al. 2006). The remaining 229 children (43.0%) did not meet all entry criteria for the study; however, in most cases, participants passed a phone screen indicating that

parents identified some level of ADHD symptoms, and other major exclusionary criteria (e.g., psychosis, major medical problems, age, etc.) were ruled out. The majority of participants who were not enrolled failed to meet the criterion requiring elevated T-scores on both the Conners' Parent Rating Scale (CPRS) and the Conners' Teacher Rating Scale (CTRS) H/I scales (n = 136). Fifty five participants did not meet diagnostic criteria for ADHD on both the (DISC) and by consensus of the study clinicians. Other children were excluded for having elevated blood pressure (n = 36) or for achieving a score below 70 on the Differential Ability Scale (DAS), a test of cognitive ability and achievment (n = 20). Eighteen children were excluded for having a rating higher than 55 on the Childrens Global Assessment Scale (CGAS). Finally, 13 participants were excluded due to co-morbid psychiatric diagnoses requiring medication, and 19 were excluded for other reasons such as prior stimulant use, history of tics, significant medical conditions, or use of excluded medications. It is important to note that participants may have failed to meet more than one criterion for enrollment. Moreover, once participants failed to meet one criterion, other criteria were not necessarily evaluated.

In general, the characteristics of the enrolled and nonenrolled children were similar with regard to age, gender, and ethnicity. As expected, however, enrolled participants were rated as having significantly higher IN and H/I symptoms by both parents and teachers (see Table 1).

It should be noted that all children used in the present analysis (i.e., both children who ultimately enrolled in PATS and those who did not) demonstrated at least some symptoms consistent with ADHD and were referred to the study by their parents or teachers. We targeted this broader sample, including the children who were not enrolled, to represent a population that is typical of young children who may present to pediatricians and mental health professionals for ADHD evaluation and treatment. Thus, our interest was on the phenomenology of how symptoms manifest in preschool children who are being evaluated for ADHD, rather than just those who are diagnosed, *per se*.

Procedures

Following initial phone screening, which, as noted, consisted of general questions about major exclusionary criteria and ADHD symptoms, participants were invited to one of the six PATS research sites. Parents of all participants first provided consent for participation in the study that involved a detailed description of all study procedures. More information about the consent procedures can be found in previous reports (Kollins et al. 2006). Basic demographic data were collected, and parents completed the CPRS. Study staff then either mailed or had parents deliver CTRS to the preschool teacher identified by the parent for completion. Because one of the inclusion criteria for enrollment in the study was an elevated score on both parent and teacher versions of the Conners' scales, the scores on these forms ruled out some children. Other children, who were not enrolled into the trial, may have not met full di-

agnostic criteria for ADHD as based on either structured (i.e., National Institute of Mental Health Diagnostic Interview Schedule for Children NIMH-DISC) or clinician interview, may have had other forms of exclusionary co-morbidity, or may have been lost to follow up. As noted, the reasons for exclusion/nonenrollment are listed in Table 2.

Measures

Conners' Parent Rating Scale. The Conners' Parent Rating Scale–Revised: Long Version (CPRS-R:L; Conners 1997) assesses parent's perception of their child's current behavioral and emotional functioning, focusing on symptoms of hyperactivity, impulsivity, somatization, anxiety, social problems, and perfectionism. The CPRS-R:L consists of 80 items rated on a four-point scale ranging from 0 ("not at all") to 3 ("almost always"). The reliability and validity of this widely used measure has been well established. The current study utilized raw scores from the 18 items that correspond to the 18 DSM-IV symptoms of ADHD.

Conners' Teacher Rating Scale. The Conners' Teacher Rating Scale–Revised: Long version (CTRS-R:L; Conners 1997) provides information about children's behavioral and emotional functioning in school and, in the present study, day-care settings. This 59-item scale assesses similar symptoms as the Parent version described above. Again, the 18 items corresponding to the DSM-IV symptoms of ADHD were used in the current study.

Statistical analysis

Confirmatory factor analysis (CFA) estimated by the diagonally-weighted least squares (DWLS) method (Jöreskog and Sörbom, 1989) was used to assess a two-factor model representing the DSM-IV dimensions of IN and H/I, a three-factor model of the theoretical constructs of inattention, hyperactivity, and impulsivity, and a single-factor model of all 18 ADHD symptoms. These three models were chosen given the desirability of testing multiple models in CFA (Biddle and Marlin 1987) and their utilization in either current

TABLE 2. DESCRIPTIVE STATISTICS FOR PARENT- AND TEACHER-RATED ADHD SYMPTOMS

ADHD symptom	Parent rating			Teacher rating		
	M	SD	n	M	SD	n
Hyperactive-Impulsive						
Always "on the go"	2.56	0.688	527	2.18	1.047	456
Runs about or climbs	2.46	0.761	527	1.85	1.156	457
Talks excessively	2.17	0.973	527	1.76	1.098	453
Difficulty waiting	2.45	0.752	526	2.11	1.003	457
Interrupts	2.44	0.772	527	2.02	1.081	455
Fidgets	2.30	0.895	527	2.04	1.094	455
Difficulty playing quietly	1.85	1.006	526	1.64	1.091	455
Blurts out answers	1.63	1.111	526	1.48	1.168	445
Leaves seat	2.40	0.806	526	2.03	1.083	450
Mean	**2.25**	**0.863**		**1.90**	**1.090**	
Inattentive						
Avoids tasks	1.71	1.063	523	1.46	1.096	439
Does not follow through	1.98	0.949	521	1.31	1.096	420
Difficulty organizing	1.63	0.971	510	1.49	1.096	436
Careless mistakes	1.63	1.015	519	1.43	1.093	432
Loses things	0.87	0.970	518	0.65	0.923	405
Forgetful	1.30	1.016	527	0.88	0.927	441
Does not listen	2.40	0.746	525	1.94	0.997	453
Difficulty sustaining attention	2.03	0.892	527	1.90	1.028	452
Easily distracted	2.28	0.846	520	2.14	1.005	451
Mean	**1.75**	**0.941**		**1.47**	**1.029**	

ADHD = Attention-deficit/hyperactivity disorder; SD = standard deviation.

(two-factor) or past (one- and three-factor) versions of the DSM. Our sample size exceeds criteria proposed by MacCallum and colleagues (MacCallum et al. 2001) of at least a 4:1 ratio of participants to variables, although other authors have noted the general lack of empirical support for such ratio rules-of-thumb in determining sample size (e.g., Muthén and Muthén 2002). On the basis of similar models examined in Monte Carlo simulation studies, we determined that a sample size of at least 400 would be needed to maximize the likelihood that parameter estimates, standard error estimates, and fit statistics would be reliably estimated (Dolan 1994; Bentler and Dudgeon 1996; Muthén et al. 1997). Data were submitted separately for parent and teachers using LISREL version 8.8; a listwise deletion procedure was used to handle missing data. Of the 532 participants, parent questionnaires were obtained for 523 (98.3%) and teacher questionnaires for 457 (87.4%). As such, for parent models, data included 476 (89.5%) cases with complete data, and, for teachers, data included just 359 (67.5%) cases. It should be noted that, whereas missing values accounted for just 0.8% ($n = 75$ missing values) of parent data and appeared random, a number of teachers ($n = 52$, 11.4% of those who provided questionnaires) failed to rate participants on the item "Loses things."

Because data from the CPRS and CTRS are ordinal, CFAs were conducted using polychoric correlation and asymptotic covariance matrices. Given that our data were also moderately multivariate nonnormal, the DWLS method of estimation was selected over the more popular maximum-likelihood (ML) method, given the tendency of the latter method to produce biased parameter estimates under conditions of multivariate nonnormality with ordinal data (Maydeu-Olivares 2001; Flora and Curran 2004). The DWLS procedure, which is similar to Muthen's (Muthén et al. 1997) robust weighted least-squares procedure, likely performs better under these conditions, even with relatively complex models and moderate sample sizes (Flora and Curran 2004).

Several widely-used fit indices were employed to assess each model's goodness-of-fit. Because violations of distributional assumptions may bias the usual chi-square statistic, we examined the Satorra–Bentler chi-square (Satorra and Bentler 1988), Additional fit indices examined included Bentler's Comparative Fit Index (CFI), the standardized root mean square residual (SRMR; Jöreskog and Sörbom 1986), root mean square errors of approximation (RMSEA; Steiger 1990; Browne and Cudeck 1993), and the Tucker–Lewis Index (TLI; Tucker and Lewis 1973). Criteria for each index of fit were as follows: SRMR $<$ 0.08, RMSEA $<$ 0.06 (Lower confidence interval [CI] near 0, upper CI $<$ 0.08), CFI and TLI $\geq$ 0.96 (Hu and Bentler 1999; Kline 2005).

Following the assessment of the fit of each model, data demonstrating poor fit were submitted to maximum likelihood exploratory factor analysis (EFA) with promax (oblique) rotation to identify latent constructs (Widaman 1993; Fabrigar et al. 1999). To determine the number of factors to extract, we used Horn's (1965) parallel analysis (PA) and Velicer's (1976) minimum average partial (MAP) analysis as recommended by recent investigators (Glorfeld 1995; Velicer et al. 2000; Hayton et al. 2004; Costello & Osborne 2005). These methods were selected over more traditional approaches [e.g., Kaiser's (1960) eigenvalue-greater-than-one rule, Cattell's (1966) Scree test] given evidence that conventional methods tend to overestimate or inconsistently identify the number of factors to extract (Zwick and Velicer 1986). Both analyses were conducted in SPSS version 14.0 using syntax specified by O'Connor (2000). The PA was conducted by first generating a random data set of the same number of observations and variables as in the observed data. Using principal components analysis, eigenvalues were extracted from the random data, and this extraction was repeated for 100 iterations. Eigenvalues from the 95th percentile of the set were then compared with those from the observed data, and only those with values greater than the random data were retained for analysis. Maximum likelihood EFA was selected over principal components analysis (PCA) because our primary aim was to identify the latent structure of the variables rather than to reduce the number of variables. All analyses related to EFAs were performed using SAS version 9.1.3.

RESULTS

Confirmatory factor analysis

Given that there were significant differences in parent and teacher ratings of ADHD symptoms between children who were enrolled and those who were not enrolled in the study, we initially conducted separate CFA analyses for enrolled and nonenrolled participants. Results for all models tested indicated similar fit regardless of enrollment status (CFA data for enrolled and nonenrolled participants are available from the first author upon request.). As such, results for the full sample of enrolled and nonenrolled participants are presented in Table 2.

For parent ratings, Satorra–Bentler chi-square statistics were significant for all models, although this was expected given our moderate sample size (Satorra and Bentler 1988). With regard to other fit indices, the two-factor model was acceptable according to the CFI, TLI, and SRMR. The RMSEA value was marginal, but taken together with the other fit indices suggested acceptable model fit (see Table 3). Factor loadings for the two-factor model were moderate (i.e., 0.4 to 0.6) to high ($>$ 0.6) for inattentive symptoms (range = 0.48 to 0.80, mean = 0.69), and moderate for hyperactive-impulsive symptoms (range = 0.50–0.70, mean = 0.59). The one-factor model fit the data less well, with none of the relevant indices meeting threshold criteria (see Table 3). Loadings were generally moderate for this model (range = 0.43–0.77, mean = 0.59). Finally, the three-factor model also demonstrated acceptable fit with our data, with similar fit indices to the two-factor model (see Table 3). In this model, factor loadings were similar to the two-factor model for inattentive (range = 0.48–0.80, mean = 0.69) and hyperactive symptoms (range = 0.51–0.66, mean = 0.59) and also moderate for impulsive symptoms (range = 0.55–0.74, mean = 0.65).

In contrast to the parent data, none of the models using teacher data was clearly a good fit for the data (see Table 3), as evidenced by failure to meet minimum thresholds on several of the identified fit indices. As with the parent data, however, the two- and three-factor mod-

TABLE 3. CFA FIT INDICES FOR ONE-FACTOR, TWO-FACTOR, AND THREE-FACTOR MODELS

Fit index	Parent-rated symptoms			Teacher-rated symptoms		
	Two-factor model	Three-factor model	One-factor model	Two-factor model	Three-factor model	One-factor model
Chi-square	390.33	373.84	693.56	597.58	528.72	1384.64
Chi-square df	134	132	135	134	132	135
p	< 0.0001	< 0.0001	< 0.0001	< 0.0001	< 0.0001	< 0.0001
SRMR	0.070	0.070	0.085	0.077	0.074	0.100
RMSEA	0.063	0.062	0.093	0.087	0.081	0.140
90% Lower CI	0.056	0.055	0.086	0.080	0.074	0.140
90% Upper CI	0.070	0.070	0.100	0.094	0.088	0.150
CFI	0.97	0.97	0.94	0.98	0.98	0.94
TLI	0.97	0.97	0.93	0.97	0.98	0.93

CFA = Confirmatory factor analysis; df = degrees of freedom; SRMR = standardized root mean square residual; RMSEA = root mean square errors of approximation; CI = confidence interval; CFI = Comparative Fit Index; TLI = Tucker–Lewis Index.

els showed similar fit, with acceptable CFI and TLI, but high RMSEA and SRMR. For all models, factor loadings ranged from moderate to high across symptom domains.

Exploratory factor analysis

Because CFAs for the parent data evidenced good fit for two models, and none of the models was a good fit with the teacher data, EFAs were conducted as described above. For parent data, results from the HPA indicated that a two-factor solution should be considered, and the MAP analysis suggested that a one-factor solution would be appropriate. Given the discrepancy between these two analyses, we also used Cattell's (1966) scree test to determine an initial solution; this test indicated a two-factor solution should be examined. The initial two-factor solution accounted for 43.2% of the variance. The first factor comprised eight of the nine inattentive symptoms (i.e., all but "does not listen"), accounting for 33.0% of the variance. An additional 10 items loaded on the second factor, which accounted for the remaining 10.2% of the variance. One item "leaves seat," failed to adequately load (> 0.4) on either factor. The decision was made to retain items with low to moderate cross-loadings (>0.2), provided that the items loaded adequately on at least one factor. We chose this approach because items with cross-loadings also were those with considerable clinical relevance (e.g., "difficulty sustaining attention," "does not listen,"

"talks excessively," "easily distracted," "blurts out answers"). The final solution accounted for 43.2% of the variance and contained 17 items, (see Table 4).

Of note, for the parent data, the first three eigenvalues were greater than 1, so according to Kaiser's conventional rule, a three-factor solution would have been initially extracted. Given that many investigators still employ this rule when making decisions about the number of factors to extract and the fact that a three-factor solution seemed to fit these data well, a three-factor model was examined for parent data. As with the two-factor solution, all IN symptoms except "does not listen" loaded at least moderately on one factor. Although the third factor was well defined, it consisted of the two verbal impulsivity items (i.e., blurts out and interrupts) as well as the item "talks excessively." Both the latter item and "interrupts" also were characterized by cross-loadings on the Hyperactive factor. Moreover, several additional items (difficulty sustaining attention, fidgets, leaves seat, loses things, and easily distracted) either loaded poorly or cross-loaded on other factors (see Table 4).

For teacher data, both the PA and the MAP indicated that extracting two factors would be appropriate for our data; a two-factor solution was also indicated by the scree plot and eigenvalues. The initial solution accounted for 57.2% of the total variance; 11 items loaded on the first factor (46.3% of the variance), which contained all nine hyperactive/impulsive items plus

TABLE 4. SUMMARY OF EXPLORATORY FACTOR ANALYSIS RESULTS FOR PARENT-RELATED ADHD SYMPTOMS ($n = 481$)

ADHD Symptom	Final 2-Factor Solution		Final 3-Factor Solution		
	Factor 1 IN	Factor 2 HI	Factor 1 IN	Factor 2 HYP	Factor 3 IMP
Hyperactive-Impulsive					
Always "on the go"	−.06	.66	−.12	.76	.02
Runs about or climbs	.08	.57	.03	.71	−.06
Difficulty waiting	.09	.59	.10	.45	.20
Interrupts	.10	.61	.12	.25	.53
Fidgets	.13	.49	.13	.36	.20
Difficulty playing quietly	.18	.50	.17	.48	.10
Talks excessively	−.21	.70	−.20	.39	.49
Blurts out answers	.08	.47	.11	−.07	.75
*Often leaves seat**	*(.24)*	*(.36)*	*(.23)*	*(.32)*	*(.11)*
Mean		**.51**		**.53**	**.59**
Inattentive					
Avoids tasks	.84	−.12	.81	.07	−.19
Does not follow through	.73	.04	.70	.09	−.01
Difficulty organizing	.82	−.01	.79	.05	−.03
Careless mistakes	.73	.04	.73	−.04	.14
Loses things	.55	−.06	.58	−.23	.22
Forgetful	.61	.10	.60	.03	.14
Difficulty sustaining attention	.51	.27	.48	.41	−.12
Does not listen	.29	.45	.28	.40	.12
Easily distracted	.49	.23	.48	.20	.08
Mean	**.57**		**.66**		
Eigenvalues	13.15	2.75	13.15	2.75	1.61
Percent of variance	33.0	10.2	33.0	10.2	7.2

*Loadings presented for this item are for the initial solution; given its poor initial loading, it was excluded from further analyses.

"easily distracted," and "does not listen." Of note, the item "often leaves seat," which loaded poorly in models using parent data, loaded well on the H/I factor for the teacher data. As with the initial solution for parent ratings, however, several moderate cross-loadings were also observed. Specifically, "often forgetful," "does not listen," "difficulty sustaining attention," "blurts out answers," and "easily distracted" had low to moderate loadings on another factor. The final, 18-item solution accounted for 60.2% of the variance. Loadings for each factor ranged from 0.45 to 0.78 (see Table 5). In the final solution, all nine theoretical H/I factors loaded well together along with "easily distracted" and "does not listen." The remaining seven IN symptoms comprised the second factor.

Finally, as with the parent data, the decision was made also to extract a three-factor solution. A very similar solution to the parent three-factor solution was obtained, again with several moderate cross-loadings and a third factor defined by the two verbal impulsivity items and "talks excessively" included five symptoms of inattention (see Table 5).

DISCUSSION

The current study assessed the factor structure of parent- and teacher-rated ADHD symptoms in a relatively large, clinically referred sample of preschoolers. To our knowledge, this is the largest sample of symptomatic children in this age group to provide data for such an analysis. We believe inclusion of data from both enrolled and nonenrolled PATS participants enriches our results, not only by increasing the sample size and variability of scores, but in enhancing the generalizability of our findings to the population of greatest relevance to clinicians—young children who present for

Table 5. Summary of Exploratory Factor Analysis Results for Teacher-Related ADHD Symptoms ($n = 356$)

ADHD Symptom	Final 2-Factor Solution		Final 3-Factor Solution		
	Factor 1 HI	Factor 2 IN	Factor 1 HYP	Factor 2 IN	Factor 3 IMP
Hyperactive-Impulsive					
Always "on the go"	.77	−.02	.65	−.09	.23
Runs about or climbs	.70	.09	.79	−.07	.05
Talks excessively	.70	−.14	.06	.01	.68
Difficulty waiting	.73	.04	.48	.04	.34
Interrupts	.76	.01	.32	.07	.51
Fidgets	.63	.12	.56	.05	.17
Often leaves seat	.67	.12	.90	−.09	−.05
Difficulty playing quietly	.61	.14	.46	.11	.24
Blurts out answers	.73	−.20	.01	−.03	.77
Mean	**.72**		**.71**		**.65**
Inattentive					
Avoids tasks	.04	.76	.17	.68	−.04
Does not follow through	.06	.69	.22	.60	−.06
Difficulty organizing	.04	.78	.15	.71	−.01
Careless mistakes	−.02	.77	−.05	.78	.09
Loses things	.09	.50	−.07	.55	.21
Forgetful	.23	.70	−.15	.69	−.05
Does not listen	.45	.37	.65	.20	−.06
Difficulty sustaining attention	.36	.52	.55	.38	−.06
Easily distracted	.56	.22	.53	.14	.16
Mean		**.61**			
Eigenvalues	17.79	3.15	17.79	3.15	1.05
Percent of variance	48.3	11.9	48.3	11.9	5.2

evaluation and treatment of ADHD symptoms. In fact, to have examined data from enrolled participants alone would have restricted our findings to those children whose symptoms may be most likely to cluster according to DSM-IV structure, and may have underestimated variance in symptom presentation seen more typically in the community or in less symptomatic children.

Overall, results suggest that the DSM-IV two-factor model of 18 inattentive and H/I symptoms is a marginal fit for preschoolers with ADHD symptoms, with better fit for parent than for teacher ratings. For both sets of raters, a one-factor model of all ADHD symptoms fit the data less well. Although a three-factor model of inattentive, hyperactive, and impulsive symptoms was a good fit for parent ratings, the same model fit the teacher data inadequately. In subsequent exploratory factor analyses, both two- and three-factor solutions were generated that provided relatively good structure for parent and teacher ratings. Of note, however, moderate cross-loadings were

present for a number of items in each model, and some items loaded relatively weakly.

Although our data suggest that both parents and teachers are able to distinguish two aspects of ADHD in children at a young age, the underlying factor structure of DSM-IV symptoms was characterized by cross-loadings or poor loadings for three inattentive items (doesn't listen, distractibility, and difficulty sustaining attention) and one to three H/I symptoms depending on reporter (blurts out, leaves seat, and talks excessively). In light of recent reports of instability of ADHD subtypes over time in children diagnosed at young ages (Lahey et al. 2004; Lahey et al. 2005), our data reinforce the notion that IN and H/I symptoms are often mixed rather than discrete and separate dimensions. This is particularly likely to be true for preschoolers who are most likely to meet criteria for the H/I or Combined type (Lahey et al. 2004).

From the extant literature alone, there are few direct comparisons to be made with our data. However, information provided by Du-

Paul and colleagues (1997, 1998) on a large, community-based (non-ADHD) sample indicate that both a one-factor and two-factor models were an adequate fit for both parent and teacher report for the 18 DSM-IV items. Interestingly, factor loadings from the current data were quite similar. In addition, the authors noted moderate cross-loadings for three parent-rated inattentive symptoms—"difficulty sustaining attention," "easily distracted," and "does not listen"—and two teacher-rated items—"does not listen," and "fidgets." These same items also loaded moderately on both factors in our sample, for both the parent and teacher reports. This suggests that these symptoms may be at least modestly associated with both IN and H/I behaviors in a wide range of children. Clinically, this makes sense given that sustained attention and focus are necessary for demonstrating organizational behaviors, and also are difficult to achieve in the presence of excessive motor activity.

Limitations

The present study is not without its limitations. First, the sample from which the data were derived was clinic referred for participation in a medication trial. As such, the representativeness of symptom presentation may be suspect compared to the general population, and even as compared to more mild cases of ADHD presenting in young children. Nevertheless, establishing the factor structure of DSM-IV symptoms in this symptomatic group of preschool children helps to define the phenomenology in this age group, which has not previously been reported. Second, compared to previous samples in which the factor structure of ADHD symptoms was studied, our study included a more ethnically diverse group of participants. The extent to which this diversity might have influenced factor structure is unclear, although there is some precedent for ADHD symptom factor structure to vary by race (Epstein et al. 1998). Given the concordance in our results with those obtained in less diverse samples (e.g., DuPaul et al.), this limitation should not drastically influence the interpretation of the results. In any case, future studies with our sample will examine race as a

moderator of factor structure for ADHD symptoms.

It is also recognized that symptom identification in this study was based entirely on parent and teacher report on the Conners' rating scales and this is a limitation for at least two reasons. First, we acknowledge that Conners' measures are not necessarily the best proxy for evaluating DSM-IV ADHD symptoms, as compared to clinician evaluation. However, given the ubiquity of these and other rating scales for symptom evaluation, we felt that the ratings from these scales were well justified. Second, such measures are subject to bias in either direction. For example, parents may over-report symptoms in an attempt to highlight a child's need for treatment, while teachers may under-report symptoms for a treatment study based upon beliefs that preschoolers should not be medicated. Moreover, error may be introduced into the data from variability seen in preschool settings affecting the demands on young children's activity levels and sustained attention, and from the decreased likelihood that preschool teachers are familiar with the use of rating scales to measure ADHD-related constructs. Nonetheless, the fact that our findings are consistent with published data from nonclinical and school-aged samples suggests that this was not a significant factor in our results.

Implications and future directions

The present study has implications for the assessment and diagnosis of ADHD in preschool-aged children. Our data suggest that for clinic-referred children, specific symptoms currently used for diagnosis may not meaningfully discriminate them according to DSM-IV-defined domains and subtypes. For example, according to current DSM-IV criteria for ADHD, a child with three IN symptoms and four H/I symptoms would not be diagnosed with this disorder. If, however, these seven symptoms include those that appear to load relatively independently on separate factors, the child may in fact demonstrate the most clearly defining symptoms of ADHD. We suspect that these children are currently told by clinicians that they have "borderline ADHD," which may not serve parents well in terms of understanding how to treat their child's impairments. Another situation to consider is the young child who demonstrates six symptoms in each domain, but three of the IN symptoms are those which tend to co-occur with hyperactive symptoms (doesn't listen, distractible, difficulty sustaining attention). This child would be diagnosed by DSM-IV criteria as Combined Type, when there may, in fact, be minimal inattention that is independently impairing. This child's future impairments and outcome may be very different from the child who demonstrates more distinct symptoms in both domains. Future work would be well served to determine whether symptoms that do not load strongly onto specific factors make unique contributions to the impairment experienced by the patients.

The current study also raises important issues to consider in the understanding of the disorder and its treatment. A number of studies have suggested that DSM-IV-defined subtypes may be differentially heritable or have different molecular genetic bases (e.g., Croes et al. 2005; Kim et al. 2005; Smoller et al. 2006); however, not all family studies find evidence for subtypes "breeding true" (Smalley et al., 2000). Our data suggest that, at least in younger children, phenotypes based on existing DSM-IV subtypes may have unwanted variance that could confound the assessment of the genetic basis of the disorders. Therefore, phenotypes based on more refined and empirically derived subtypes could enhance future genetic studies. In a similar manner, it has been suggested that ADHD subtypes may respond differentially to psychopharmacological treatment (e.g., Diamond 2005). Especially because only limited data are available on the safety and efficacy of medications in preschool children (Greenhill et al. 2006), it is imperative that additional work be done to identify predictors of treatment response. Using refined approaches to defining factors in this age group may serve that role, although the conceptual and analytic approaches for studying these phenotypes would differ from what we have described in the present study.

Collectively, these findings lend further support to the notion that DSM-IV subtypes may not be valid clinical descriptors of the disorder in the preschool-aged group. The results also have implications for the development of future classification of symptoms, particularly for younger children, but perhaps across ages as well. Indeed, it may be that other symptoms not routinely assessed in this age group are more saliently associated with ADHD in the preschool years. Identification of any such symptoms may aid in improving our ability to diagnose the disorder in young children.

DISCLOSURES

The following financial disclosures indicate potential conflicts of interest among the PATS investigators and industry sources for the period 2000–2007. [1]Honoraria/consultant, [2]research support, [3]speaker's bureau, [4]significant equity (>$50,000). Dr. Murray: Eli Lilly,[2] Pfizer.[2] Dr. Kollins: Athenagen,[1,2] Cephalon,[1] Eli Lilly,[1,2] McNeil, New River Pharmaceuticals,[2] Pfizer,[2] Psychogenics,[2] Shire.[1,2] Dr. Greenhill: Alza,[2] Aventis,[1] Celltech,[2] Cephalon,[2] Eli Lilly,[1,2] Glaxo Wellcome,[2] Janssen,[1] McNeil,[2] Medeva,[2] Novartis Corporation,[2] Noven,[2] Otsuka,[1] Sanofi, Shire,[1,2] Solvay,[1] Somerset,[2] Thomson Advanced Therapeutics Communications,[1] Wyeth Ayerst.[2] Dr. Swanson: Alza,[1,2] Celgene,[1,2] Celltech,[1,2,3] Cephalon,[1,2,3] Eli Lilly,[1,2] Gliatech,[1,2] Janssen,[1,2,3] McNeil,[1,2,3] Novartis,[1,2] Shire,[1,2] UCB. Dr. Sharon Wigal: Celltech,[1,2,3] Cephalon,[1,2,3] Eli Lilly,[2] Janssen,[3] McNeil,[1,2,3] New River Pharmaceuticals,[2] Novartis,[1,2,3] Shire.[1,2,3] Dr. Abikoff: Abbot Labs,[1] Celltech,[2] Cephalon,[1] Eli Lilly,[1,2] McNeil,[1,2] Novartis,[2] Pfizer,[2] Shire.[1,2] Dr. McCracken: Abbott, Bristol Meyers Squibb,[1] Eli Lilly,[1,2,3] Gliatech,[2] Janssen,[1,3] Johnson & Johnson, McNeil,[1,2] Novartis, Noven,[1] Pfizer,[1,2] Shire,[1,2] UCB, Wyeth. Dr. Riddle: Astra-Zeneca,[1] Glaxo-Smith-Kline,[1] Janssen,[1] Pfizer,[2] Shire.[1] Dr. McGough: Eli Lilly,[1,2,3] McNeil,[1,2,3] New River Pharmaceuticals,[2] Novartis,[1,2,3] Pfizer,[1,2,3] Shire.[1,2,3] Dr. Posner: Abbott Laboratories, AstraZeneca Pharmaceuticals, Aventis, Bristol-Meyers Squibb, Cephalon, Eisai, Forest Laboratories, GlaxoSmithKline, Johnson & Johnson, Novartis, Organon USA, Sanofi-Shire,[1,2] Wyeth Research, UCB. Dr. Tim Wigal: Celltech,[2] Cephalon,[2] Eli Lilly,[2,3] Janssen,[2] McNeil,[2,3] Novartis,[2]

Shire.[2,3] Mr. Davies: Amgen,[4] Bard, Glaxo-SmithKline,[4] Johnson & Johnson,[4] Merck,[4] Pfizer,[4] Wyeth.[4] Dr. Ghuman: Bristol Myers-Squibb,[2] Drs. Vitiello and Cunningham and Ms. Chuang and Skrobala have no conflicts of interest or financial ties to report as they have not received support from companies manufacturing medications.

REFERENCES

American Psychiatric Association. Diagnostic and Statistical Manual of Mental Disorders, 4th ed. (DSM-IV). Washington, DC, American Psychiatric Association, 1994.

Bentler PM: Comparative fit indices in structural models. Psycholog Bull 107:238–246, 1990.

Bentler PM, Bonett DG: Significance tests and goodness-of-fit in the analysis of covariance structures. Psycholog Bull 88:588–606, 1980.

Bentler PM, Dudgeon P: Covariance structure analysis: Statistical practice, theory, and directions. Ann Rev Psychol 47:563–592, 1996.

Biddle BJ, Marlin MM: Causality, confirmation, credulity, and structural equation modeling. Child Dev 58:4–17, 1987.

Browne MW, Cudek R: Alternative ways of assessing model fit. In: Testing Structural Equation Models. Edited by Bollen KA, Long, JS. Newbury Park (California), Sage, 1993, pp 445–455.

Cattell RB: The scree test for the number of factors. Multivariate Behav Res 1:245–276, 1966.

Collett BR, Crowley SL, Gimpel GA, Greenson JN: The factor structure of DSM-IV attention deficit-hyperactivity symptoms: A confirmatory factor analysis of the ADHD-SRS. J Psychoed Assess 18:361–373, 2000.

Conners CK: Conners' Rating Scales–Revised: Technical Manual. North Tonawanda (New York), Multi-Health Systems, 1997.

Conners CK, Sitarenios G, Parker JD, Epstein JN: The revised Conners' Parent Rating Scale (CPRS-R): factor structure, reliability, and criterion validity. J Abnorm Child Psychol 26:257–268, 1998a.

Conners CK, Sitarenios G, Parker JD, Epstein JN: Revision and restandardization of the Conners' Teacher Rating Scale (CTRS-R): Factor structure, reliability, and criterion validity. J Abnorm Child Psychol 26:279–291, 1998b.

Costello AB, Osborne JW: Best practices in exploratory factor analysis: four recommendations for getting the most from your analysis. Practical Assessment Research & Evaluation, 10. Accessed at http://pareonline.net/getvn.asp?v=10&n=7, 2005.

Croes EA, El Galta R, Houwing-Duistermaat JJ, Ferdinand RF, Lopez Leon S, Rademaker TA, Dekker MC, Oostra BA, Verhulst F, Van Duijn CM: Phenotypic subtypes in attention deficit hyperactivity disorder in an isolated population. Eur J Epidemiol 20:789–794, 2005.

Diamond A: Attention deficit disorder (attention deficit hyperactivity disorder without hyperactivity): A neurobiologically and behaviorally distinct disorder from attention deficit hyperactivity disorder (with hyperactivity). Dev Psychopathol 17:807–825, 2005.

Dolan CV: Factor analysis of variables with 2, 3, 5, and 7 response categories: A comparison of categorical variable estimators using simulated data. Br J Math Statist Psychol 47:309–326, 1994.

DuPaul, GJ, Power, TJ, Anastopoulos, AD, Reid R, McGoey KE., Ikeda MJ: Teacher ratings of attention deficit hyperactivity disorder symptoms: Factor structure and normative data. Psycholog Assess 9:436–444, 1997.

DuPaul GJ, Power TJ, Anastopoulos AD, Reid R: ADHD Rating Scale-IV: Checklists, Norms, and Clinical Interpretations. New York, Guilford Press, 1998.

DuPaul GJ, McGoey KE, Eckert TL, VanBrakle J: Preschool children with attention-deficit/hyperactivity disorder: Impairments in behavioral, social, and school functioning. J Am Acad Child Adolesc Psychiatry 40:508–515, 2001.

Epstein JN, March JS, Connors CK, Jackson DL: Racial differences on the Connors' Teacher Rating Scale. J Abnormal Child Psychol 26:109–118, 1998.

Fabrigar LR, Wegener DT, MacCallum RC, Strahan EJ: Evaluating the use of exploratory factor analysis in psychological research. Psycholog Methods, 3:272–299, 1999.

Flora DB, Curran PJ: An empirical evaluation of alternative methods of estimation for confirmatory factor analysis with ordinal data. Psycholog Meth 9:466–491, 2004.

Gomez R, Harvey J, Quick C, Scharer L, Harris G: DSM-IV ADHD: Confirmatory factor models, prevalence, gender and age differences based on parent and teacher ratings of Australian primary school children. J Child Psychol Psychiatry 40:265–274, 1999.

Glorfeld LW: An improvement on Horn's parallel analysis methodology for selecting the correct number of factors to retain. Educ Psycholog Meas 55:377–393, 1995.

Greenhill L, Kollins SH, Abikoff H, McCracken J, Riddle M, Swanson J, McGough J, Wigal S, Wigal T, Vitiello B, Skrobala A, Posner K, Ghuman J, Cunningham C, Davies M, Chuang S, Cooper T: Efficacy and safety of immediate-release methylphenidate treatment for preschoolers with ADHD. J Am Acad Child Adolesc Psychiatry 45:1284–1293, 2006.

Hayton JC, Allen DG, Scarpello V: Factor retention decisions in exploratory factor analysis: A tutorial on parallel analysis. Organiz Res Methods 7:191–205, 2004.

Horn JL: A rationale and test for the number of factors in factor analysis. Psychometrika 32:179–185, 1965.

Hu L, Bentler, PM: Cutoff criteria for fit indexes in covariance structure analysis: Conventional criteria versus new alternatives. Struct Equation Model 6:1–55, 1999.

Jöreskog K, Sörbom D. LISREL 7 User's Reference Guide. Mooresville (Indiana), Scientific Software, 1989.

Kaiser HF: The application of electronic computers to factor analysis. Educ Psycholog Meas 20:141–151, 1960.

Kim YS, Leventhal BL, Kim SJ, Kim BN, Cheon KA, Yoo

HJ, Kim SJ, Badner J, Cook EH: Family based association study of DAT1 and DRD4 polymorphism in Korean children with ADHD. Neurosci Lett 390:176–181, 2005.

Kline RB. Principles and Practices of Structural Equation Modeling, 2nd ed. New York, Guilford Press, 2005.

Kollins SH., Greenhill L, Swanson J, Wigal S, Abikoff H, McCracken J, Riddle M, McGough J, Vitiello B, Wigal T, Skrobala A, Posner K, Ghuman J, Davies M, Cunningham C, Bauzo A: Rationale, design, and methods of the Preschool ADHD Treatment Study (PATS). J Am Acad Child Adolesc Psychiatry 45:1275–1283, 2006.

Lahey BB, Applegate B, McBurnett K, Biederman J, Greenhill L, Hynd GW, Barkley RA, Newcorn J, Jensen P, Richters J, Garfinkel B, Kerdyk L, Frick PJ, Ollendick T, Perez F, Hart EL, Waldman I, Shaffer D: DSM-IV field trials for attention deficit hyperactivity disorder in children and adolescents. Am J Psychiatry 151:1673–1685, 1994.

Lahey BB, Pelham WE, Loney J, Kipp H, Ehrhardt A, Lee SS, Willcutt EG, Hartung CM, Chronis A, Massetti G: Three-year predictive validity of DSM-IV attention deficit hyperactivity disorder in children diagnosed at 4–6 years of age. Am J Psychiatry 161:2014–2020, 2004.

Lahey BB, Pelham WE, Loney J, Lee SS, Willcutt E: Instability of the DSM-IV Subtypes of ADHD from preschool through elementary school. Arch Gen Psychiatry 62:896–902, 2005.

MacCallum RC, Widaman KF, Preacher KJ, Hong S: Sample size in factor analysis: The role of model error. Multivar Behav Res 36:611–637, 2001.

Maydeau-Olivares A: Limited information estimation and testing of Thurstonian models for paired comparison data under multiple judgment sampling. Psychometrika 66:209–228, 2001.

Molina BS, Smith BH, Pelham WE: Factor structure and criterion validity of secondary school teacher ratings of ADHD and ODD. J Abnorm Child Psychol 29:71–82, 2001.

Murray DW, Kollins SH, Hardy KK, Abikoff HB, Swanson JM, Cunningham C, Vitiello B, Riddle MA, Davies M, Greenhill LL, McCracken JT, McGough JJ, Posner K, Skrobala AM, Wigal T, Wigal SB, Ghuman JK, Chuang SZ: Parent versus teacher ratings of attention-deficit/hyperactivity disorder symptoms in the Preschoolers with Attention-Deficit/Hyperactivity Disorder Treatment Study (PATS). J Child Adolesc Psychopharmacol 17:605–619, 2007.

Muthén LK, Muthén, BO: How to use a Monte Carlo study to decide on sample size and determine power. Struct Equation Model 9:599–620, 2002.

Muthén BO, du Toit SHC, Spisic, D: Robust inference using weighted least squares and quadratic estimating equations in latent variable modeling with categorical and continuous outcomes. Unpublished manuscript, 1997.

O'Connor BP: SPSS and SAS programs for determining the number of components using parallel analysis and Velicer's MAP test. Behav Res Methods, Instrument Computers 32:396–402, 2000.

Satorra A, Bentler PM: Scaling corrections for chi-square statistics in covariance structure analysis. In: American Statistical Association 1988 Proceeding of the Business and Economic Section. Alexandria (Virginia), American Statistical Association, 1988.

Smalley SL, McGough JJ, Del'Homme M, NewDelman J, Gordon E, Kim T, Liu A, McCracken JT: Familial clustering of symptoms and disruptive behaviors in multiplex families with attention deficit hyperactivity disorder. J Am Acad Child Adolesc Psychiatry 39:1135–1143, 2000.

Smoller JW, Biederman J, Arbeitman L, Doyle AE, Fagerness J, Perlis RH, Sklar P, Faraone SV: Association between the 5HT1B receptor gene (HTR1B) and the inattentive subtype of ADHD. Biol Psychiatry 59:460–467, 2006.

Steiger JH: Structural model evaluation and modification: An interval estimation approach. Multivar Behav Res 25:173–180, 1990.

Tucker LR, Lewis C: A reliability coefficient for maximum likelihood factor analysis. Psychometrika 38:1–10, 1973.

Velicer WF: Determining the number of components form the matrix of partial correlations, Psychometrika 41:321–327, 1976.

Velicer WF, Eaton CA, Fava JL: Construct explication through factors or component anlaysis: A review and evaluation of alternative procedures for determining the number of factors or components. In: Problems and Solutions in Human Assessment: Honoring Douglas N. Jackson at seventy. Edited by Goffin RD, Helmes E. Norwell (Massachusetts), Kluwer Academic, 2000.

Widaman KF: Common factor analysis versus principal component analysis: Differential bias in representing model parameters? Multivar Behav Res 28:263–311, 1993.

Wilens TE, Biederman J, Brown S, Tanguay S, Monuteaux MC, Blake C, Spencer TJ: Psychiatric comorbidity and functioning in clinically referred preschool children and school-age youths with ADHD. J Am Acad Child Adolesc Psychiatry 41:262–268, 2002.

Zwick WR Velicer WF: Factors influencing five rules for determining the number of components to retain. Psycholog Bull 99:432–442, 1986.

ADVANCES IN PRESCHOOL PSYCHOPHARMACOLOGY
© 2009 Mary Ann Liebert, Inc.
140 Huguenot Street, 3rd Floor
New Rochelle, NY 10801-5215

Effects of Source of DNA on Genotyping Success Rates and Allele Percentages in the Preschoolers with Attention-Deficit/Hyperactivity Disorder Treatment Study (PATS)

James M. Swanson, Ph.D.,[1] Robert K. Moyzis, Ph.D.,[2] James J. McGough, M.D.,[3]
James T. McCracken, M.D.,[3] Mark A. Riddle, M.D.,[5] Scott H. Kollins, Ph.D.,[6]
Laurence L. Greenhill, M.D.,[4] Howard B. Abikoff, Ph.D.,[7] Tim Wigal, Ph.D.,[1]
Sharon B. Wigal, Ph.D.,[1] Kelly Posner, Ph.D.,[4] Anne M. Skrobala, M.A.,[4]
Mark Davies, M.P.H.,[4] Jaswinder K. Ghuman, M.D.,[8] Charles Cunningham, Ph.D.,[9]
Benedetto Vitiello, M.D.,[10] Annamarie Stehli, M.P.H.,[1] Susan L. Smalley, Ph.D.,[3]
and Deborah Grady, Ph.D.[2]

ABSTRACT

Objective: **In children diagnosed with attention-deficit/hyperactivity disorder (ADHD) and their parents, who were participants of the Preschool ADHD Treatment Study (PATS), we as-**

[1]University of California Irvine Child Development Center, Irvine, California.
[2]University of California Irvine Department of Biological Chemistry, Irvine, California.
[3]UCLA Semel Institute for Neuroscience and Human Behavior, Los Angeles, California.
[4]Department of Psychiatry, New York State Psychiatric Institute, Columbia University, New York, New York.
[5]Johns Hopkins University Division of Child Psychiatry, Baltimore, Maryland.
[6]Duke University Division of Child Psychiatry, Durham, North Carolina.
[7]New York University Child Study Center, New York, New York.
[8]University of Arizona Department of Psychiatry, Tucson, Arizona.
[9]McMaster University Department of Psychology, Hamilton, Ontario, Canada.
[10]National Institute of Mental Health, Bethesda, Maryland.
[11]New York State Psychiatric Institute/Columbia University, New York, New York.
This research was supported by a cooperative agreement between the National Institute of Mental Health and the following institutions: University of California Irvine (U01-MH60833); Duke University Medical Center (U01 MH60848); NYSPI/Columbia University (UO1 MH60903); New York University Child Study Center (U01 MH60943); University of California Los Angeles (U01 MH60900); Johns Hopkins University (U01 MH60642) and was conducted at the Departments of Psychiatry, Divisions of Child and Adolescent Psychiatry, New York State Psychiatric Institute, New York University Child Study Center, Johns Hopkins University, Duke University, University of California at Los Angeles, and the University of California at Irvine.
PATS Study Group. The authors wish to acknowledge the following members of the PATS Study Group: University of California Irvine, Marc Lerner, M.D., Ken Steinhoff, M.D., Robin Epstein, M.D. Steve Simpson, M.A., Ron Kotkin, Ed.D., Audrey Kapelinsky, L.C.S.W., Joey Trampush, Ben Thorp; Duke University Medical Center, Allan Chrisman, M.D., Ave Lachiewicz, M.D., Priscilla Grissom, Ph.D., Desiree Murray, Ph.D., Rebecca McIntyre, M.A.; NYSPI/Columbia University, Janet Fairbanks, M.D., Pablo H. Goldberg. M.D., John K. Burton, M.D., Lena S. Kessler, Tova Ferro, Ph.D.; New York University Child Study Center, Tracey Rawls, M.A., Roy Boorady, M.D.; Mark Krushelnycky, M.D.; Melvin Oatis, M.D., Daphne Anshel, Ph.D.; Lori Evans, Ph.D.; University of California Los Angeles, Caroly Pataki, MD; Robert Suddath, MD, Melissa Del'Homme, PhD, Jennifer Cowen, M.A., Keri Vasquez, Cynthia Whitham, M.S.W.; Eleanor Zamora-Paja; Frederick Frankel, Ph. D. Johns Hopkins University, Golda Ginsburg, Elizabeth Kastelic, Alexander M. Scharko, MD, Deidre Everist; Nathan Kline Institute, Thomas Cooper, M.A., Jim Robinson, M.Ed., Terri DeSouza, R.N., M.P.A., Rita Lindberg, M.S.; National Institute of Mental Health, Joanna Chisar.

sessed the effect of source of DNA (from buccal or blood cells) on the genotyping success rate and allele percentages for the five polymorphisms in three candidate genes (DAT1, *DRD4*, and SNAP 25) investigated in the PATS pharmacogenetic study of response to stimulant medication.

Method: At baseline assessment, 241 individuals (113 probands and 128 parents) consented to participate; 144 individuals (52 probands and 92 parents) provided blood samples from venipuncture, and 97 individuals (61 probands and 36 parents) provided buccal samples from cheek swab as specimens for isolation of DNA. Three types of polymorphisms—variable number of tandem repeat (VNTR) polymorphism, tandem duplication polymorphism (TDP), and single nucleotide polymorphism (SNP)—were evaluated, including the *DRD4* gene 48-bp VNTR in exon III, the DAT1 gene 40-bp VNTR in 3'-untranslated region, the *DRD4* gene TDP 120-bp duplication in the promoter region, the SNAP-25 gene TC-1069 SNP, and the SNAP-25 gene TG-1065 SNP. Standard procedures were used to genotype individuals for each of these five polymorphisms.

Results: Using the methods available in 2004, the genotyping success rate was on the average much greater for DNA from blood cells than buccal cells (e.g., 91% vs. 54% in probands). For some polymorphisms (*DRD4*-VNTR, *DRD4*-TDP, and SNAP25-TC SNP), allele proportion also varied by blood versus buccal source of DNA (e.g., 26.5% vs. 18.6% for the 7-repeat allele of the *DRD4* gene).

Conclusions: The much lower success rate for genotyping based on DNA from buccal than blood cells is likely due to the quality of DNA derived from these two sources. The observed source differences in allele proportion may be due to self-selection related to choice of how specimens were collected (from cheek swab or venipuncture), or to a selective detection of some alleles based on differences in DNA quality.

INTRODUCTION

A PRIMARY OBJECTIVE of most molecular genetic studies of attention-deficit/hyperactivity disorder (ADHD) is to relate variation in phenotype to variation in genotype. Investigations using candidate gene and genome scan approaches have identified several genes associated with the diagnosis of ADHD, but estimates of strengths of association (odds ratio or relative risk) are too low to justify use of genetic tests in clinical practice (see Thapar et al. 2006). Another objective is to relate response to treatment to genotype. Pharmacogenetic studies have indicated that some genes may be useful in predicting response to stimulant medication or side effects to this treatment, and reviews of this area related to ADHD are provided by McGough (2005) and McGough et al. (2006). Current issues are related to uncertainty about which allele might be the risk allele for a given gene and small effect sizes for comparison of response across subgroups with and without the hypothesized risk allele. On this basis, the consensus is that pharmacogenetic information is not yet sufficient to be applied in clinical practice (McGough 2005). However, rapid advances in specification and use of genetic information is expected, and the potential clinical utility of this information has been given as the rationale for much of the past, current, and proposed research on genetics (see Collins et al. 2004).

Systematic nongenetic or random variation in either phenotype or genotype may distort or mask underlying genotype–phenotype relationships. Reliable methods have been developed for specifying phenotype (e.g., assessment of symptoms based on interviews and rating scales), but the information from these methods is from subjective reports, which may vary over time or over different conditions of observation. In contrast, the methods for the specification of genotype are considered to be objective and the result definite. However, many methodological factors affect the specification of genotype (Walsh et al. 1992; Kaiser et al. 2002). Here we provide additional evaluation of the genotypes described in the report by McGough et al. (2006) on the pharmacogenetics in the Preschoolers with ADHD Treatment Study (PATS).

Some variation in the ADHD phenotype depends on the criteria and decision rules used [see Santosh et al. 2005 for a comparison of phenotypes based on International Classification of Diseases and Related Health Problems, 10th revision (ICD-10) and *Diagnostic and Statistical Manual of Mental Disorders,* 4th edition (DSM-IV) criteria] (American Psychiatric Association, 1994). For any given set of criteria, variation may also occur due to source of information for diagnosis. According to DSM-IV criteria, symptom presence is obtained from subjective reports about the child's behavior from two sources, typically the parents and teachers of the child. In school-aged children, information at the symptom level is often discrepant for these two sources (see Swanson et al. 1999). We will not address variation in phenotype here, because this issue has been addressed elsewhere. For example, in a methodological evaluation of the ADHD phenotype in the PATS, Kollins et al. (2006) used factor analysis to address source differences in the factor structure of ADHD in preschool children, and suggested that " . . . parents may over-report symptoms in an attempt to highlight a child's need for treatment, while teachers may under-report symptoms for a treatment study based upon beliefs that preschoolers should not be medicated" and " . . . at least in younger children, phenotypes based on existing DSM-IV subtypes may have unwanted variance that could confound the assessment of the genetic basis of the disorders". Because "unwanted variance" may also be present in genotype as well as phenotype, here we address a methodological factor (source of DNA) that may affect variation in genotype.

For any given phenotype (e.g., PATS diagnosis of ADHD), multiple genotypes could be considered within and across the many genes in the human genome. McGough et al. (2006) provided the rationale for addressing five specific genotypes from three candidate genes. Two of these were based on findings from the initial molecular genetic studies of ADHD (Cook et al. 1995; LaHoste et al. 1996), which focused on candidate genes suggested by the dopamine hypothesis of ADHD (see Wender 1971) and the site of action of stimulant medications considered to be dopamine agonists (see Volkow et al. 1995). Cook et al. (1995) evaluated a polymorphism generated by a variable

number of tandem repeat (VNTR) segment of DNA in a noncoding region—the 3' untranslated region (3'-UTR)—of the dopamine transporter (DAT1) gene. In a typical sample of individuals with European ancestry, this polymorphism produces two primary alleles based on length, with a 10-repeat variant representing about 70% of alleles and the 9-repeat variant representing most of the other alleles. LaHoste et al. (1996) evaluated a polymorphism generated by a VNTR in a coding region (exon III) of the dopamine receptor D4 (*DRD4*) gene, which in a given sample of European ancestry produces multiple alleles based on 2–11 repeats of the VNTR, with the four-repeat variant representing about 70% of alleles, the seven-repeat variant about 15%, the two-repeat about 10%, and other repeat variants the remainder of the alleles. Since these two initial reports, many studies have attempted to replicate these associations, with remarkable success (see Faraone et al. 2005) that is seldom observed in psychiatric genetics. However, there remain unexplained failures to replicate (see Swanson et al. 2002; Li et al. 2006).

Other polymorphisms specified by McGough et al. (2006) were based on the findings of McCracken et al. (2000), who reported association of ADHD with another polymorphism in the *DRD4* gene generated by a 120-bp tandem duplication polymorphism (TDP) in a noncoding (promoter) region that produces a 120-bp allele or a 240-bp allele, and the findings of Barr et al. (2000) who reported association of ADHD with single nucleotide polymorphisms (SNPs) at two locations within the SNAP-25 gene, due to the presence of the nucleotide T or C at locus 1,065 and the presence of the nucleotide T or G at locus 1,069. The *DRD4* 120-bp TDP polymorphism is in strong linkage with the exon III 48-bp VNTR (Ding et al. 2002; Wang et al. 2004). Some attempts to replicate these associations have been successful, but unexplained nonreplications also have been reported.

McGough et al. (2006) described how genotypes were established based on each of these five polymorphisms (*DRD4*-VNTR, DAT-VNTR, *DRD4*-TDP, SNAP-SNP-TC, and SNAP-SNP-TG) for a subset ($n = 81$) of the PATS sample. Successful genotyping was obtained for an average of only 70% of the 81 individuals (52 for the *DRD4*-VNTR, 55 for the DAT1-VNTR, 55 for the *DRD4*-promoter, 58 for the SNAP25-T1069C, and 61 for SNAP-T1065G). Possible reasons for this failure to amplify DNA in about 30% of the individuals and subsequent sample reduction, which were mentioned but not discussed in detail by McGough et al. (2006), will be addressed here.

The initial step in genotyping is the extraction of DNA from the nucleus of cells. In the literature of the molecular genetics of ADHD, two sources predominate: buccal cells and blood cells. The intrusiveness and cost of the typical methods to collect these specimens differ. Buccal cells are usually obtained using relatively noninvasive methods to collect a specimen (e.g., cheek swab or saliva), whereas blood cells are usually obtained using a relatively invasive method (e.g., venipuncture). The collection of DNA from buccal cells may be preferred by some investigators under the assumption that this will maximize the number of subjects who will participate in study, require less effort and training of staff, and lower cost. However, DNA from blood cells is preferred by other investigators because of some problems with using DNA from buccal cells, which may be contaminated by DNA from residual food and bacteria in the mouth. Also, most buccal cells are dead, and thus DNA in these cells may be degraded by the action of enzymes in the mouth. Other factors may affect the decision to use venipuncture or cheek swabs/saliva to collect blood cells or buccal cells as a source of DNA in a given study. For example, if venipuncture is required for clinical purposes (e.g., to obtain a blood sample for standard clinical chemistry tests), provisions can be considered for obtaining an additional small blood sample at the same time as a source of DNA for research. Some studies use one of these methods for specimens, either from blood samples from venipuncture (e.g., LaHoste et al. 1996; Swanson et al. 1998; Moffitt et al 2001) or from buccal cells from cheek swabs (e.g., Fossella et al. 2002; Moffitt et al. 2001; Cornish et al. 2005), and others use both in the same individuals (e.g., Hamarman et al. 2004) or in different subgroups or cohorts (e.g., Mill et al. 2006).

In the 81 probands of the PATS in the phar-macogenetic study reported by McGough et al. (2006), 30 donated a specimen via cheek swab that provided buccal cells and 51 donated a specimen via venipuncture that provided blood cells for this first step. McGough et al. (2006) noted blood–buccal differences in amplification of DNA and success in obtaining information for genotyping, but the sample was too small to evaluate methodological issues about source of DNA. To expand the sample, we used DNA from all 113 probands (including the 32 that did not enter the medication titration trail) and from 128 parents of these children who elected to participate in the molecular genetic component of the PATS. This provided a sample of $n = 241$ individuals for this methodological study of the effects of source of DNA on genotype.

In the PATS protocol, either a specimen was collected by venipuncture or cheek swab to provide a source for DNA, and only rarely were specimens collected by both methods in the same individual (see McGough et al. 2006). Choice and decisions by investigators at the six PATS sites as well as by the individual participants resulted in an approximately equal mixture of specimens as sources (blood cells and buccal cells) of DNA for amplification and determination of genotype. This aspect of the PATS dataset offers an opportunity to evaluate fundamental properties of DNA processing (amplification success rate and allele percentage) and to determine whether there are difference in subgroups of subjects with DNA derived from different sources (blood or buccal cells). This report does not address the usual questions of molecular genetic studies of ADHD, such as possible association of ADHD with genetic polymorphisms or differences in response to stimulant medication that may depend on these polymorphisms, but it does address issues related to the collection of DNA that may become relevant to clinicians in the future. At the present time, clinicians are unlikely to request a genetic test, but as new information accumulates from research on diagnostic genetics and pharamcogenetics, clinical applications are likely to emerge. In the future, when clinicians request genetic tests, the specification of source of DNA (e.g., from the standard procedures based on blood or buccal cells, or perhaps from other sources or methods that are now topics of investigation) may be relevant and important.

METHODS

The PATS protocol employed a pretreatment with parent training to screen out children who responded to nonpharmacological intervention before entering the medication titration trial phase of the study (see Greenhill et al. 2006; Kollins et al. 2006). At the postparent training baseline assessment, subjects enrolled in PATS were invited to participate in optional molecular genetic studies of ADHD, including a pharmacogenetic investigation of methylphenidate (MPH) treatment response that has been reported elsewhere (see McGough et al. 2006). Written consent was provided by parents for their child's participation following procedures approved by Institutional Review Boards of each of the sites of the study. At each site, the choice to rely on cheek swabs (to obtain DNA from buccal cells) or venipuncture (to obtain DNA from blood cells) was partially determined by local conditions, including clinical requirements and availability of staff for obtaining blood samples, and by individual choice to participate in the molecular genetic component of the study.

DNA isolation and purification

Lymphoblastoid cell lines were established for all blood samples with methods for transformation, cell culture, and DNA purification that have been described previously (Chang et al. 1996; Ding et al. 2002; Grady et al. 2003). DNA from buccal samples was isolated by lysis and extraction with the Qiagen Kit using the manufacturer's protocol (Qiagen, Valencia, CA).

Candidate genes, polymorphisms, major alleles, and genotypes

Selection of candidate genes and polymorphisms for the PATS pharmacogenetic study (DRD4-VNTR, DAT1-VNTR, DRD4-TDP, SNAP25-SNP-TC, and SNAP25-SN-TG) was based on the literature, which has been reviewed elsewhere (see McGough 2005) and will not be repeated here. For the pharmacogenetic study, genotype was defined based on homozygosity or heterozygosity of the most frequent or major allele of each of these polymorphisms (see Table 2 in McGough et al. 2006). Specifically, this provided a genotype based on homozygous versus nonhomozygous status of each participant for the DRD4 exon III four-repeat allele, the DAT1 3'-UTR 10-repeat allele, the DRD4 promoter 240 allele, the SNAP25-TC T allele, and the SNAP25 TG T allele. Here we follow the lead of McGough et al. (2006) and focus on the major allele for these polymorphisms, which maximizes the number of alleles for comparison of source of DNA.

Statistical analyses

Source of DNA (blood or buccal cells) was the primary independent variable in exploratory analyses to determine if a difference was present for each polymorphism for two outcome measures and analyses. The first outcome measure was success of genotyping (success or blank), and the Fisher exact test was used to compare the percentage of blanks for the two sources. The second outcome measure was the observed percentage of each allele generated by the polymorphism, and the Fisher exact test was used to compare the percentages of major alleles for the two sources. To examine the possibility that there may also be an effect of family status (child or parent) on the percentage of major alleles, logistic regression was performed with source, family status, and the source–family status interaction as factors. An alpha level of 0.05 was used to evaluate statistical significance in all tests.

RESULTS

Participants

Of the 183 families who entered the medication titration phase of the PATS, 241 individuals (113 probands and 128 parents) consented to participate also in the additional molecular genetics component of the study. From these families, 144 individuals (52 probands and 92 parents) provided blood samples via venipunc-

TABLE 1. DISPOSITION OF PARTICIPANTS IN THE PATS

Status	Duke	JHU	NYSPI	NYU	UCI	UCLA	Totals
Passed caseness	51	44	50	47	68	43	303
Enrolled in PT	45	40	44	45	67	38	279
Completed PT	39	38	44	42	64	34	261
Enrolled in lead-in	30	19	28	26	56	24	183
Completed lead-in	30	19	25	23	52	20	169
Proband in genetics							113

PATS = Preschool ADHD Treatment Study; JHU = John's Hopkins University; NYSPI = New York State Psychiatric Institute; NYU = New York University; UCI = University of California, Irvine; UCLA = University of California, Los Angles; PT = parent training.

ture and 97 individuals (61 probands and 36 parents) provided buccal samples via cheek swab as the source for DNA. The disposition of the total sample is outlined in Table 1.

DNA amplification

The rate of successful DNA amplification for all five polymorphisms differed by source, with a large overall advantage for blood cells over buccal cells. This advantage was present in all five polymorphisms for probands (for DAT1, 100% vs. 43%, $p < 0.001$; for $DRD4$-TDP, 88% vs. 52%, $p < 0.001$; for $DRD4$-VNTR, 94% vs. 39%, $p < 0.001$; for SNAP T1065G, 85% vs. 67%, $p < 0.03$; for SNAP T1069C, 88% vs. 69%, $p < 0.01$) and in three of the polymorphisms for parents (for DAT1, 87% vs. 61%, $p < 0.0011$; for $DRD4$-TDP, 86% vs. 58%, $p < 0.007$; for $DRD4$-VNTR, 95% vs. 53%, $p < 0.0001$). For the SNP polymorphisms in the SNAP25 gene, the amplification rates were about the same for SNAP-SNP-TG (80% vs. 81%, NS) and for SNAP-SNP-TC (83% vs. 81%, NS).

Effect of source on allele proportions

For each gene and polymorphism, the allele frequencies are shown in Table 2, with allele percentages shown on one line for all alleles including blanks and on another line for all nonblank alleles. The Fisher exact test was used to compare the percentages of nonblank major allele across the subgroups defined by DNA source (blood vs. buccal). The difference was significant for three of the five polymorphisms ($DRD4$-VNTR-4-repeat, 59.5% vs. 73.2%, $p < 0.048/0.096$; $DRD4$_promoter-240, 76.6% vs. 46.67%, $p < 0.0001/0.0001$; SNAP25-T1069C,

89.29% vs. 78.81%, $p < 0.01/0.02$), but not for the other two polymorphisms (DAT1-VNTR-10, 73% vs. 69%, $p = 0.357/0.714$; SNAP25-T1065G, 77% vs. 84%, $p < 0.065/0.130$).

The purpose of combining probands and parents was to establish groups as large as possible for comparison of source. When smaller subgroups are formed separately for probands and parents, similar patterns were apparent in each subgroup (i.e., in the separate subgroups for probands or parents, there is a much greater rate of successful amplification of DNA from blood than buccal cells, and both subgroups show similar differences in allele percentages for each source). Logistic regression analyses were performed that incorporated family status as a two-level factor, and neither the main effect for this factor nor the interaction with Source was significant (see Table 3).

An alternative method to test the hypothesis of source difference in genotyping success is to use a chi-square test to contrast the entire distribution of alleles instead of just the major allele. These tests were performed for each polymorphism, and the same pattern was observed: $DRD4$ (2, 4, 7, or other), chi-square (3) = 8.2422, $p < 0.0413$; DAT-VNTR (9, 10, or other), chi-square (4) = 3.8731, $p = 0.4235$; $DRD4$-TDP (120 or 240), chi-square (1) = 30.2550, $p < 0.0001$; SNAP-SNP-TG (T or G), chi-square (1) = 2.5152, $p < 0.1128$; SNAP-SNP-TC (T or C), chi-square (1) = 6.7395, $p < 0.0094$.

DISCUSSION

One reason often given for use of DNA derived from buccal cells rather than blood cells is that the acquisition of specimens from cheek

TABLE 2. ALLELE PROPORTIONS FOR FIVE POLYMORPHISM OF THREE CANDIDATE GENES

DRD4 VNTR	Blank	2	3	4	5	6	7	8	
Blood	16	21	6	162	9	1	72	1	n = 144
288	5.56	7.29	2.08	56.25	3.13	0.35	25.00	0.35	% for 288 alleles
272		7.72	2.21	59.56	3.31	0.37	26.47	0.37	% for 272 nonblank alleles
Buccal	108	2	4	63	1	0	16	0	n = 97
194	55.67	1.03	2.06	32.47	0.52	0.00	8.25	0.00	% for 194 alleles
86		2.33	4.65	73.26	1.16	0.00	18.60	0.00	% for 86 nonblank alleles

DAT VNTR	Blank	3	7	9	10	11	
Blood	24	1	0	68	192	3	n = 144
288	8.33	0.35	0.00	23.61	66.67	1.04	% for 288 alleles
264		0.38	0.00	25.76	72.73	1.14	% for 264 nonblank alleles
Buccal	98	0	1	27	66	2	n = 97
194	50.52	0.00	0.52	13.92	34.02	1.03	% for 194 alleles
96		0.00	1.04	28.13	68.75	2.08	% for 96 nonblank alleles

DRD4 TDP	Blank	120	240	
Blood	40	58	190	n = 144
288	13.89	20.14	65.97	% for 288 alleles
248		23.39	76.61	% for 248 nonblank alleles
Buccal	89	56	49	n = 97
194	45.88	28.87	25.26	% for 194 alleles
105		53.33	46.67	% for 105 nonblank alleles

SNAP-TG	Blank	T	G	
Blood	44	188	56	n = 144
288	15.28	65.28	19.44	% for 288 alleles
244		77.05	22.95	% for 244 nonblank alleles
Buccal	52	119	23	n = 97
194	26.80	61.34	11.86	% for 194 alleles
142		83.80	16.20	% for 142 nonblank alleles

SNAP-TC	Blank	T	C	
Blood	52	186	50	n = 144
288	18.06	64.58	17.36	% for 288 alleles
236		78.81	21.19	% for 236 nonblank alleles
Buccal	54	125	15	n = 97
194	27.84	64.43	7.73	% for 194 alleles
140		89.29	10.71	% for 140 nonblank alleles

VNTR = variable number of tandem repeat; TDP = tandem duplication polymorphism.

swabs is less intrusive compared to venipuncture, and this would increase the participation of subjects in molecular genetic studies. In the PATS, more probands (preschool children) did opt for the less invasive procedure (61 vs. 51). The procedures for specimen collection differed across site, which may have operated to reduce this difference. The site with the greatest number of subjects in the PATS required a blood test for clinical chemistry tests as part of standard procedures for participation in a clinical trial, and this provided an opportunity for acquiring a blood sample from the probands without an additional venipuncture. It is interesting that for parents, the opposite pattern was observed, with more adults opting to provide a specimen via venipuncture than via cheek swab.

When only a subset of the total sample volunteers for an addition to a protocol, as was the case in the PATS molecular genetic study reported here, selection bias is a threat to validity of the addition. In the PATS, several potential selection biases should be considered. Possible biases include the selection of cases by inclusion and exclusion criteria, the volunteer rate for the molecular genetic addition, and the decision to rely on source of specimens for DNA (venipuncture vs. cheek swabs). Of 183 probands who entered the PATS lead-in phase, only 113 (62%) agreed to participate in the molecular genetics study. Of these children, 46%

TABLE 3. LOGISTIC REGRESSION ANALYSIS OF SOURCE AND FAMILY STATUS

		DF	Chi-square	P > Chi-square
DRD4 VNTR	Source	1	5.02	0.0250
	Family status	1	0.11	0.7376
DRD4 TDP	Source	1	24.37	0.0001
	Family status	1	3.02	0.0821
DAT VNTR	Source	1	0.35	0.5536
	Family status	1	1.09	0.2970
SNAP25-TG	Source	1	1.75	0.1858
	Family status	1	1.52	0.2179
SNAP25-TC	Source	1	7.02	0.0081
	Family status	1	0.03	0.8718

DF = Degrees of freedom; VNTR = variable number of tandem repeat; TDP = tandem duplication polymorphism; P = probability.

opted to provide a specimen via venipuncture and 53% via cheek swab as a source of DNA. On the average, the amplification rate was 94% for DNA from blood cells derived from venipuncture and 40% from buccal cells derived from cheek swab. It is possible that selection bias may have operated to produce differences in the findings reported here, with more adventuresome or less anxious individuals opting for the more invasive procedure.

There were significantly higher rates of failure for DNA amplification in samples derived from buccal cells versus blood cells, but this depended on the genetic assay required to genotype the polymorphism of the candidate gene. For assays based on short DNA segments, such as for the SNPs in the SNAP25 gene, source did not matter, but for assays based on long DNA segments, such as for the VNTR polymorphisms in the DAT1 and *DRD4* genes, amplification rate differed by source. The overall effect was large, and the source difference was greatest for the most complex VNTR (the 48-bp repeat of the exon III VNTR). Another interesting but unexplained difference was the lower amplification rate for the short SNP polymorphisms from blood cells (about 80%) than for the long VNTR polymorphisms from blood cells (about 95%).

These differences are likely related to the amount and/or quality of DNA derived from the two sources. A greater amount of DNA is usually obtained from blood cells than from buccal cells. Because the eventual amplification by PCR depends on the initial phase that may be randomly biased for some alleles over others in small amounts of DNA, the larger amount of DNA from blood cells may provide a better estimate of alleles proportion than the smaller amount of DNA from buccal cells (see Walsh et al. 1992). New methods for collecting buccal cells have been proposed (e.g., from saliva samples rather than from buccal cells collected by cheek swabs, as in the PATS), and may produce greater amounts of DNA.

The quality of DNA is different when derived from blood cells and buccal cells. When DNA is isolated from a blood sample, the cells are alive, but not all contain DNA. The red blood cells without nuclei are removed, so only white blood cells with nuclei and DNA are used. This may remove a source of noise when amplifying the DNA. When DNA is isolated from buccal cells, the cells are dead, but cells from bacteria that are present are alive and may increase over time (Sigurdson et al. 2006). Also, enzymes in the mouth start to degrade the dead cells, which cuts DNA into short fragments. This degradation may selectively complicate the amplification of alleles that consist of long DNA segments. Thus, the amplification of long polymorphisms may be greater in intact DNA from blood cells than from degraded DNA from buccal cells.

The difference in allele proportion documented here may be due to one or more of these potential selection biases. However, differences in DNA derived from buccal and blood samples, due to differential bacterial contamination, DNA degradation, allele length, or other factors, may account for the observed difference. Within the relatively long polymorphisms of the *DRD4* gene, amplification of short alleles may be favored over long alleles in degraded DNA, which could account for the higher percentage of the four-repeat alleles of the *DRD4* exon III VNTR from DNA derived from buccal cells than from blood cells. Of course, the observed difference may be due to chance rather than selection bias or differences in DNA derived from blood or buccal cells.

On the basis of the results of the exploratory analyses reported here, several recommendations seem warranted for planning future research. First, if the genetic component is an inseparable part of a study instead of an elective addition, then it may be reasonable to have consent for the genetic component as part of the entry criteria. This would avoid some possible selection biases, although it may exclude some individuals and thus restrict overall entry into the study. Second, if missing data on genotype are a major concern, then it may be reasonable to offer only one procedure (venipuncture for collection of blood cells) instead of offering a choice of two procedures (venipuncture or cheek swabs, as in the PATS). Then, for those individuals who elect to participate, on whom other data is collected (e.g., on phenotype, demographics, outcome, etc.) at considerable investment of time, effort, and expense, the current best source of DNA (from blood cells) would be provided that would maximize genotype data available for analysis. Third, studies of DNA from blood cells and buccal cells from the all participants would be valuable. In the present study, comparisons of the two sources DNA were based on different individuals, some of whom provided blood cells and others buccal cells. If the comparison were made based on the same individuals, with all providing blood and buccal cells, then data would be available to address the next set of questions about possible differences due to the source of DNA in future studies of the molecular genetics of ADHD.

DISCLOSURES

Financial Disclosures: The following financial disclosures indicate potential conflicts of interest among the PATS investigators and industry sources for the period 2000–2007. [1]Honoraria/consultant, [2]research support, [3]speaker's bureau, [4]significant equity (>$50,000). Dr. Posner: As part of an effort to help execute the FDA suicidality classification mandates, Dr. Posner has had research support (2) GlaxoSmithKline, Forest Laboratories, Eisai, AstraZeneca Pharmaceuticals, Johnson & Johnson, Abbott Laboratories, Wyeth Research, Organon USA, Bristol-Meyers Squibb, Sanofi-Aventis, Cephalon, Novartis, UCB Pharma, Shire.[1,2] Dr. Murray: Eli Lilly,[2] Pfizer.[2] Dr. Abikoff: Abbott Labs,[1] Celltech,[2] Cephalon,[1] Eli Lilly,[1,2] McNeil,[1,2] Novartis,[2] Pfizer,[2] Shire.[1,2] Dr. Ghuman: Bristol Myers-Squibb.[2] Dr. Kollins: Athenagen,[1,2] Cephalon,[1] Eli Lilly,[1,2] McNeil, New River Pharmaceuticals,[2] Pfizer,[2] Psychogenics,[2] Shire.[1,2] Dr. Sharon Wigal: Celltech,[1,2,3] Cephalon,[1,2,3] Eli Lilly,[2] Janssen,[3] McNeil,[1,2,3] New River Pharmaceuticals,[2] Novartis,[1,2,3] Shire.[1,2,3] Dr. Tim Wigal: Celltech,[2] Cephalon,[2] Eli Lilly,[2,3] Janssen,[2] McNeil,[2,3] Novartis,[2] Shire.[2,3] Dr. McCracken: Abbott, Bristol Meyers Squibb,[1] Eli Lilly,[1,2,3] Gliatech,[2] Janssen,[1,3] Johnson & Johnson, McNeil,[1,2] Novartis, Noven,[1] Pfizer,[1,2] Shire,[1,2] UCB, Wyeth. Dr. McGough: Eli Lilly,[1,2,3] McNeil,[1,2,3] New River Pharmaceuticals,[2] Novartis,[1,2,3] Pfizer,[1,2,3] Shire.[1,2,3] Dr. Boorady: Shire.[1,3] Mr. Davies: Amgen,[4] Bard, GlaxoSmithKline,[4] Johnson & Johnson,[4] Merck,[4] Pfizer,[4] Wyeth.[4] Dr. Swanson: Alza,[1,2] Celgene,[1,2] Celltech,[1,2,3] Cephalon,[1,2,3] Eli Lilly,[1,2] Gliatech,[1,2] Janssen,[1,2,3] McNeil,[1,2,3] Novartis,[1,2] Organon,[1] UCB, Shire.[1,2] Dr. Riddle: Astra-Zeneca,[1] Glaxo-Smith-Kline,[1] Janssen,[1] Pfizer,[2] Shire.[1] Dr. Greenhill: Alza,[2] Sanofi Aventis,[1] Celltech,[2] Cephalon,[2] Eli Lilly,[1,2] Glaxo Wellcome,[2] Janssen,[1] McNeil,[2] Medeva,[2] Novartis Corporation,[2] Noven,[2] Otsuka,[1] Shire,[1,2] Solvay,[1] Somerset,[2] Thomson Advanced Therapeutics Communications,[1] Wyeth Ayerst.[2] Drs. Vitiello, Cunningham, Kastelic, and Fisher, and Ms. Chuang and Ms. Skrobala have no conflicts of interest or financial ties to disclose as they have not received support from companies manufacturing medications.

REFERENCES

American Psychiatric Association: *Diagnostic and Statistical Manual of Mental Disorders,* 4th edition. Washington (D.C.): American Psychiatric Association, 1994.

Barr CL, Feng Y, Wigg K, Bloom S, Roberts W, Malone M, Schachar R, Tannock R, Kennedy JL: Identification of DNA variants in the SNAP-25 gene and linkage study of these polymorphisms and attention-deficit/hyperactivity disorder. Mol Psychiatry 5:405–409, 2000.

Chang F-M, Kidd JR, Livak KJ, Pakstis AJ, Kidd KK: The world-wide distribution of allele frequencies of the human dopamine D4 receptor locus. Hum Genet 98:91–101, 1996.

Collins FS: The case for a US prospective cohort study of genes and environment. Nature 429:475–477, 2004.

Cook EH Jr., Stein MA, Krasowski MD, Cow NJ, Olkon DM, Kieffer JE, Leventhal BL: Association of attention deficit disorder and the dopamine trasporter gene. Am J Hum Genet 56:993–998, 1995.

Cornish KM, Manly T, Savage R, Swanson J, Morisano D, Butler N, Grant C, Cross G, Bentley L, Hollis CP: Association of the dopamine transporter (DAT1) 10/10-repeat genotype with ADHD symptoms and response inhibition in a general population sample. Mol Psychiatry 10:686–98, 2005.

Ding YC, Chi HC, Grady DL, Morishima A, Kidd JR, Kidd KK, Flodman P, Spence MA, Schuck S, Swanson JM, Zhang YP, Moyzis RK: Evidence of positive selection acting at the human dopamine receptor D4 gene locus. Proc Natl Acad Sci USA 99:309–314, 2002.

Faraone SV, Perlis RH, Doyle AE, Smoller JN, Goralnick JJ, Holmgren MA, Sklar P: Molecular genetics of attention-deficit/hyperactivity disorder. Biol Psychiatry 57:1313–1323, 2005.

Fosella J, Posner MI, Fan J, Swanson JM, Pfaff DW. Attentional phenotypes for the analysis of higher mental function. Scientif World J 2:217–223, 2002.

Greenhill L, Kollins S, Abikoff H, McCracken J, Riddle M, Swanson J, McGough J, Wigal S, Wigal T, Vitiello B, Skrobala A, Posner K, Ghuman J, Cunningham C, Davies M, Chuang S, Cooper T: Efficacy and Safety of Immediate-release Methylphenidate Treatment for Preschoolers with ADHD. J Am Acad Child Adolesc Psychiatry 45:1284–1293, 2006.

Grady DL, Chi HC, Ding YC, Smith M, Wang E, Schuck S, Flodman P, Spence MA, Swanson JM, Moyzis RK: High prevalence of rare dopamine receptor D4 alleles in children diagnosed with attention-deficit hyperactivity disorder. Mol Psychiatry 8:536–545, 2003.

Hamarman S, Fossella J, Ulger C, Brimacombe M, Dermody J: Dopamine receptor 4 (DRD4) 7-repeat allele predicts methylphenidate dose response in children with attention deficit hyperactivity disorder. J Child Adolesc Psychopharmacol 14:564–574, 2004.

Kaiser R, Tremblay P-B, Roots I, Brockmoller J: Validity of PCR with emphasis on variable number of tandem repeat analysis. Clin Biochem 35:49–56, 2002.

Kirley A, Lowe N, Hawi Z, Mullins C, Daly G, Waldman I, McCarron M, O'Donnell D, Fitzgerald M, Gill M: Association of the 480 bp DAT1 allele with methylphenidate response in a sample of Irish children with ADHD. Am J Med Genet 121B:50–54, 2003.

Kollins S, Greenhill L, Swanson J, Wigal S, Abikoff H, McCracken J, Riddle M, McGough J, Vitiello B, Wigal T, Skrobala A, Posner K, Ghuman J, Davies M, Cunningham C, Bauzo A: Rationale, Design, and Methods of

the Preschool ADHD Treatment Study (PATS). J Am Acad Child Adolesc Psychiatry 45:1275–1283, 2006.

LaHoste GJ, Swanson JM, Wigal SB, Glabe C, Wigal T, King N, Kennedy JL: Dopamine D4 receptor gene polymorphism is associated with attention deficit hyperactivity disorder. Molecular Psychiatry 1:121–124, 1996.

Li Dm Sham PC, Owen MJ, He L: Meta-analysis shows significant association between dopamine system genes and attention deficit hyperactivity disorder (ADHD). Hum Mol Genet 15:2276–2284, 2006.

McCracken JT, Smalley SL, McGough JJ, Crawford L, Del Homme M, Cantor RM, Liu A, Nelson SF: Evidence for linkage of a tandem duplication polymorphism upstream of the dopamine D4 receptor gene (DRD4) with attention deficit hyperactivity disorder (ADHD). Mol Psychiatry 5:531–536, 2000.

McGough JJ: Attention-deficit/hyperactivity disorder pharmacogenomics, Biol Psychiatry 57:1367–1373, 2005.

McGough JJ, McCracken JT, Swanson JM, Riddle M, Kollins SH, Greenhill LL, Abikoff H, Davies M, Chuang S, Wigal TL, Wigal SB, Posner K, Skrobala A, Kastelic E, Ghuman J, Cunningham C, Shigana S, Moyzis RK, Vitiello B: Pharmacogenetics of methylphenidate response in preschoolers with ADHD. J Am Acad Child Adolesc Psychiatry, 45:1314–1322, 2006.

Mill J, Caspi A, Williams, BS, Craig I, Taylor A, Polo-Torres M, Berridge CW, Poulton R, Moffit TE: Prediction of heterogeneity in intelligence and adult prognosis by genetic polymorphisms in the dopamine system among children with attention-deficit/hyperactivity disorder. Arch Gen Psychiatry, 63:462–469, 2006.

Moffit TE, Moffit TE, Caspi A, Rutter M, Silva PA: Sex differences in antisocial behavior: conduct disorder, delinquency, and violence in the Dunedin Longitudinal Study. Cambridge, England, Cambridge University Press, 2001.

Schaffer D, Fisher P, Lucas, C: The NIMH diagnostic interview schedule for children version 4.0 (DISC-4.0). New York: Ruane Center for Early Diagnosis, Division of Child Psychiatry, Columbia University, 1996.

Santosh P, Taylor E, Swanson JM, Wigal S, Chuang S, Davies M, Greenhill L, Newcorn J, Arnold L, Jenson P, Vitiello B, Elliott G, Hinshaw S, Hechtman L, Abikoff H, Pelham W, Hoza B, Molina B, Wells K, Epstein J, Posner M: Refining the diagnoses of inattention and overreactivity syndromes: a reanalysis of the Multimodal Treatment study of attention deficit hyperactivity disorder (ADHD) based on ICD-10 criteria for hyperkinetic disorder. Clin Neurosci Res 5:304–314, 2005.

Sigurdson AJ, Ha M, Consentino M, Franklin T, Haque KA, Qi Y Glaser C, Reid Y, Vaught JB, Bergen AN : Long-term storage and recovery of buccal cell DNA from treated cards. Cancer Epidemiol Biomarkers Prev 15:385–388, 2006.

Swanson JM, Wigal S, Greenhill L, Brown R, Waslick B, Lerner M, Williams L, Flynn D, Agler D, Crowley KL,

Fineberg E, Regino R, Baren M, Cantwell D: Objective and subjective measures of the pharmacodynamic effects of Adderall in the treatmeant of children with ADHD in a controlled laboratory classroom setting. Psychopharmocol Bull 34:55–60, 1998.

Swanson JM, Lerner M, March J, Gresham F: Assessment and intervention for attention-deficit/hyperactivity disorder in the schools: Lessons from the MTA Study. Pediatr Clin N Am 46:993–1009, 1999.

Swanson JM, Moyzis R, Fossella J, Fan J, Posner M: Adaptionism and molecular biology: An example based on ADHD. Behav Brain Sci 25:530–531, 2002.

Thapar A, O'Donovan M, Owen MJ. The genetics of attention deficit hyperactivity disorder. Hum Mol Genet 14:R275–R282, 2006.

Volkow ND, Ding YS, Fowler JS, Wang GJ, Logan J, Gatley JS, Dewey S, Ashby C, Lieberman J, Hitsemann R, Wolf AP: Is methylphenidate like cocaine? Studies on their pharmacokinetics and distribution in the human brain. Arch Gen Psychiatry 52:456–463, 1995.

Walsh S, Erlich HA, Higuchi, R: Preferential PCR amplification of alleles: Mechanisms and solutions. PCR Methods Applic 1:241–250, 1992.

Wang E, Ding YC, Flodman P, Kidd JR, Kidd KK, Grady DL, Ryder OA, Spence MA, Swanson JM, Moyzis RK: The genetic architecture of selection at the human dopamine receptor D4 (DRD4) gene locus. Am J Hum Genet 74:931–944, 2004.

Wender P: Minimal brain dysfunction in children. Wiley-Liss, New York, 1971.

ADVANCES IN PRESCHOOL PSYCHOPHARMACOLOGY
© 2009 Mary Ann Liebert, Inc.
140 Huguenot Street, 3rd Floor
New Rochelle, NY 10801-5215

Pharmacokinetics of Methylphenidate in Preschoolers with Attention-Deficit/Hyperactivity Disorder

Sharon B. Wigal, Ph.D.,[1] Suneel Gupta, Ph.D.,[2] Laurence L. Greenhill, M.D.,[3]
Kelly Posner, Ph.D.,[3] Marc Lerner, M.D.,[1] Kenneth Steinhoff, M.D.,[1] Tim Wigal, Ph.D.,[1]
Audrey Kapelinski, LCSW,[1] Jonathan Martinez, B.A.,[1] Nishit B. Modi, Ph.D.,[2]
Annamarie Stehli, MPH,[1] and James Swanson, Ph.D.[1]

ABSTRACT

Objective: The aim of this study was to compare the pharmacokinetics of immediate-release methylphenidate (MPH) in preschool and school-aged children with attention-deficit/hyperactivity disorder (ADHD).

Methods: Preschool children 4–5 years ($n = 14$) and school-aged children 6–8 years ($n = 9$) with diagnoses of ADHD were titrated to an effective dose of MPH based on parent, teacher, and clinician ratings in a protocol specified by the Preschoolers with ADHD Treatment Study (PATS) and then attended a laboratory school where the single morning dose of immediate release MPH was administered. Blood samples for measurement of MPH concentrations were obtained predose, and at 1, 2, 4, and 6 hours postdose. A nonlinear model was used to derive three pharmacokinetic (PK) values for analysis: Peak plasma concentration (C_{max}), half-life ($t_{1/2}$), and clearance (CL).

Results: The two groups did not differ in the mean mg dose of MPH ($p = 0.33$), or in the weight-adjusted mg/kg dose ($p = 0.20$). Dose-normalized C_{max} was significantly higher ($p = 0.003$), and clearance was significantly slower ($p = 0.0002$) in preschool than in school-aged children.

Conclusions: In this sample, age significantly affected absorption and metabolism of MPH, so that preschool children had greater exposure than school-aged children to the same weight-adjusted dose. These data suggest additional studies should be performed to characterize age-related differences in PK properties of MPH that may inform practitioners about dosing strategies based on the age and size of children being treated.

---

[1]University of California, Irvine, Irvine, California.
[2]ALZA Corporation, Mountainview, California.
[3]New York State Psychiatric Institute/Columbia University, New York, New York.
Statistical Experts: Nishit Modi, Ph.D., and Annamarie Stehli, MPH, Child Development Center, Department of Pediatrics, University of California, Irvine, Irvine, California.
This research was supported by NIMH contract MH60833, MH02042, and PHS M01RR00827 from the National Center for Research Resources under the direction of Dr. Dan Cooper.
Disclaimer: The opinions and assertions contained in this report are the private views of the author and are not to be construed as official or as reflecting the views of the National Institute of Mental Health, the National Institutes of Health, or the Department of Health and Human Services.

INTRODUCTION

METHYLPHENIDATE (MPH) is the most commonly prescribed psychotropic medication for the treatment of attention-deficit/hyperactivity disorder (ADHD) in children, including the subgroup of preschool children, even though it does not have Food and Drug Administration (FDA) approval for use in children under 6 years of age. Because of the increasing use of stimulant medication in this group, the National Institute of Health Consensus Development Conference on the Diagnosis and Treatment of Attention-Deficit Hyperactivity Disorder (1998) identified a need for studies of the risks and benefits associated with treatment of preschool-aged children with stimulant medication, including pharmacokinetic (PK) properties to evaluate age-related effects on drug absorption and metabolism, pharmacodynamic (PD) properties to evaluate onset, peak, and duration of behavioral effects, dose–response characteristics, and side effects related to short- and long-term exposure to stimulants.

Although some controlled clinical trials have been performed with preschool children with ADHD as subjects, to our knowledge there have been no prior PK studies of MPH in this age group. Recently, age-related differences in the PK properties of MPH were documented in an industry-sponsored comparison of Concerta™, a controlled-release formulation of MPH, in school-aged and adolescent subjects (Food and Drug Administration, 2005). The finding indicated that clearance of MPH depended on age and was greater (faster) in adolescents, which was sufficient to warrant a change in the package insert for Concerta™ to guide clinical treatment of different age groups (McNeil 2004).

The primary objective of this small, preliminary study was to compare the plasma concentrations and associated pharmacokinetic parameters (maximum concentration, half-life, and clearance) after administration of a clinically-titrated morning dose of MPH in preschool and school-aged children with ADHD from one of the six sites of the Preschoolers with ADHD Treatment Study (PATS) who were evaluated in the context of a laboratory school protocol (Swanson et al. 2000; Wigal and Wigal 2006) and to relate the findings of the literature in age-related effects on the PK properties of MPH.

METHODS

Single site of the PATS

Challenges were encountered in the groundbreaking PATS protocol that required some modifications as it was implemented. One modification was to restrict the overall PATS to preschool children, because recruitment challenges and limited funding made the evaluation of school-aged children impractical. The University of California, Irvine (UCI) site had accelerated recruitment, and school-aged children were entered into the PATS protocol before it was modified. Another modification was to eliminate the laboratory school component from the protocol, which was intended for implementation at each of the six sites after the titration phase (Kollins et al. 2006). Accelerated recruitment at the UCI site (Greenhill et al. 2006), prior experience with the laboratory school protocol (Swanson et al. 2003; Wigal and Wigal, 2006), and extra funding to one of the UCI investigators made it feasible to implement this component partially at the UCI site.

The PK study was an add-on component to the PATS protocol, but the design requirements of a school-aged comparison group and the implementation of the laboratory school protocol precluded execution at all sites. Therefore, it was a single-site study implemented at one of the PATS sites with a small sample size. In this paper we present preliminary information from a small sample to guide future work on age-related differences in the PK properties of MPH.

Subjects

The subjects for this study met the general entry criteria for the multisite PATS described in detail by Greenhill et al. (2006) and followed the same overall protocol also described in detail by Kollins et al. (2006), which will not be repeated here. The additional entry criteria and protocol methods of this single-site PK study will be described in detail.

Children were required to meet the criteria for ADHD, Combined Type or Predominantly Hyperactive-Impulsive Type as defined by the criteria in the *Diagnostic and Statistical Manual of Mental Disorders*, 4th edition (DSM-IV; diagnostic code 314.01) (American Psychiatric Association, 1994), to be between the ages of 36–65 months old (for the preschool groups) and 72–96 months old (for the school-aged group), and to be able to tolerate catheter insertion for the collection of blood samples to be used for the measurement of plasma concentrations of MPH.

In the overall PATS protocol (Kollins et al. 2006) subjects participated in prebaseline (3-week, open-label, lead-in) assessments of tolerability to doses of immediate release MPH from 1.25 mg to 7.5 mg, followed by a double-blind, placebo-controlled medication titration trial of those doses administered three times a day (t.i.d.), a parallel, between-group comparison of the best dose chosen during titration versus placebo, and a 10-month, open-label follow-up starting at the best dose with monthly clinic visits in which dose adjustments were allowed. For the single-site PK study, participants were given their morning dose of the clinically optimized t.i.d. MPH regimen established during the maintenance phase of the PATS.

Study design

This study was conducted at UCI in accordance with the principles of the Declaration of Helsinki and its amendments, and approved by the UCI Institutional Review Board. At a screening visit, parents provided written consent for their child's enrollment, and all subjects provided either written or verbal assent. Subjects who met study eligibility requirements were scheduled to attend the Saturday session for PK data collection. Figure 1 shows the laboratory classroom schedule for the PK study day. Subjects were instructed not to eat or to take study medication prior to coming to the laboratory school. Subjects were prescribed EMLA® cream (2.5% lidocaine and 2.5% prilo-

caine) for local, topical anesthesia at the catheter insertion site, and parents were instructed to apply this immediately prior to arrival for maximal numbing action on site. Children were fed a standardized, regular breakfast consisting of cereal, 1% milk, and fresh fruit at about 7 a.m. and were given their morning dose of MPH by 8 a.m. Thus, food intake was controlled to exclude potential effects of food on the PK properties of MPH (Chan et al. 1983; Gonzalez et al. 2002).

The PK samples were obtained via a catheter placed in the antecubital vein in each subject's forearm. Subjects participated in various distracter techniques including viewing "I Spy" books and listening to songs on tape during catheter insertion and PK sampling. Blood samples prior to dosing and at four times after dosing (1, 2, 4, and 6 hours) were collected into EDTA Vacutainer® tubes. The blood samples were processed immediately by centrifugation, and the plasma samples were stored at approximately $-20°C$ before frozen shipment on dry ice to National Medical Services (NMS), where they were analyzed by high-performance liquid chromatography/mass spectrometry (LC/MS) to determine the concentrations of *d-threo-* and *l-threo*-MPH, as well as *d-* and *l*-ritalinic acid, the principal MPH metabolites (data on file at NMS). The quantification limits of the assay were as follows: For *l-threo*-MPH in plasma, the lower limit of quantification (LLOQ) defined as the lowest concentration achieving an acceptable coefficient of variation (C.V.) of ±20% at the LLOQ was a value of 0.5 ng/mL and the upper limit of quantification (ULOQ) was defined as the highest concentration achieving an acceptable C.V. of ±15% at the ULOQ with a value of 100 ng/mL; for ritalinic acid in plasma, the C.V.'s were similar in value, with the LLOQ of 5.0 ng/mL and the ULOQ of 400 ng/mL.

PK profiles were analyzed by noncompartmental methods (WinNonlin version 4.1, Pharsight Corporation). The maximum MPH plasma concentration (C_{max}) and time to reach the maximum concentration (T_{max}) were recorded as the observed values. The elimination half-life was estimated using the terminal portion of the concentration profile, and the area under the concentration-time curve ex-

Hour	Time	Activity	Hour	Time	Activity
	7:45	Arrival & Vitals/Temp Catheter & Breakfast & PK		12:15	Lunch
				12:30	Nap/Quiet Time
0 Hour	9:00	Class #0		1:20	Vitals
	9:30	Dosing			
	9:40	Snack	**4 Hour**	1:30	PK & Class #3
	9:50	Outdoor Play		2:00	Outdoor Free Play
	10:20	Vitals		2:30	Snack
				2:40	Indoor Activity
1 Hour	10:30	PK & Class #1		3:20	Vitals
	11:00	Indoor Free Play			
	11:10	Vitals	**6 Hour**	3:30	PK & Class #4
				4:00	RECESS Play
2 Hour	11:30	PK & Class #2		4:15	Clean Up/Prizes
	12:00	RECESS Play		4:30	Dismissal

FIG. 1. Study day schedule.

trapolated to infinity (AUC$_{inf}$) was calculated by a linear trapezoidal method. The apparent clearance is the clearance (CL) divided by the fraction (F) of the dose determined by bioavailability (F) or (CL/F), and in both absolute and weight-adjusted terms the apparent clearance was estimated as the quotient of the dose and AUC$_{inf}$. Four subjects in the school-aged group had insufficient data to allow estimation of a half-life or AUC$_{inf}$. PK parameter estimates for the school-aged and preschool groups were based on prospective estimates of sample size and were compared using a two-tailed t-test.

Because the sample sizes for the preschool ($n = 14$) and school-aged ($n = 9$) children were small, for the reasons outlined above, we present effect sizes with confidence intervals of our comparisons as well as significance levels. Estimates of effect size can be used to make informed estimates about the sample size and power requirements for future studies.

RESULTS

Patients

Basic demographic information including gender and ethnicity for the two age groups are shown in Table 1. Of 18 preschool children who consented to the study, a total of 14 subjects were enrolled, 1 subject would not comply with study procedures on the practice day preceding the PK study day and was withdrawn from participation, 1 subject withdrew consent due to excessive fear of needles, and 2 subjects participated in classroom measurements only on the PK day to maintain adequate classroom size, with no blood samples collected. Of 10 school-aged subjects who consented to the study, 9 were enrolled. One child was ill and unable to attend the study day. Of the preschool children, 1 child received 2.5 mg, 8 children received 5 mg, 4 children received 7.5 mg, and 1 child received 10 mg of MPH. Of the school-aged children, 2 children received 2.5 mg, 2 children received 5 mg, 1 child received 7.5 mg, and 4 children received 10 mg of MPH.

As expected, the preschool-aged group was significantly ($p < 0.0001$ for each) younger (5.3 versus 7.4 years of age), shorter (112 versus 129 cm), and weighed less (19 versus 28 kg) than the school-aged group (see Table 1).

Pharmacokinetic effects

Table 2 shows the comparison of weight, clearance, and other variables of the preschool-aged and school-aged children who completed the PK protocol. A total of 115 blood samples were collected across the multiple observations within each of the subjects. d-MPH was quantified in all samples; l-MPH typically was negligible and could not be quantified by analysis as is typically found in PK studies of oral administration (Srinivas et al. 1992; Srinivas et al. 1993; Quinn et al. 2004), which accounts for the maximum bioavailability (50%) of oral doses of the racemic mixture of MPH (see Chan et al. 1983). Ritalinic acid concentrations were high and quantifiable in all samples. The ratio of the d-ritalinic acid to d-MPH was the same for all samples and, therefore, only the MPH is presented and discussed here. There was considerable variability in the estimated PK parameters (%CV ranging from 32 to 72). At time 0 hour, when blood levels of MPH were not expected due to the short half-life of the drug and the overnight washout period, only 1 out of 23 subjects had a quantifiable blood sample, and this value was very small (<0.5 ng/ml).

The range of titrated dose levels (i.e., 2.5–7.5 mg t.i.d.) was identical for both age groups (see Fig. 2). The average total morning dose was 5.89 mg for preschoolers and 6.94 mg for

TABLE 1. SUMMARY OF DEMOGRAPHIC DATA

	Preschool children (n = 14)	School-aged children (n = 9)
Gender		
% Male	64.3	44.4
% Female	35.7	55.6
Diagnosis		
% Combined	71.4	100
% Hyperactive/impulsive	28.6	
Age		
Mean	5.3 years	7.4 years
Range	4–6 years	7–8 years
Weight		
Mean	19.2 kg	28.3 kg
Range	14.6–22.7 kg	21.2–39.8 kg
Height		
Mean	112 cm	129.43 cm
Range	98–119 cm	121–140 cm
Dose level		
Median	5.0 mg	7.5 mg
Range	2.5–10.0 mg	2.5–10.0 mg

TABLE 2. COMPARISONS OF PRESCHOOLERS AND SCHOOL-AGED SUBJECTS

	Preschoolers	School-aged	Difference in effect size	p value	95% Confidence interval
Age	5.33 ± 0.56	8.00 ± 0.56	4.77	<0.001	(3.03, 6.17)
Weight (kg)	19.2 ± 2.6	28.3 ± 5.8	2.22	<0.001	(1.10, 3.19)
Dose (mg)	5.89 ± 1.9	6.94 ± 3.3	0.42	0.33	(−0.44, 1.25)
Dose/weight (mg/kg)	0.311 ± 0.09	0.252 ± 0.13	−0.54	0.20	(−1.37, 0.33)
CL/F (L/hour)	99.5 ± 44	232.6 ± 75	2.52	<0.001	(1.13, 3.68)
CL/F weight (L/hour per kg)	5.12 ± 1.9	7.91 ± 1.6	1.52	0.01	(0.33, 2.57)
V/F (L)	457.8 ± 210	737.8 ± 296	1.2	0.034	(0.062, 2.23)
$t_{1/2}$ (hour)	3.82 ± 2.7	2.18 ± 0.3	−0.53	0.32	(−1.5, 0.53)
AUC (ng.h/mL)	75.2 ± 54	41.8 ± 22	−0.53	0.32	(−1.5, 0.53)
AUC/D (hour/L)	0.012 ± 0.005	0.0047 ± 0.002	−1.54	0.009	(−2.60, −0.35)
C_{max} (ng/mL)	10.2 ± 5.0	7.6 ± 4.2	−0.55	0.22	(−1.38, 0.33)
1,000 C_{max}/D (1/L)	1.72 ± 0.5	1.10 ± 0.3	−1.44	0.003	(−2.31, −0.46)
T_{max} (hour)	2.57 ± 0.9	2.56 ± 1.1	−0.01	0.98	(−0.85, 0.83)

CL = clearance; F = fraction of dose determined by bioavailability; AUC = area under the curve; V = volume; L = liter; D = dose normalized. CL/F = apparent clearance; V/F = apparent volume of distribution; $t_{1/2}$ = half-life; T_{max} = time to maximum plasma concentration; C_{max}, maximum plasma concentration.

school-aged children (see Table 2), but this difference was not significant in a comparison of the absolute mg dose ($p = 0.33$) or the relative mg/kg dose adjusted for weight ($p = 0.20$).

As shown in Fig. 3, clearance and dose-normalized C_{max} were strongly correlated with age. This was expected, because weight is a function of age and apparent clearance and dose-normalized C_{max} would be expected to

vary directly with weight (and correspondingly with age).

The dose-normalized maximum concentration was significantly ($p = 0.003$) higher for the preschool-aged group (1.72 L^{-1}) than the school-aged group (1.1 L^{-1}). Similarly, the dose-normalized AUC was significantly higher ($p = 0.009$) for the preschool-aged group (0.012 L/hour) than for the school-aged group (0.0047

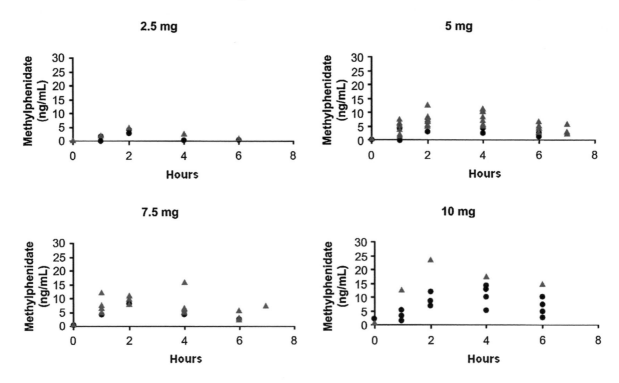

FIG. 2. Identical range of titrated dose levels by age group. ▲ Preschoolers ● School-aged.

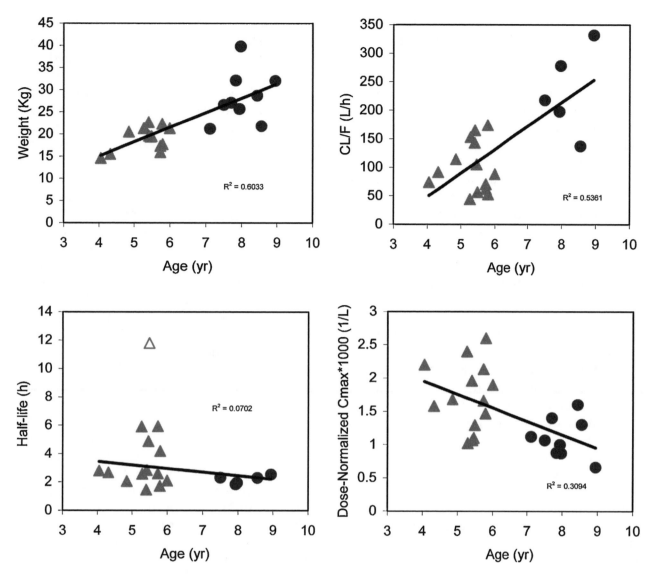

FIG. 3. Correlations with age in years. The preschool-aged child with the apparently long half-life was excluded from the regression. Inclusion of this datum did not influence the regression. CL/F = apparent clearance; L/h = liters per hour; R^2 = correlation.

L/hour). The half-life for MPH was 3.82 hours for the preschool-aged group and 2.18 hours for the school-aged group. This difference was not statistically significant ($p = 0.46$), but the effect size was -0.69, (-1.70, 0.38).

The preschool-aged group had a significantly ($p < 0.0001$) decreased apparent clearance of MPH than the school-aged group (99.5 L/hour compared to 232.6 L/hour), and the effect size was 2.52 (1.13, 3.68). When controlled for weight, the clearance for the preschool-aged group (5.12 L/hour per kg) was still lower than for the school-aged group (7.91 L/hour per kg), and this difference remained statistically sig-

nificant ($p = 0.01$), and the effect size was 1.52 (0.33, 2.57).

DISCUSSION

To our knowledge, this is the first study to present a preliminary comparison of PK characteristics of MPH in preschool children with ADHD to another age group. The primary finding of this preliminary study is the slower clearance of MPH in the group of preschool-aged children compared to the same PK parameter in school-aged children. Of the various PK parameters, clearance is thought to be the most relevant to clinical practice because it serves as a surrogate for dose-adjusted exposure. Clearance represents the sum of individual clearance processes [hepatic (biliary and metabolic), renal, etc.] and is expected to change in relation to factors that influence these processes. Our estimates of clearance are consistent with the few reports in the literature, which provide estimates of clearance in school-aged children from a small sample in a traditional repeated measures PK protocol: $n = 4$, 5.47 L/hour per kg (Hungund et al. 1979) and a large sample in a population PK protocol with one measure from each individual: $n = 213$, 5.4 L/hour per kg (Shader et al. 1999). These values as depicted in Fig. 4 fall between the values we observed from our preschool (5.12 L/hour per kg) and school-aged (7.91 L/hour per kg) groups constrained to narrow age ranges.

In an early publication about the PK properties of MPH, comparison of school-aged children with adults suggested that clearance was not related to age (Wargin et al. 1983). However, recent evidence suggests that apparent clearance of MPH does vary with age (Food and Drug Administration, 2005). This led to a change in the package insert for Concerta®, a controlled-release formulation of MPH, which now states, "Increase in age resulted in increased apparent oral clearance" (CL/F) (58% increase in adolescents compared to children (McNeil 2004). Some of these differences could be explained by body weight differences among these populations. This suggests that subjects with higher body weight may have lower exposures of total methylphenidate at

similar doses." The data from the present study are consistent with this statement and suggest that younger and smaller preschool-aged children may have greater exposure to MPH than older and heavier school-aged children at similar doses. A similar PK effect was reported for mixed amphetamine salts extended release (MAS SR; Adderall XR®) between child, adolescent, and adult age groups (Kramer et al. 2005).

The faster clearance of MPH by school-aged children compared to preschool children may be due to the increase in size and maturation of the metabolic enzymes in the older group. There are many implications of these ontogenetic differences, but little information is published in the literature to answer basic questions about this (Coffey 1983). Ginsberg et al. (2002) reviewed PK parameters of children and adults for 45 therapeutic drugs with a wide range of indications and PK factors and analyzed for systematic differences across age groups. They noted, in general, shorter half-lives with more rapid clearance in the older child age groups as seen in the present study. However, information on age differences in the PK properties of MPH was not included in their review, because there was very little data published on the PK properties of MPH (particularly in young children).

Another possible explanation of the difference in clearance may be that preschool-aged children may have less fully developed metabolic enzymes such as esterases and organ functioning than school-aged children, which would result in a slower clearance in the younger age group. This result is counterintu-

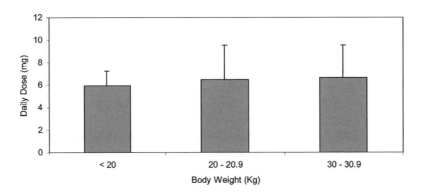

FIG. 4. Mean MPH dose in relation to body weight.

itive, but has been reported with other drugs with increasing age in the lower age range. An example of a drug that shows an increase in clearance from preschool to school-aged children is the antiepileptic drug, topiramate (Dahlin and Ohman 2004).

In the present study, the mean dose for the school-aged group was higher (but not significantly, due to the small sample size), but the MPH plasma concentration was lower than for the preschool-aged group. Because the doses were titrated for both groups to achieve good clinical effect, this suggests that younger and lighter children may require higher plasma concentrations for maximum efficacy than older and heavier children. However, there are at least two speculations to consider. In the PATS, the doses included in the titration process were limited to 7.5 mg t.i.d. or less, compared to 20 mg t.i.d. or less in the Multimodality Treatment Study of ADHD or MTA. The degree of efficacy (ES) was related to dose in the PATS, so at high doses the relationship of efficacy to plasma level may have been different. Also, the finding in the current study is based on systemic concentrations of MPH, not brain levels or central nervous system effects at the site of action of MPH, which is primarily blockade of the dopamine transporter (DAT) in the striatum (Volkow 1995; Volkow et al. 2002). The age- and weight-related differences in transport into the brain might result in similar brain levels of MPH and similar degree of DAT inhibition despite age- and weight-related differences in plasma concentrations in MPH.

The MPH dose and plasma concentration data presented in the current investigation also are consistent with published reports on MPH. Shader et al. (1999) characterized the population PK of b.i.d. and t.i.d. MPH in children with ADHD. In their study, the mean age of the children ranged from 5.4 to 18 years, and their weights ranged from 17 to 142 kg. The mean total daily dose was 33.6 mg (range = 10–60). In their study, they also noted that the total daily dose increased with body weight for both the b.i.d. and t.i.d. dosing regimens. In contrast, the plasma MPH concentrations decreased with body weight ($p > 0.1$ for the b.i.d. regimen and 0.1 ($p < 0.05$ for the t.i.d. regimen). These results are consistent with the observations noted in the present study. Additionally, the clearance value of 5.4 L/hour per kg reported by Shader et al. (1999) is comparable to that noted in the present investigation.

PK variables (such as distribution and clearance, which affect optimal dose titration of drugs) are related to body water, muscle mass, organ blood flow, and organ function (Rowland and Tozer 1989). Statistically controlling for body weight would be expected to cause nonsignificant PK effects unless it reflects some other physiological organ function—maturation of metabolic enzymes systems involved in metabolism or central processing changes in site utilization of the drug. The metabolism of MPH is through hydrolysis/de-esterification and some oxidation (Markowitz et al. 2003), but the hydrolyzing enzymes such as human carboxylesterase CES1A1 (Zejin et al. 2004) may have a different pattern in this process in preschoolers than in school-aged children. If these age-related differences do exist, it may have implications for pharmacologic treatment (including MPH) of preschoolers with ADHD.

Preschool children have higher circulating levels of MPH than school-aged children for the same weight-adjusted dose. The half-life of MPH was nonsignificantly longer for preschool-aged children than school-aged children in this study probably due to the small sample size. The design of the present study could not address whether more sleep problems or loss in appetite correlated with higher plasma MPH concentrations later in the day because all of these children already were maintained on an efficacious dose. This would have to be addressed in future studies with laboratory school assessments in preschoolers occurring during initial exposure to stimulant treatment.

LIMITATIONS

The primary limitation of this study is the small number of subjects in each age group. Some reasons for the small sample (discussed above) were due to recruitment issues related to accumulating a group of participants in the laboratory school protocol and the age of the children. This issue should be addressed in future studies to ensure a larger sample size.

Another limitation was the number of blood samples per subject and the short time interval covered by these samples. This limitation was related to the young age of the preschool children, which made participation in the usual 8- to 12-hour laboratory school day impractical. Another primary limitation was the relatively short sampling period (i.e., only 6–7 hours following oral dosing) used in this study. This provides the minimum required for a reasonable estimate of $t_{1/2}$—approximately one half-life following the expected value of T_{max}. Given these two primary limitations, the estimates of the half-life and clearance must be interpreted cautiously. The preliminary findings from this initial study need to be replicated with larger samples to establish generalizability of the results.

Also, as typical in studies of the influence of age on PK, this was a cross-sectional study of different children at separate points in development, and, therefore, does not reflect how an individual may change with age. The results from this study in small groups of children merit further investigation in larger studies, in which children are followed from an early age to adulthood and PK characteristics are measured at multiple time points during development.

CLINICAL IMPLICATIONS

The primary finding of this preliminary study suggests that preschool children with ADHD may absorb, distribute, metabolize, or eliminate MPH differently than school-aged children with ADHD. The full report of the efficacy data from the PATS (Greenhill 2006) suggests that clinical titration may result in similar absolute doses but higher relative (mg/kg) doses in preschool children than in school-aged children. This, along with possible differences in PK characteristics, may suggest differences in dose and dosing rate for preschool children compared to school-aged children. The clinician is faced with two questions when prescribing IR MPH for a child with ADHD: (1) "What dose is required for this patient?" (which typically is chosen based on titration) and (2) "How often and when should the dose be administered?" (which is traditionally set at 3- to 4-hour intervals for b.i.d. and t.i.d. regimens).

Are the same plasma concentrations needed in preschool-aged children and school-aged children to achieve the same clinical effect? The present study suggests not, since both age groups were titrated to maximum clinical effect (based on subjective ratings) but had different plasma concentrations. The findings from the present study suggest that preschool-aged children may need higher concentrations to achieve the same effect as school-aged children. These findings also are consistent with the clinical practice of generally using absolute MPH dose rather than weight-adjusted (mg/kg) dosees. If the range of doses is about the same for preschool and school-aged children, then the smaller size (and volume of distribution) will result in a higher concentration of MPH in plasma. However, as discussed earlier in this paper and in Kollins et al. (2006), the absolute dose as well as the effect size for efficacy for this end point (derived from the crossover titration trial) were lower for the preschool-aged group than is typical for school-aged children with ADHD treated with MPH.

Is the same dosing rate appropriate for preschool and school-aged children? The present study suggests not, because the concentration at the titrated dose appears to be higher and the clearance decreased in preschool children than in school-aged children. On the basis of the standard use of PK information, for a given average concentration, the dosing rate would be proportional to clearance.

Practitioners may want to consider using a different target dose regimen of MPH (stated as a range of absolute or mg/kg doses) for preschoolers and school-aged children due to the possible age-related differences in clearance. This would be similar to and consistent with the different targets for school-aged children and adolescents, which has been noted by the FDA (Food and Drug Administration 2005) and has been acknowledged in the package insert for the most commonly prescribed formulation of MPH in current clinical practice (McNeil 2004), which noted that clearance is related to weight and may suggest adjustments in the dosing regimen. The FDA (Food and Drug Administration, 2005) report provided information on estimates of clearance for school-aged children (243 L/hour), adolescents (384 L/hour), and adults (497 L/hour), which provide a context for the estimates of clearance for the present study for preschool children (99 L/hour) and school-aged children (232 L/hour). Even though these estimates depend on the assay used for determining MPH concentrations and other factors that may vary across studies, this does clearly indicate that clearance of MPH in plasma is related to age and/or size and varies considerably from early childhood (about 100 L/hour) to adulthood (about 500 L/hour).

Additional information on the PK characteristic of MPH is needed to use this basic information to guide clinical practice for selecting and optimizing the doses for the treatment of all ages of children diagnosed with ADHD.

DISCLOSURES

The following financial disclosures indicate potential conflicts of interest among the investigators and industry sources for the period 2000–2005: [1]Honoraria/Consultant, [2]Research Support, [3]Speaker's Bureau, [4]Significant Equity. Dr. Sharon Wigal: ALZA,[2,3] Celltech,[1,2,3] Cephalon,[1,2,3] Eli Lilly,[1,2] Janssen,[3] McNeil,[1,2,3] New River Pharmaceuticals,[1] Novartis,[1,2,3] Shire.[1,2,3] Drs. Gupta and Modi: Employees of ALZA Corporation, which is a wholly owned subsidiary of Johnson and Johnson; Dr. Greenhill: ALZA,[2] Celltech,[2] Cephalon,[2] Eli Lilly,[1,2] Glaxo Wellcome,[2] Janssen,[1] McNeil,[2] Medeva,[2] Novartis,[2] Noven,[2] Otsuka,[1] Sanofi Aventis,[1] Shire,[1,2] Solvay,[1] Somerset,[2] Thomson Advanced Therapeutics Communications,[1] Wyeth Ayerst.[2] Dr. Posner: Shire.[1,2] Drs. Lerner and Steinhoff: ALZA,[2,3] Celltech,[1,2,3] Cephalon,[1,2,3] Eli Lilly,[2,3] Janssen,[3] McNeil,[1,2,3] Novartis,[1,2,3] Shire.[1,2,3] Dr. Tim Wigal: Celltech,[2] Cephalon,[2] Eli Lilly,[2] McNeil,[2] Novartis,[2] Shire.[1,2] Ms. Kapelinski, Mr. Martinez, and Ms. Stehli have no conflict of interest as they have not received support from companies manufacturing medications. Dr. Swanson: ALZA,[1,2,3] Celgene,[1,2,3] Celltech,[1,2,3] Cephalon,[1,2,3] Eli Lilly,[1,2,3] Janssen,[1,2,3] McNeil,[1,2,3] Novartis,[1,2,3] Shire,[1,2,3] Targacept.[1]

REFERENCES

American Psychiatric Association: *Diagnostic and Statistical Manual for Mental Disorders.* 4th edition Washington, D.C., American Psychiatric Association, 1994.

Chan Y, Swanson J, Soldin S, Thiessen J, MacLeod S, Logan W: Methylphenidate hydrochloride given with or before breakfast: II. Effects on plasma concentration of methylphenidate and ritalinic acid. Pediatrics 72:56–59, 1983.

Coffey B, Shader RI, Greenblatt DJ: Pharmacokinetics of benzodiazepines and psychostimulants in children. J Clin Psychopharma 3:217–225, 1983.

Dahlin M, Ohman I: Age and antiepileptic drugs influence topiramate plasma levels in children. Pediatr Neurol 31:248–253, 2004.

Food and Drug Administration: Clinical Pharmacology/Biopharmaceutics Review BPCA Summary Review, 2005. Available at www.fda.gov/cder/foi/esum/2004/21121se1-008 Concerta_BPCA_pharm_biopharm.pdf/.

Ginsberg G, Hattis D, Sonawane B, Russ A, Banati P, Kozlak M, Smolenski S, Goble R: Evaluation of child/adult pharmacokinetic differences from a database derived from the therapeutic drug literature. Toxicol Sci 66:185–200, 2002.

Gonzalez M, Pentikis H, Anderl N, Benedict M, DeCory H, Dirksen S, Hatch S: Methylphenidate bioavailability from two extended release formulations. Int J Clin Pharmacol Ther 40:175–184, 2002.

Greenhill L, Kollins S, Abikoff H, McCracken J, Riddle M, Swanson J, McGough J, Wigal S, Wigal T, Vitiello B, Skrobala A, Posner K, Ghuman J, Cunningham C, Davies M, Chuang S, Cooper T: Efficacy and safety of immediate-release methylphenidate treatment for preschoolers with ADHD. J Am Acad Child Adolesc Psychiatry 45:1284–1293, 2006.

Hungund B, Perel JM, Hurwic MJ, Sverd J, Winsberg BG: Pharmacokinetics of methylphenidate in hyperkinetic children. Br J Clin Pharmacol 8:571–576, 1979.

Kollins S, Greenhill LL, Swanson J, Wigal S, Abikoff H, McCracken JT, Riddle M, McGough JJ, Vitiello B, Wigal T, Skrobala AM, Posner K, Ghuman JK, Davies M, Cunningham C, Bauzo A: Rationale, design, and methods of the preschool ADHD treatment study (PATS). J Am Acad Child Adolesc Psychiatry 45:1275–1283, 2006.

Kramer WG, Read SC, Mays DA: Effect of body weight, age, and sex on the pharmacokinetics of MAS XR in children, adolescents, and adults. Presented in poster form at the *45th Annual National Clinical Drug Evaluation Unit Meeting,* Boca Raton (Florida), 2005.

Markowitz JS, Straughn AB, Patrick KS: Advances in the pharmacotherapy of attention-deficit-hyperactivity disorder: focus on methylphenidate formulations. Pharmacotherapy 23:1281–1299, 2003.

McNeil: Concerta (methylphenidate HCl) Extended-release tablets. Mountain View, California ALZA Corporation, 2004.

National Institute of Health Consensus Development Conference: Diagnosis and Treatment of Attention

Deficit Hyperactivity Disorder: Revised Master Draft Statement. In: National Institute of Health Consensus Development Conference, 1998.

Quinn D, Wigal S, Swanson J, Hirsch S, Ottolini Y, Dariani M, Roffman M, Zeldis J, Cooper T: Comparative pharmacodynamics and plasma concentrations of *d*-threo-methylphenidate hydrochloride after single doses of d-threo-methylphenidate hydrochloride and *d,l*-threo-methylphenidate hydrochloride in a double-blind, placebo-controlled, crossover laboratory school study in children with attention-deficit/hyperactivity disorder. J Am Acad Child Adolesc Psychiatry 43:1422–1429, 2004.

Rowland M, Tozer TN: Clinical Pharmacokinetics. Concepts and Applications, 2nd edition. Philadelphia, Lea & Febiger, 1989.

Shader RI, Harmatz JS, Oesterheld JR, Parmelee DX, Sallee FR, Greenblatt DJ: Population pharmacokinetics of methylphenidate in children with attention-deficit hyperactive disorder. J Clin Pharmacol 39:775–785, 1999.

Srinivas N, Hubbard J, Korchinski E, Midha K: Stereoselective urinary pharmacokinetics of dl-threo-methylphenidate and its major metabolite in humans. J Pharm Sci 81:747–749, 1992.

Srinivas N, Hubbard J, Korchinski E, Midha K: Enantioselective pharmacokinetics of dl-threo-methylphenidate in humans. Pharm Res 10:14–21, 1993.

Swanson JM, Agler D, Fineberg E, Wigal S, Flynn D, Quintana Y, Talebi H: UCI Laboratory School Protocol for PK/PD Studies. In: Ritalin: Theory and Practice, 2nd edition. Edited by Greenhill L, Osman B. Mary Ann Liebert, Inc., 2000, pp 405–430.

Swanson JM, Gupta S, Lam A, Shoulson I, Lerner M, Modi N, Lindemulder E, Wigal S: Development of a new once-a-day formulation of methylphenidate for the treatment of attention-deficit/hyperactivity disorder: proof-of-concept and proof-of-product studies. Arch Gen Psychiatry 60:204–211, 2003.

Volkow ND: Is methylphenidate like cocaine? Studies on their pharmacokinetics and distribution in the human brain. Arch Gen Psychiatry 52:456–463, 1995.

Volkow ND, Wang G-J, Fowler JS, Logan J, Franceschi D, Maynard L, Ding Y-S, Gatley SJ, Gifford A, Zhu W, Swanson JM: Relationship between blockade of dopamine transporters by oral methylphenidate and the increases in extracellular dopamine: Therapeutic implications. Synapse 43:181–187, 2002.

Wargin W, Patrick K, Kilts C, Gualtieri CT, Ellington K, Mueller RA, Kraemer G, Breese GR: Pharmacokinetics of methylphenidate in man, rat and monkey. J Pharmacol Exp Ther 226:382–386, 1983.

Wigal SB, Wigal TL: The Laboratory School Protocol: Its origin, use and new applications. J Att Disord 10:92–111, 2006.

Zejin S, Murry D, Sanghani S, Davis W, Kedishvilli N, Zou Q, Hurley T, Bosron W: Methylphenidate is stereoselectively hydrolyzed by human carboxylesterase CES1A1. J Pharmacol Exp Therapeut 310:469–476, 2004.

PART 3

Review of Treatments for Attention-Deficit/
Hyperactivity Disorder in Preschoolers

ADVANCES IN PRESCHOOL PSYCHOPHARMACOLOGY
© 2009 Mary Ann Liebert, Inc.
140 Huguenot Street, 3rd Floor
New Rochelle, NY 10801-5215

Psychopharmacological and Other Treatments in Preschool Children with Attention-Deficit/Hyperactivity Disorder: Current Evidence and Practice

Jaswinder K. Ghuman, M.D.,[1] L. Eugene Arnold, M.D.,[2] and Bruno J. Anthony, Ph.D. [3]

ABSTRACT

Objective: This article reviews rational approaches to treating attention-deficit/hyperactivity disorder (ADHD) in preschool children, including pharmacological and nonpharmacological treatments. Implications for clinical practice are discussed.

Data Sources: We searched MEDLINE, PsychINFO, Cumulative Index to Nursing & Allied Health, Educational Resources Information Center, Cochrane Database of Systematic Reviews and Database of Abstracts of Reviews of Effects for relevant literature published in English from 1967 to 2007 on preschool ADHD. We also reviewed the references cited in identified reports.

Study Selection: Studies were reviewed if the sample included at least some children younger than 6 years of age or attending kindergarten, the study participants had a diagnosis of ADHD or equivalent symptoms, received intervention aimed at ADHD symptoms, and included a relevant outcome measure.

Data Extraction: Studies were reviewed for type of intervention and outcome relevant to ADHD and were rated for the level of evidence for adequacy of the data to inform clinical practice.

Conclusions: The current level of evidence for adequacy of empirical data to inform clinical practice for short-term treatment of ADHD in preschool children is Level A for methylphenidate and Level B for parent behavior training, child training, and additive-free elimination diet.

INTRODUCTION

ATTENTION DEFICIT/HYPERACTIVITY disorder (ADHD) frequently begins between 2 and 4 years of age (Connor 2002; Egger and Angold 2006). It is associated with significant impairment in terms of emotional distress for the preschool child and the caregivers (DuPaul et al. 2001), expulsion from daycare or early education settings (Blackman 1999), demands on

---

[1]Department of Psychiatry, University of Arizona, Tucson, Arizona.
[2]Nisonger Center, Ohio State University, Columbus, Ohio.
[3]Center for Child and Human Development, Department of Pediatrics, Georgetown University, Washington, D.C.
This paper was supported by a grant from the National Institute of Mental Health K23 MH01883 and an award from the Arizona Institute of Mental Health Research to JKG and a grant from National Institute of Mental Health K23 MH01899 to BJA.

the caregiver's time, exclusion from family events, and accident proneness and other safety concerns (Lahey et al. 2004; Rappley et al. 1999). Children with ADHD have comorbid mental health and chronic health problems and are frequent users of the healthcare system (Rappley et al. 2002). As shown by several prospective longitudinal follow up studies, behavior problems in preschool children persist to school-age years and continue to be associated with significant impairment (Campbell and Ewing 1990; Campbell et al. 2000; Egeland et al. 1990; Fischer et al. 1984; Lahey et al. 2004; Lavigne et al. 1998; McGee et al. 1991; Richman et al. 1982). In a recent study, 79.2% of the preschool children who met full diagnostic criteria for ADHD and 34.5% of the preschool children who met criteria in one situation only at initial assessment continued to meet full ADHD diagnostic criteria and exhibited global academic and social impairment three years later (Lahey et al. 2004).

Impairment from ADHD and persistence of problems at later ages underscores the need for early intervention in preschool children with ADHD (Beckwith 2000; Bierman et al. 2007; Campbell 2002; Conduct Problems Prevention Research Group 1999; Elliot et al. 2002; Petras et al. 2008; Shure et al. 2001). Recently, the Preschool Psychopharmacology Working Group (PPWG) reviewed pharmacological treatment studies in preschool children and proposed treatment algorithms for preschool psychiatric disorders (Gleason et al. 2007), however the nonpharmacological treatments for ADHD were not reviewed in detail. The primary objective of this paper is to review rational approaches to pharmacological and nonpharmacological treatment of ADHD in preschoolers and the implications for clinical practice. For the purposes of this paper, we define preschool age as prior to starting formal schooling, i.e., first grade. Hence, we reviewed studies that included children in kindergarten and/or younger than 6 years of age. The Food and Drug Administration (FDA) provides additional demarcation for children younger than 6 years. Most of the pharmacological agents for treatment of ADHD are approved by the FDA only for children older than 6 years (with the excep-

tion of amphetamines), and the FDA considers their use in children younger than 6 years as "off-label."

METHODS OF REVIEW

We searched MEDLINE, PsychINFO, Cumulative Index to Nursing & Allied Health, Educational Resources Information Center, Cochrane Database of Systematic Reviews and Database of Abstracts of Reviews of Effects for relevant literature on treatment of preschool ADHD. We also reviewed the references cited in identified reports to locate other relevant studies. Due to limited literature in this area, we reviewed both controlled and non-controlled studies. The reviewed studies met the following inclusion criteria: Published in English in the past 40 years (between 1967 to 2007); included at least some children younger than 6 years of age and/or attending kindergarten who had a diagnosis of ADHD; or exhibited behavior problems that are part of the ADHD diagnostic criteria, involved intervention aimed at ADHD symptoms, and included an outcome measure to monitor ADHD symptoms. To determine the level of evidence to inform clinical practice, we adapted the International Psychopharmacology Algorithm Project criteria (Jobson and Potter 1995) previously used by Judice and Mayes (2003) to categorize psychopharmacology treatments in preschool children. Since most of the reviewed child training studies were single case design experiments (state of current evidence for child training studies), based on the Task Force on Promotion and Dissemination of Psychological Procedures guidelines (Task Force on Psychological Intervention Guidelines 1995) previously used by Chorpita et al. (2002) to assess efficacy of psychosocial treatment studies in children and adolescents, we modified the criteria to include single case design experiments in addition to randomized controlled trials.

A treatment was considered to have evidence at Level A, if it demonstrated a significant difference on an ADHD outcome variable in a sample of preschoolers with a Diagnostic and Statistical Manual (DSM) diagnosis of ADHD in at least two randomized controlled trials (RCT) or two series of single case design experiments comparing randomly assigned active treatment to a comparison treatment or placebo. A treatment was considered to have evidence at Level B, if it demonstrated a significant difference on an ADHD outcome variable in a sample of preschoolers with a DSM diagnosis of ADHD in one RCT, two or more RCTs with mixed results, or one series of single case design experiments comparing randomly assigned active treatment to a comparison treatment or placebo. Level C was assigned to a treatment to indicate that data were based on uncontrolled trials, case reports, retrospective chart reviews, or informed clinical opinion.

TREATMENT OF PRESCHOOL ATTENTION-DEFICIT/ HYPERACTIVITY DISORDER

Here we review the current available evidence for psychopharmacological and nonpsychopharmacological interventions (psychosocial and alternative treatments) and clinical implications for preschool children with ADHD. Prior to starting any treatment, it is important to conduct a comprehensive assessment that is contextually relevant and takes into account the rapid developmental changes occurring during preschool years. Because a comprehensive discussion of the assessment process for diagnosing ADHD in preschool children is beyond the scope of this paper, the reader is referred to several excellent reviews addressing preschool nosology, diagnosis, and assessment (Angold et al. 2004; Campbell 2002; Carter et al. 2004; Egger and Angold 2006; Emde et al. 1993; Task Force on Research Diagnostic Criteria: Infancy and Preschool 2003). In general, a multi-method and multi-informant evaluation extending over multiple appointments to assess symptomatology and impairment in multiple environments and caregiving contexts is recommended (Carter et al. 2004; Gleason et al. 2007). A combination of diagnostic interviews and parent and teacher rating scales, with psychometric data in preschoolers, are commonly employed to aid in the diagnostic and assessment process. Examples of the parent and teacher rating scales

include Conners' Rating Scales-Revised (CRS-R) (Conners 2001), Swanson, Nolan and Pelham (SNAP) rating scale (Swanson 1992), Child Behavior Checklist-$1^1/_2$ (CBCL-$1^1/_2$) (Achenbach and Rescorla 2000), and ADHD Rating Scale (ADHD-RS) (DuPaul 1998; Gimpel and Kuhn 2000). The Preschool Age Psychiatric Assessment (PAPA) (Egger et al. 2006) is a reliable and valid semi-structured diagnostic parent-interview that is widely used in research studies of preschool pathology. However, clinical settings may find the cost and length of the PAPA training and administration to be a barrier for its use in routine clinical practice. Nonetheless, adequate history, mental status examination, and collateral information are important for developing an appropriate treatment plan that addresses the biopsychosocial issues specific to each family.

Psychopharmacological treatment

There are several challenges to psychopharmacological treatment of preschool children with ADHD. Preschool age is a period of continued rapid neuronal maturation including synaptic remodeling and construction. Cortical synaptic density reaches its maximum at age 3 and is substantially modified by the pruning process from ages 3 to 7 years (Huttenlocher 1990). Cerebral metabolic rate peaks between 3 and 4 years of age (Chugani 1987). Aminergic systems play an important role in neurogenesis, neuronal migration, axonal outgrowth, and synaptogenesis (Coyle 1997) and are also the targets of action for many psychopharmacological agents as indicated by studies in preclinical models. Thus, clinicians are faced with a dilemma. On one hand, whether it is prudent to recommend exposing the rapidly developing brain of a preschool child to psychopharmacological agents. On the other hand, clinicians also need to consider the consequences of an untreated disorder. Early exposure to adverse environmental circumstances and stress has been shown to result in long-lasting impact on the brain and emotional regulation of animals and humans (Graham et al. 1999; Matthews 2002; Nemeroff 2004).

Information about the use of psychopharmacological agents for treatment of ADHD is available mostly for school age children. In school age children, psychostimulants are the mainstay of treatment for ADHD; nonstimulant psychopharmacological agents are frequently recommended as a second-line treatment if a school age child's ADHD symptoms do not adequately respond to stimulants (Dulcan and Benson 1997). Recently, a nonstimulant psychopharmacological agent, atomoxetine, has been shown to be a safe and effective treatment of ADHD in school age children (Kratochvil et al. 2004; Michelson et al. 2001). Comparatively, there is limited information on the use of psychopharmacological agents for treatment of ADHD in preschool children. No pharmacokinetic and dose finding studies to identify dosage and frequency of drug administration in preschool children are available. Until recently, clinicians were left to extrapolate findings from older children to preschool children. However, medications used in older children may have specific toxicities in preschool children (Wigal et al. 2006), and there may be differences in efficacy in preschool children compared to school age children (Greenhill et al. 2006). Additionally, extrapolation to preschool children of data collected in older children is not always possible due to differences in development.

There are over 250 published studies of psychopharmacological agents in school age children with ADHD (Wilens et al. 2002). In contrast, there are a total of 24 published reports (blinded and open-label studies) on the use of psychopharmacological agents involving over 495 preschool children with ADHD. Of the 24 published reports (Tables 1 and 2), 20 published reports are on the use of stimulants, 2 published case reports on the use of α2 agonists, 1 published case report on the use of atomoxetine, and 1 published case report on the use of fluoxetine in preschool children with ADHD.

Psychostimulant studies. Of the 20 published studies on the use of stimulants in preschool children, 12 double-blind group treatment studies (one parallel groups, 10 crossover and 1 ABA design) included 417 preschool children treated with methylphenidate (MPH). Two double-blind MPH/placebo crossover studies

included both preschool and older children, but did not specify the number of preschool participants (Barkley 1988; Fischer and Newby 1991); and one blinded time series treated one preschool child with dextroamphetamine (Speltz et al. 1988). The remaining five published reports are open-label studies or case reports involving a total of 61 preschool children treated with MPH or dextroamphetamine (Alessandri and Schramm 1991; Byrne et al. 1998; Cohen et al. 1981; Ghuman et al. 2001; Stiefel and Dossetor 1998).

Twelve of the fifteen blinded MPH studies treated typically developing preschool children with ADHD; seven studies included only preschool children (Barkley 1988; Conners 1975; Firestone et al. 1998; Greenhill et al. 2006; Musten et al. 1997; Schleifer et al. 1975; Short et al. 2004; Speltz et al. 1988), while the other six studies included both preschool and older children (Barkley et al. 1988; 1985; 1984; Chacko et al. 2005; Cunningham et al. 1985; Fischer and Newby 1991). Of the other two studies, one included a mixture of inpatient or outpatient preschool and school age children with ADHD who were either typically developing or had autism or other developmental disorders (Mayes et al. 1994), and the one remaining blinded study treated preschool children with developmental disorders (Handen et al. 1999). The diagnostic procedure used most frequently included a combination of clinical interview and dimensional rating scales. With the exception of the recent PATS study, sample size was small ranging from 11–59, duration of the psychostimulant trials ranged from 3–9 weeks, and stimulant dose ranged from 0.15–0.6 mg/kg. Mixed outcomes were reported for efficacy. Based on direct observation of the preschool children's nursery school behavior, one study reported no improvement with MPH compared to placebo (Schleifer et al. 1975). Positive response to MPH was reported by other investigators in 80%–83% of typically developing preschool children (Conners 1975; Greenhill et al. 2006; Short et al. 2004) and 71%–73% of preschool children with developmental disorders (Handen et al. 1999). Data on side effect profile in preschool children was also divergent. Rates of side effects ranged from minimal or clinically negligible (Conners 1975) to 89%

TABLE 1. PUBLISHED BLINDED STUDIES OF STIMULANT TREATMENT OF ATTENTION-DEFICIT/HYPERACTIVITY DISORDER IN PRESCHOOL CHILDREN

Authors	Age Range (Mean ± SD)	N/ n < 6 years	Procedure for ADHD Diagnosis	Intervention Medication/ Dose	Study Design/ Duration	Outcome Assessment (for ADHD and disruptive behaviors)	Study Outcome	Side Effects/Safety
Conners, 1975	<6 years (57.7 ± 13.2 months)	59/59	Clinical interview, parent questionnaire	(MPH 11.8 mg/day (1.5 mg/kg/day)	Double-blind, 2 parallel groups (MPH, placebo) / 6 weeks	Parent Behavior Rating Scale, Global Clinical Improvement Rating, measures of vigilance, seat activity & impulsivity	Significant clinical improvement (93% improved on MPH, 11.5% improved on placebo) as rated by the physician on the Global Clinical Improvement Rating, significant reduction in restlessness and disruptive behavior as rated by the parents on the Parent Behavior Rating Scale. Measures of vigilance, seat activity & impulsivity did not show significant difference between MPH and placebo	Minimal side effects, trend towards elevated blood pressure in the MPH group
Schleifer et al., 1975	40–58 months (49 ± months[1])	26/26	Clinical interview	MPH 2.5–30 mg/day on a qd or bid schedule	Double-blind, crossover (placebo & MPH "optimal dose") / 4–6 weeks	Nursery school observation, Hyperactivity Rating Scale measures of reflectivity-impulsivity, field independence and motor impulsivity	Improvement based on caregiver report, no improvement on nursery school observation or psychological measures	Dysphoria, social withdrawal, poor appetite, difficulty getting to sleep
Barkely et al., 1984	48–119 months (60.8 ± 7.6 months)	54/18	Clinical interview, Conners' Rating Scale-Parent (CRS-P), WWPARS	MPH 0.15 mg/kg bid, 1.5 mg/kg bid	Double-blind, crossover (placebo & 2 MPH doses) / 3 weeks	Mother-child interaction	Significant improvement in child compliance and off-task behavior with MPH, "normalizing" effect of MPH on mother-child interactions	More frequent side effects on high MPH dose than low dose or placebo
Barkley et al., 1985	5–9 years (89 months[1])	60/12	Psychiatric assessment, CRS-P, Werry Weiss Peters Activity Rating Scale (WWPARS), Home Situations Questionnaire (HSQ)	MPH 0.3 mg/kg bid. 0.7 mg/kg bid	Double-blind, crossover (placebo & 2 MPH doses) / 4 weeks	Mother-child interaction during free play and task periods	Child compliance and length of sustained compliance improved with the higher dose during the task period, drug effects did not differ during free play or across age levels	Greater number of side effects on MPH compared to placebo

(continued)

Authors	Age Range (Mean ± SD)	N/ n < 6 years	Procedure for ADHD Diagnosis	Intervention Medication/ Dose	Study Design/ Duration	Outcome Assessment (for ADHD and disruptive behaviors)	Study Outcome	Side Effects/Safety
Cunningham et al., 1985	4–6 years (68 months[1])	42/**12**	Clinical diagnosis CRS-P	Single dose of MPH 0.15 mg/kg, 0.50 mg/kg	Double-blind, crossover (placebo & 2 MPH doses)/ 4 sessions	Videotaped observations during freeplay, co-operative task, and simulated school setting	↓ actometer readings & ↑ on-task behavior during the simulated school setting, linear dose response, optimal ↓ in controlling and domineering interactions observed at 0.15 mg/kg dose with no incremental benefit on 0.50 mg/kg dose	Side effects were not monitored
Barkley, 1988	31–59 months (46.8 ± 6.7 months)	27/**27**	Clinical interview, CRS-P, WWPARS, HSQ	MPH 0.15 mg/kg bid, 1.5 mg/kg bid	Triple-blind, crossover (placebo & 2 MPH doses)/ 3 weeks	Mother-child interaction	↑ rates of compliance and length of sustained compliance with maternal commands, and on task behavior on higher dose during the task period	Trend for more frequent side effects on MPH compared to placebo
Barkley, at al, 1988	5–12 years (8.5 ± 2.3 years)	23/**not specified**	Semistructured parent interview, CRS-P or CRS-Teacher (CRS-T)	MPH 0.3 mg/kg bid, 0.5 mg/kg bid	Double-blind, crossover (placebo & 2 MPH doses)/ 3 weeks	Gordon Diagnostic System (GDS) for vigilance and impulse control, playroom observation during a restricted academic situation, CRS-P, CRS-T, HSQ, School Situations Questionnaire (SSQ)	80% of the children responded positively to MPH on parent and teacher ratings of hyperactivity and disruptive behaviors, and ↓ off-task and hyperactivity ratings during playroom observation (restricted academic situation). Significant main drug effects for 16 of the 31 outcome measures, mostly on teacher ratings and observations during the restricted academic situation, both doses were equally effective	No difference in the number or severity of side effects. Two children discontinued the study due to development of tics in response to the medication and were excluded from the study analysis
Speltz et al., 1988[2]	51 months	1/**1**	Clinical interview, CRS-T	Dextroamphetamine (DEX) 2.5 mg bid DEX 5 mg bid and Day Program	Double-blind time series (placebo & 2 DEX doses in counterbalanced order)/ 11 weeks	Daily observations of 15-minute work periods and 20-minute free play for frequency of on-task behavior, and teacher ratings of aggressive and disruptive behaviors and reports of side effects	↓ off-task and aggressive behavior on DEX compared to placebo. Behavior gains maintained at follow up 2 years later	↑ whining, listlessness, solitary play, stomachache ↓ appetite, more frequent during 5 mg bid dose

Study	Age	N (treated/placebo)	Assessment	Medication/Dose	Design	Outcome measures	Results	Side effects
Fischer & Newby, 1991	2–17 years (8.9 ± 2.9 years)	161/**not specified**	Semistructured parent interview, CRS-P, CRS-T, Child Behavior Checklist (CBCL), Teacher Rating Form (TRF)	MPH 0.2 mg/kg & 0.4 mg/kg BID	Double-blind crossover (placebo & 2 MPH doses) / 3 weeks	CRS-P, CRS-T, HSQ SSQ, reaction time, GDS viligance task	Significant positive medication response on parent and teacher ratings of hyperactivity and laboratory measures of viligance and off-task behaviors, higher dose was most effective	No side effects reported
Mayes et al., 1994[3]	2–13 years (7.1 years[1])	69/14	Clinical interview	MPH 7.5–30 mg/day on a tid schedule	Double-blind, ABA (placebo & MPH "optimal dose")/3 weeks	Conners' 10-item ADHD Parent Rating Scale	79.4% improved on MPH based parent ratings on the Conners' scale	50.7% experienced side effects irritability, ↓ appetite, lethargy
Musten et al., 1997; Firestone et al., 1998	48–70 months (58.1 ± 8.2 months)	31/31	Diagnostic Interview for Children and Adults-Parents (DICA-P), Swanson, Nolan and Pelham checklist (SNAP), CRS-P, attention task	MPH 0.3 mg/kg bid, 0.5 mg/kg bid	Double-blind, crossover (placebo & 2 MPH doses) / 3 weeks	Parent-child interaction tasks, CRS-P, GDS Delay and Vigilance Tasks	↑ attention and on-task during laboratory observation, ↓ impulsivity and hyperactivity as rated by parents on the CRS-P, no improved in compliance to parent requests	10% experienced severe side effects: social withdrawal, sadness. ↑ number & ↑ severity of side effects with the higher dose
Handen et al., 1999[4]	48–71 months (58.9 ± 8.2 months)	11/11	Clinical interview, Preschool Behavior Questionaire (PBQ), CRS-P	MPH 0.3 mg/kg/dose & 0.6 mg/kg/dose qd to tid	Double-blind, crossover (placebo & 2 MPH doses) / 3 weeks	CRS-T, PBQ, direct behavior observation	72.7% improved on MPH based on at-least 40% reduction in teacher ratings of hyperactivity and inattention, significant improvement on clinic-based observations of activity level and compliance, more improvement on the higher dose	45% experienced side effects (social withdrawal and irritability); side effects more frequent at the higher dose
Short et al., 2004	<6 years (63 months[1])	28/28	Diagnostic Interview Schedule for Children-Parent (DISC-P) or clinical interview, Conners' Abbreviated Symptoms Questionnaire (CASQ), ADHD Rating Scale (ADHD-RS)	MPH 5 mg, 10 mg, 15 mg bid or mixed amphetamine salts (MAS; Adderal) 5 mg, 10 mg & 15 mg qd	Double-blind, crossover (placebo & 2 or 3 MPH or MAS doses) / 3–4 weeks	ASQ, ADHD-RS, HSQ	Improved parent and teacher ratings of ADHD on either stimulant by at least 1 SD in 82% of the children and by 2 SD in 50% of the children. Clinical ratings of normalized behavior on best dose in 82% of the children	↓ appetite, crying & rebound effects

(continued)

TABLE 1. Published Blinded Studies of Stimulant Treatment of Attention-Deficit/Hyperactivity Disorder in Preschool Children (Cont'd)

Authors	Age Range (Mean ± SD)	N/ n < 6 years	Procedure for ADHD Diagnosis	Intervention Medication/ Dose	Study Design/ Duration	Outcome Assessment (for ADHD and disruptive behaviors)	Study Outcome	Side Effects/Safety
Chacko et al., 2005	5–6 years (6.1 ± 0.57 months)	36/14	Structured parent interview, parent and teacher Disruptive Behavior Disorder rating scales	MPH 0.3 mg/kg & 0.6 mg/kg bid and Behavior Modification System in a Summer Treatment Program	Double-blind, crossover (placebo & 2 MPH doses)/ 8 weeks	Point system, classroom rules, productivity and accuracy of class work	Improved classroom behavior for following rules and non-compliance and class work completion on both MPH doses compared to placebo, little incremental improvement in classroom measures on the higher MPH dose compared to the lower MPH dose. 28% children improved with classroom behavioral intervention & showed no incremental benefit of MPH	↓ appetite
Greenhill et al., 2006	3–5.5 years (53 ± 8 months)	165/165	Clinical assessment for DSM-IV diagnosis of ADHD, unanimous consensus by the panel of investigators, CRS-P, CRS-T	MPH 1.25 mg, 2.5 mg, 5.0 mg, 7.5 mg tid	Double-blind, crossover (placebo & 4 MPH doses) after 10 weeks of parent training/ 5 weeks	Swanson, Kotkin, Atkins, M-Flynn, and Pelham (SKAMP), Conners, Loney and Milch (CLAM) rating scales	Significant ↓ in parent- and teacher-rated ADHD symptoms on the 3 higher doses	↓ appetite stomachache, and sleep difficulties, ↑ rates of social withdrawal and lethargy, ↓ growth velocity, 8.3% discontinued due to MPH side effects

[1]SD not provided.
[2]Individualized weekly parent training sessions, classroom behavior management program and social skills training group were also administered concurrently.
[3]Included inpatient or outpatient preschool and school age children with autism, other developmental disorders or no developmental disorders.
[4]Included preschool children with mental retardation.
ADHD = attention-deficit/hyperactivity disorder; MPH = methylphenidate.

TABLE 2. PUBLISHED OPEN-LABEL STUDIES OF STIMULANT TREATMENT OF ATTENTION-DEFICIT/HYPERACTIVITY DISORDER IN PRESCHOOL CHILDREN

Authors	Age Range (Mean ± SD)	N/n < 6 years	Diagnostic Procedure for Eligibility	Medication/ Dose	Study Design/ Duration	Outcome Assessment (for ADHD and disruptive behaviors)	Study Outcome	Side Effects/Safety
Cohen et al., 1981	Kindergarten aged[1]	24/24	Clinical interview, CRS-T	MPH 10–30 mg/day	Three randomized parallel groups (MPH, Cognitive Behavior Management [CBM], and CBM + MPH), open-label treatment/ 10 weeks	Cognitive and motor impulsivity tasks, parent and teacher behavior rating scales, classroom observation	No treatment effect in any of the groups	4 of the 14 (29%) children on MPH stopped medication due to side effects and were reassigned to either CBT or no treatment
Alessandri & Scharmm, 1991	50 months	1/1	Clinical interview, CPRS	DEX 2.5 mg bid	Open-label A-B-A-B reversal design/ 16 weeks	Blinded ratings of off-task behavior, level of cognitive play and social participation during structured activity and unstructured play; teacher rated PBQ, CTRS	↓ off-task behavior, ↑ attention, ↑ developmentally appropriate goal-directed, organized and symbolic play, & improved social functioning on direct observation ratings of behavior during structured activity and unstructured play	↑ solitary & parallel play
Byrne et al., 1998	62 months[1]	8/8	Clinical interview, Continuous Performance Test for Preschoolers— Visual (CPTP-V), CPT-Auditory (A), CRS-P, CBCL	MPH 15–20 mg/day or DEX 7.5–15 mg/day on qd-tid schedule	Open-label/ 5 months	CPTP-V, CPT-A, CRS-P, CBCL	↑ attention & social relations, ↓ problem behaviors	No information
Stiefel & Dossetor, 1998	5 years	1/1	Clinical interview	DEX 5 mg bid	Open-label/ 4 years	Clinical assessment	Improved behavior	Initial problem with reduced appetite and getting to sleep ameliorated with time
Ghuman et al., 2001	40–70 months (56.4 ± (9.6 months)	27/27	Clinical interview	MPH 0.55 mg/kg/day or DEX 0.43 mg/kg qd-qid	Chart review/ 24 months	Clinical Global Impression-Severity (CGI-S) and CGI-Improvement	74% experienced improvement at 3 months and 70% at 12 and 24 months	63% experienced side effects; poor appetite, stomachache, irritability, dysphoria, sleep disturbance, headache, dull/tired; 11% stopped stimulants due to side effects

[1]Mean age not provided.
MPH = methylphenidate; DEX = dextroamphetamine.

in typically developing preschool children (Schleifer et al. 1975) and 45%–50% in preschool children with developmental disorders (Handen et al. 1999; Mayes et al. 1994). Dysphoria, crying, whining, irritability, and solitary play were more frequently reported in preschool children than seen in older children.

The 6-site PATS study randomized 165 preschool children (3–5.5 years) diagnosed with ADHD in a placebo-controlled, double-blind crossover design, to one week each of 4 MPH doses (1.25 mg, 2.5 mg, 5 mg and 7.5 mg TID) and placebo. With the exception of the lowest MPH dose, improvements in parent- and teacher-rated ADHD symptoms were reported with MPH compared to placebo; the 7.5 mg TID dose was found to be the most effective. The effect sizes (Cohen's d) in the intent-to-treat sample ranged from 0.4–0.8 and were smaller than those reported for school age children treated with MPH (Greenhill et al. 2006). Interestingly, secondary analyses of the PATS efficacy data showed that preschoolers with ADHD with no or one comorbid disorder (primarily oppositional defiant disorder [ODD]) had treatment responses (Cohen's d = 0.89 and 1.00, respectively) at the same level as found in school age children (Ghuman et al. 2007). Preschoolers with 2 comorbid disorders had moderate treatment response (Cohen's d = 0.56) and preschoolers with 3 or more comorbid disorders did not respond to MPH (Ghuman et al. 2007). However, caution is needed in the generalization of the findings as there were only 15 preschoolers (9% of the sample) with 3 or more comorbid disorders compared to 150 preschoolers with two comorbid disorders (n = 34, 21% of the sample), one comorbid disorder (n = 69, 42% of the sample) or no comorbid disorders (n = 47, 28% of the sample). In addition to decreased appetite, stomach ache, and sleep difficulties usually seen in school age children, increased rates of social withdrawal and lethargy were reported especially at higher doses. A higher discontinuation rate (8.3%) due to MPH side effects was reported in the PATS study than the 0.5% discontinuation rate in the National Institute of Mental Health (NIMH) Multimodal Treatment of ADHD (MTA) study with school-age ADHD children (Wigal et al. 2006). Compared with the

Center for Disease Control (CDC) norms, the preschool children with ADHD in the PATS were 2.0 cm taller and 1.8 kg heavier at baseline. A 20% less than expected annual height gain (−1.38 cm/year) and 55% less than expected annual weight gain (−1.32 kg/year) was reported for the children who continued MPH for a year in the open-label follow up phase (Swanson et al. 2006). Decrease in weight velocity was evident at the end of the 5-week double-blind crossover phase. Most preschoolers with ADHD were able to maintain improvement over 10 months of open-label follow up treatment (Vitiello et al. 2007).

Two of the open-label stimulant studies were prospective open-label treatment trials, two were case reports, and one was a retrospective chart review. Positive response to stimulants (MPH or dextroamphetamine) was reported in four of the open-label studies; one prospective treatment trial reported no treatment effect and reported a 30% discontinuation rate due to MPH adverse effects (Cohen et al. 1981).

Non-stimulant studies. The two published case reports of open-label treatment with α2 agonists in 5 preschool children with ADHD reported improvement in hyperactive and impulsive behavior (Cesena et al. 1995; Lee 1997), one published case report of open-label treatment with atomoxetine in 10 preschool children reported improvement in hyperactive, impulsive and inattentive symptoms (Kratochvil et al. 2007), and one published case report of open-label treatment with fluoxetine in one preschool child with ADHD reported improvement in attention span (Campbell et al. 1995) (Table 3).

Prescribing patterns. Despite controversy and scarcity of empirical information regarding dose guidelines, safety, and efficacy, psychopharmacological agents are being prescribed to preschool children.

This is a serious public health concern and was identified as a research priority by the Surgeon General (National Institutes of Health 2000; US Public Health Service 2000) and the White House (Pear 2000).

In 1994, 226,000 MPH prescriptions were written for children under 6 years of age (US

TABLE 3. PUBLISHED REPORTS OF NON-STIMULANT TREATMENT OF ATTENTION-DEFICIT/HYPERACTIVITY DISORDER IN PRESCHOOL CHILDREN

Authors	Age Range (Mean ± SD)	N/n < 6 years	Diagnostic Procedure for Eligibility	Medication/ Dose	Study Design/ Duration	Outcome Assessment (for ADHD and disruptive behavior)	Study Outcome	Side Effects/Safety
Campbell et al., 1995	3 years	1/1	Clinical interview	Fluoxetine 10 mg qd	Open-label/ 6 weeks	Clinical assessment	Improved attention even-tempered, ↓ aggression	No significant side effects
Cesena et al., 1995[1]	56 months (4.8 years)	1/1	Clinical interview	Clonidine 0.025 mg tid	Open-label/ 5 months	ASQ, CGI-ADHD	Normalization of hyperactivity & attention on teacher ASQ, improved sleep	Sedation early in treatment, was resolved later in the course of treatment
Lee, 1997	31–42 months	4/4	Clinical interview, CBCL/2-3, CPRS	Guanfacine 0.25 mg bid-1.25 mg/day	Open-label/ 2–6 months	Clinical assessment	↓ impulsive hyperactive and aggressive behavior, ↓ tantrums, improved mother-child relations	Sedation and transient benign chest pain
Kratochvil et al., 2007	5–6 years (6.1 ± 0.58 years)	22/10	DISC-4, clinical interview, ADHD Rating Scale (ADHD-RS)	Atomoxetine 10–45 mg/day qd or bid	Open-label/ 8 weeks	ADHD-RS, CGI	Improved ADHD-RS scores and CGI	Mood lability, reduced appetite, weight loss (mean = 1.04 ± 0.8 kg)

[1]Child's ADHD symptoms were seen as manifestation of HIV encephalopathy.
ADHD = attention-deficit/hyperactivity disorder.

Food and Drug Administration 1997). A three-fold increase in MPH use in 2–4 year old children was reported from 1991–1995 (Zito et al. 2000); Marshall (2000) reported that 150,000 to 200,000 children between the ages of 2 and 4 years were estimated to be taking MPH. Out-patient prescription data from 7 state Medicaid programs revealed 67.3% stimulant and 26% α-agonist use in 2001 in 2–4 year old children treated with psychotropic agents (Zito et al. 2007).

Pre-school children with ADHD symptoms are more often treated with stimulants in the community than with any other drug. Those not treated with stimulants, are often given other psychotropic medications, including those that have not been shown to have any efficacy in ADHD, such as selective serotonin reuptake inhibitors (SSRIs) (Rappley et al. 2002) and those with some efficacy for ADHD but leading to severe long-term adverse events (e.g., tardive dyskinesia), such as neuroleptics (Minde 1998; Rappley et al. 2002). Health Maintenance Organization (HMO) and Medicaid database surveys in 1995 showed frequent use of psychotropic medications in preschool children diagnosed with ADHD. Frequency of psychotropic drug prescription in 1–3 year old children diagnosed with ADHD (N = 223) in the Michigan Medicaid system was 57% (n =127) compared to 26% (n = 47) for psychosocial intervention (Rappley et al. 1999). Psychotropic medications alone as a sole intervention strategy were utilized in 40% children (n = 89); comparatively psychosocial intervention as a sole treatment was utilized in only 9% (n = 21). Stimulants were prescribed for 93.7%, α2 agonists for 44.9%, tricyclic antidepressants for 33.1%, neuroleptics for 15.7%, and SSRIs for 11% of the preschool children receiving psychotropic medications. More than half of the children received treatment for longer than 6 months. Medication monitoring was inadequate—for 75 children (59%) follow-up visits occurred every 3 months and for 25 children (19%) at intervals greater than 6 months (Rappley et al. 2002).

Summary of psychopharmacological treatments. There is evidence for short-term efficacy and long-term effectiveness and tolerability of psy-

chostimulants, especially MPH, in preschool children with ADHD. Response is reported to be less robust and response rate is reported to be lower in preschool children with ADHD compared to older children. Preschool children with ADHD are sensitive to developing more side effects especially at higher doses and have unique adverse effect profile including more irritability and mood changes. This sensitivity to stimulant adverse effects may be a limiting factor in achieving an adequate and/or robust response in preschool children with ADHD. Only open-label information is available regarding effectiveness and tolerability of one non-stimulant, atomoxetine, in preschool children with ADHD. Additionally, pharmacological interventions may be effective in reducing core ADHD symptoms such as impulsivity, overactivity, and inattention among preschool children with ADHD (Greenhill et al. 2006); however, there is little evidence to suggest that psychostimulants improve long-term interpersonal relationships known to be important in predicting outcomes for children displaying disruptive behaviors (Coie and Dodge 1998; Pelham et al. 1998; Rubin et al. 2006). Moreover, no information is available about long-term safety and effects of psychopharmacological agents on brain development in preschool children.

Psychosocial treatments

Concerns about the short- and long-term safety of psychopharmacological agents especially on the developing brain of preschool children, coupled with ethical, societal, and political beliefs about manipulating behavior through medication and perceived overprescription (Jensen et al. 1999) often lead families and providers to favor other interventions for preschoolers (Dulcan and Benson 1997). In this section, we will review current evidence for success of psychosocial treatments in preschool children with ADHD.

There is evidence from studies in school-age children that long-term behavioral improvements may require psychosocial interventions (Ialongo et al. 1993). Inhibitory processes play a critical role in impaired functioning in children with ADHD (Barkley 1997; Barkley 1998;

Barkley 2003; Nigg 2001; Nigg 2003; Quay 1997) and these, although rudimentary, are developing rapidly during the preschool period (Davidson et al. 2006; Diamond and Taylor 1996; Espy et al. 1999; Garon et al. 2008; Jones et al. 2003; Rueda et al. 2005). Psychosocial interventions targeting key executive functions, especially inhibitory processes, may be particularly helpful (Diamond et al. 2007; Dowsett and Livesey 2000).

Limited psychosocial intervention research has been conducted with preschool samples of children formally diagnosed with ADHD (Bryant et al. 1999; McGoey et al. 2002); however, there is considerable evidence that parent, child, and parent-child interventions can reduce problem behaviors in young children displaying a range of disruptive behaviors, including excessive hyperactivity and inattention as reviewed in the following section. We have grouped the psychosocial intervention studies into those that train parents in behavioral techniques and use the parents as the primary agent of change, and those that train children in a classroom setting to reduce problematic behaviors.

Parent training. Among psychosocial interventions, parent training to help parents learn and implement behavioral treatment has the strongest evidence base showing positive effects for school age children with ADHD (Chorpita and Daleiden 2002). For preschool children with ADHD, parent training in behavior management is an especially helpful and the most appropriate psychosocial intervention (Stanley and Stanley 2005; Webster-Stratton et al. 2001). When children are young, parents have an enormous impact on their child's behavior (Capage et al. 1998; Eyberg et al. 1995; Funderburk et al. 1998; Hembree-Kigin and McNeil 1995) creating a window of opportunity to teach parents how to be positive and consistent in their parenting responses, help reduce noncompliant and aggressive behaviors, and help their child persist at a difficult task and provide successful experiences for their child, thus reducing risk for continued problems in later years. Parent behavior training programs for preschool children have been modeled after efficacious programs developed with older chil-

dren (Anastopoulos et al. 1993; Dishion and McMahon 1998), and draw upon both social-learning and attachment theories to varying extent. Parent training programs may include sessions with parents, parent-child dyad, or a combination of parent sessions and work with the parent-child dyad to improve parent-child relationship, and increase the child's prosocial behaviors and decrease negative behaviors.

There are 15 published reports of parent behavior training treatment trials (either controlled, case series or case reports) that monitored outcomes in ADHD symptoms in preschool children with a DSM diagnosis of ADHD or preschool children displaying ADHD symptoms (Tables 4 and 5). However, there was a wide variation in the study design, type of control groups, inclusion criteria, diagnostic measures, type of psychosocial intervention, method of intervention delivery, and outcome measures employed in the studies. Nine studies used a randomized parallel groups design with control groups ranging from wait-list, community treatment, combination treatment to minimal treatment (Barkley et al. 2000; Bor et al. 2002; Corrin 2004; Jones et al. 2007; McGoey et al. 2005; Pisterman et al. 1992; 1989; Sonuga-Barke et al. 2001; Strayhorn and Weidman 1989; Strayhorn and Weidman 1991) and six studies did not employ any control group (Chang et al. 2004; Danforth 1999; Drash et al. 1976; Erhardt and Baker 1990; Henry 1987; Huang et al. 2003). Eight of the nine controlled studies included only preschool children and four of these eight studies selected the preschoolers based on a DSM diagnosis of ADHD through clinical or structured parent interview (Bor et al. 2002; Pisterman et al. 1992; 1989; Sonuga-Barke et al. 2001), and the other four selected preschoolers based on a rating scale cutoff. The ninth controlled study included both preschool-age and school-age children with a DSM diagnosis of ADHD. Sample sizes ranged from 20-50 per group. Most studies employed group-training sessions except for three studies that employed individual training sessions with the parents (Bor et al. 2002; Henry 1987; Sonuga-Barke et al. 2001). Training was conducted over 8–12 sessions, each parent training session lasting 1–3 hours. Most studies included both teaching/modeling sessions with

TABLE 4. PUBLISHED CONTROLLED STUDIES OF PSYCHOSOCIAL TREATMENTS IN PRESCHOOL CHILDREN WITH ATTENTION DEFICIT HYPERACTIVITY DISORDER: PARENT TRAINING

Authors	Age range in years (Mean age ± SD)	N/n < 6 years	Procedure for ADHD Diagnosis; Inclusion Criteria	Psychosocial intervention	Study Design/ Duration	Outcome Assessment (for ADHD and disruptive behaviors)	Study Outcome
Strayhorn & Weidman, 1989; 1991	2–5 (3.9[1])	96/96	No clinical assessment, parent questionnaire based on DSM III-R diagnostic criteria; At-risk for behavior problems (complaints of ADHD, disruptive behaviors or emotional difficulties, low socioeconomic status), 40% parents endorsed ≥ 8 of 14 ADHD symptoms	Group parent training and individual sessions work with the parent-child dyad	Two randomized parallel groups: parent behavior training (PBT) or minimal treatment control group, open-label treatment/ 12 sessions	Parent and teacher ratings on ADHD, compliance, and internalizing symptoms on the Behar Preschool Behavior Questionnaire; direct observation of parent and child behaviors, parenting practices	Improvement in the PBT group in parent-rated ADHD and internalizing symptoms, and child and parent behaviors on direct observation. No improvement in teacher ratings, or verbal ability measures. Improved parent behavior correlated positively with improved child behavior Improvement in teacher-rated classroom behavior at 1 year follow-up
Pisterman et al., 1989	3–6 (4.15 ±0.78)	50/50	Structured screening interview, >1 SD on the Conners' Hyperactivity Index; DSM-III criteria for ADDH	Group parent training and 2 individual sessions with the parent-child dyad	Two randomized parallel groups: immediate treatment or delayed treatment group, open-label treatment/ 12 weeks	Parent ratings on the Conners' Hyperactivity Index, direct behavioral assessment of child attention, child compliance and parental style of interaction	No treatment effect on child attention or parent-rated Conners' Hyperactivity Index. Improvement in the immediate treatment group in child compliance; improved parental style of interaction. Outcome reported only for 46 of the 50 randomized children; four children (8%) dropped out after group assignment. Five children received methylphenidate during the study. Improvement maintained at 3 month follow up

Study	Age (mean ± SD)	N	Diagnosis	Treatment design	Outcome measures	Results
Pisterman et al., 1992	3–6 (3.9 ± 0.62)	57/**57**	Semi-structured screening interview, cutoff threshold for parent or teacher Swanson, Nolan and Pelham (SNAP) rating scale and Conners' Hyperactivity Index; DSM-II criteria for ADDH	Group parent training and 2 individual sessions with the parent-child dyad	Two randomized parallel groups: immediate treatment or delayed treatment group, open-label treatment/ 12 weeks	Direct behavioral assessment of child attention, child compliance and parental style of interaction	No treatment effect on child attention on direct observation Improvement in child compliance and parental style of interaction in the immediate treatment group. Outcome reported only for 45 of the 57 randomized children; 12 children (21%) dropped out after group assignment with a higher drop-out rate for less educated parents. Four children received stimulants during the study. Improvement maintained at 3 month follow up
Barkley et al., 2000; Shelton et al., 2000	4.5–6 (48 ± 0.5)	158/ **158**	Diagnostic Interview Schedule for Children-Parent (DISC-P), Conners' rating Scale-Parent (CRS-P); Cutoff dimensional threshold for Hyperactive, Oppositional &/or Conduct Problem factors on CRS-P, no clinical diagnosis of ADHD required for inclusion, 66% children met ADHD criteria on the DISC-P	10 weekly group parent training sessions followed by 6 monthly booster sessions, special treatment classroom	Four randomized parallel groups; Parent Training (PT) Special Treatment Classroom (STC), combined (PT and STC) or no treatment control groups, open-label treatment/ 9 months (school year)	DISC-P, parent and teacher ratings of child behavior on Child Behavior Checklist (CBCL), Home Situations Questionnaire (HSQ), School Situations Questionnaire (SSQ), Self-Control Rating Scale (SCRS); Continuous Performance Test (CPT); parent self-report on parenting practices and competence; clinic observation for disruptive behavior and parent-child interaction; and classroom observation	No improvement and poor attendance in the PT group. STC produced improvement in parent ratings of adaptive behavior, teacher ratings of social skills, attention and aggression; and classroom observation ratings of externalizing behavior. No improvement in academic achievement or parent ratings of home behavior; and no improvement in laboratory measures of attention, impulse control or parent-child interaction in any of the treatment groups. No difference in the groups at 2 year follow-up

(continued)

Authors	Age range in years (Mean age ± SD)	N/n < 6 years	Procedure for ADHD Diagnosis; Inclusion Criteria	Psychosocial intervention	Study Design/ Duration	Outcome Assessment (for ADHD and disruptive behaviors)	Study Outcome
Sonuga-Barke et al., 2001	3²	78/78	Structured clinical interview (Parental Account of Childhood Symptoms (PACS), Werry-Weiss-Peters Activity Scale (WWPAS); Cutoff threshold for the ADHD Hyperkinesis scale of the PACS and cutoff threshold on the WWPAS	Eight 1-hour weekly in-home individual parent training sessions and work control with the mother-child dyad	Three randomized parallel groups: parent training (PT), parent counseling and support (PC&S) or waiting-list (WLC) groups, open-label treatment/ 8 weeks	Clinician ratings of ADHD based on parent interview using the PACS; play observation for attention/parent self-engagement: Parenting report on the Satisfaction and Parenting Efficacy scales of the Parental Sense of Competence (PSOC) scale	PT more effective than PC&S and WLC in improving ADHD symptoms both on parent interview and play observation, and improvement in mothers' sense of well-being Improvement maintained at 23 weeks
Bor et al., 2002	3–4 (3.42 ± 0.31)	87/87	Structured diagnostic interview, Eyberg Child Behavior Inventory (ECBI); DSM IV diagnosis of ADHD, >90th percentile on the Inattentive Behavior subscale of the ECBI and at least 1 family adversity factor	Ten 60–90-minute individual sessions (7 parent training sessions and 3 parent-child sessions) for the Standard and 12 for the Enhanced Behavior Family Intervention (SBFI and EBFI)	Three randomized parallel groups: SBFI, EBFI, waitlist (WL) control group. open-label treatment/ 15–17 weeks	Parent ratings on the ECBI, Parent Daily Report (PDR), Parenting Sense of Competency (PSOC) scale, Parenting Scale (PS), Parent Problem Checklist (PPC), observation of mother-child behavior	No treatment effect on parent-rated inattentive behavior. Improvement in parent-reported child behavior problems, dysfunctional parenting, and parental competence with both SBFI and EBFI; significantly less observed child negative behavior with EBFI; no difference in SBFI and EBFI conditions. Outcome reported only for 63 of the 87 randomized children; 24 children did not complete intervention and post-assessment. Gains maintained at 1-year follow-up
Corrin, 2004	4.5–8.5 (6.6 ± 1.25)	55/9	Structured parent interview, CRS-P; DSM diagnosis of ADHD	Ten weekly group child and parent training sessions	Two randomized parallel groups: child group training or combined parent and child training, open-label treatment/ 10 weekly sessions	CBCL, CRS-P, HSQ	Improvement in CRS-P Hyperactivity scale in both treatment groups, 17 children were on stimulant medication

Study	Age[2]	N	Diagnostic criteria	Intervention	Study design	Measures	Outcomes
McCoey et al., 2005	3–5 (4.04 ± 0.72)	57/57	Semi-structured parent interview for DSM-IV criteria for ADHD, and cutoff threshold for parent and teacher Hyperactivity or Inattention subscale of the CRS; at-risk for ADHD	Multi-component intervention including 12 weekly group parent training sessions & 9 monthly booster sessions, preschool consultation, and medication consultation as needed	Two randomized parallel groups: Early Intervention (EI) or a Community Treatment Control (CTC) group, open-label treatment/ 12 months	Preschool and Kindergarten Behavior Scales (PKBS), direct observation of classroom behavior and parent-child interaction, Medical Outcomes and Service Utilization, Consumer knowledge ratings	No treatment effect reported on parent- and teacher-rated Attention problems/Overactivity subscale of the PKBS, improvement in on-task performance, compliance, self-control, and social skills; increased positive parenting behaviors, reductions in negative parent behavior, and positive changes in family coping were seen in both groups. Outcome reported for completers (21 out of the 30 children (70%) randomized to EI) only. Four children were prescribed stimulants or clonidine.
Jones et al., 2007; 2008	3–4 (3.86 ± 0.51)	79/79	No clinical assessment, cutoff threshold for parent Hyperactivity subscale of the Strengths and Difficulties Questionnaire (SDQ); cutoff threshold for parent problem or intensity subscale of the ECBI and Hyperactivity subscale of the SDQ	Twelve 2.5 hour-weekly Incredible Years Basic Parent Training (IY-BPT) group sessions and weekly telephone calls	Two randomized parallel groups: IY-BPT or waitlist (WL) control group, open-label treatment/ 12 weeks	Parent ratings on the Conners' Abbreviated Parent Rating Scale (CAPRS), and Child Deviance (negative and destructive behavior and non-compliance) subscale score of the Dyadic Parent-Child Interaction Coding System (DPICS) based on observation of mother-child behavior	Parents reported greater reduction on the CAPRS scores in the IY-BPT group compared to the WL group, and improvement was significant even after controlling for co-occurring conduct problems as measured by the Child Deviance subscale scores of the DPICS

Gains maintained at 6 months, 12 months and 18 months post-intervention. |

[1]SD not provided.
[2]Mean age not provided.
ADHD = attention-deficity/hyperactivity disorder.

TABLE 5. PUBLISHED NON-CONTROLLED STUDIES OF PSYCHOSOCIAL TREATMENTS IN PRESCHOOL CHILDREN WITH ATTENTION DEFICIT HYPERACTIVITY DISORDER: PARENT TRAINING

Authors	Age range in years Mean age ± SD)	N/n < 6 years	Procedure for ADHD Diagnosis & Inclusion Criteria	Psychosocial intervention	Study Design/ Duration	Outcome Assessment (for ADHD and disruptive behaviors)	Study Outcome
Drash et al., 1976	2–4.8 (2.8[1])	5/5	Clinical diagnosis of ADHD	Weekly 3-hour parent classes (two mother-child pairs also received direct training), child group training in a classroom setting	Case series, prospective, no control group. open-label treatment/ 9 months	Parent-rated Behar Preschool Behavior Questionnaire (BPBQ), direct behavior observation during group classroom situation and a standardized task completion activity	Parent-rated BPBQ Hyperactivity and Distractibility subscale scores, decreased from 90th percentile to 52nd percentile, high rates of compliance rates across settings Two children received psychotropic medication
Henry, 1987	4.5–10.5 (7.3[1])	6/n < 6 years not spec- ified	DSM-III diagnosis of ADHD by a psychiatrist and a psychologist, stabilized on psychostintulant medication	Four 20-minute symbolic modeling sessions with the child followed by six 60-minute combined symbolic modeling and parent training sessions administered	Case study, prospective, no control group, open-label treatment/ 10 weeks	Parent Conners' Symptom Questionnaire, observation of child compliance to parental task during a structured task	3/5 children improved on the parent ratings of the Conners' Symptom Questionnaire. A combination of medication, symbolic modeling and parent training was more effective than a combination of medication and symbolic modeling or medication alone in reducing noncompliance. Parent training for time-out procedure was most effective. Combined symbolic modeling and medication was not any more effective than medication alone. Gains maintained at 6 months
Erhardt and Baker, 1990	5.2–5.8	2/2	Diagnosed as being hyperactive by the pediatrician. parent score of >15 on the Abbreviated Symptom Questionnaire (CASQ)	Six 2-hour group parent training and four 1-hour individual consultation and parent-child interactive sessions	Case study, prospective, no control group, open-label treatment/ 10 sessions	Parent ratings on the CASQ, Iowa Conners' Rating Scale. Werry-Weiss-Peters Activity Scale (WWPAS), Child Behavior Checklist (CBCL)	Improved parental ratings of hyperactivity, tantrums, aggression, compliance and social functioning

Study	Age	N	Diagnosis	Intervention	Design	Measures	Outcomes
Danforth, 1999	4.0 (Twins)	2/2	DSM IV diagnosis of ADHD and oppositional defiant disorder (ODD), clinical diagnosis by the referring pediatrician	Eight 1-hour weekly parent training sessions using the Behavior Management Flow Chart	Case study, prospective, no control group, open-label treatment/8 sessions	Conners' Rating Scale-Parent (CRS-P), CBCL, Parent Daily Report telephone checklist, direct observation of mother-child interaction	CRS-P Hyperactive Index T scores decreased from 80 to 50 for one twin and remained unchanged for the other twin; increased compliance and decreased aggressive behavior on direct observation of mother-child interaction
Huang et al., 2003	3–6 (5.42 ± 1.1)	23/23	Diagnosis of ADHD on Barkley's semistructured interview questionnaire	Nine 1-hour weekly group parent training sessions and 1 booster session 4 weeks later	Prospective, no control treatment condition, open-label treatment/10 sessions	Disruptive Behavior Rating Scale-Parent Form, Child Attention Profile, and Home Situations Questionnaire	Improved parental ratings for ADHD and ODD symptoms, significant decline in the severity of symptoms and problem behaviors at home. Outcome reported for completers (n = 14, 61% of the recruited sample) only Four children were also taking stimulants during the trial
Chang et al., 2004	4–6 (6 ± 0.8)	8/8	DSM IV diagnosis of ADHD by 2 child psychiatrists	Eight 2-hour weekly group parent training and joint parent-child social skills training group sessions	No control group/8 sessions	No information provided regarding how outcome assessment was conducted	Parents reported improved ADHD behaviors in 3 (37.5%) children; improvement in emotional expression/regulation, less parental frustration and increased satisfaction regarding child's behavior at home.

[1]SD not provided.
ADHD = attention-deficit/hyperactivity disorder.

the parents and work with the parent-child dyad with the exception of one study that included parent training sessions only (Jones et al. 2007), one study that included parent and/or child training sessions separately (Corrin 2004) and two studies that included only didactic teaching sessions with the parents (Barkley et al. 2000; Huang et al. 2003). Outcome assessments varied among the studies and included parent ratings of ADHD and disruptive behaviors, and direct behavior observation by independent raters for on-task behavior, child compliance with maternal commands, and parent-child interaction quality during structured play.

Improvements in ADHD symptoms were reported in three of the eight controlled studies that included only preschool children (Jones et al. 2007; Sonuga-Barke et al. 2001; Strayhorn and Weidman 1989) and only one of these studies (Sonuga-Barke et al. 2001) was in preschoolers formally diagnosed with ADHD. Preschoolers diagnosed with ADHD (N = 78) were randomized to 8 weeks of parent training, parent counseling and support, or a wait-list group (Sonuga-Barke et al. 2001). Improvements in ADHD symptoms were reported with parent training compared to the other two conditions; positive effects were maintained at 6 month follow-up. No improvement in hyperactive, impulsive and/or inattentive symptoms on parent ratings or direct observation was reported in the remaining 5 controlled studies that included only preschool children. Improvements in ADHD symptoms were also reported in most of the non-randomized non-controlled case series (Drash et al. 1976; Erhardt and Baker 1990; Huang et al. 2003).

With the exception of Barkley et al (2000), most investigators reported improvements in parenting skills, parenting style of interaction, and child compliance. Barkley et al. (2000) reported poor treatment response with parent behavior training in kindergarteners (N = 158) who met dimensional rating scale cutoff criteria for hyperactive, impulsive, inattentive, and aggressive behavior. The kindergarteners were assigned to one of four treatment groups: parent training only, classroom day treatment only, a combined condition, or a no treatment control group. The parent training intervention produced no effects.

There may be several reasons for the poor treatment response in this study. Inclusion criteria for the study were based on a rating scale cutoff and no clinical or structured diagnostic interviews were conducted for a diagnosis of ADHD. Most important, neither the children's caregivers nor their teachers had indicated impaired functioning in the kindergartners included in the study. There is evidence that psychosocial treatment approaches have greater impact on those children rated with higher levels of problems (Kellam et al. 1998; Wilson and Lipsey 2007). Furthermore, only 25% of the parents attended more than four parent behavior training sessions, and, finally, the parent behavior training was delivered in a didactic format.

Parent-Child Interaction Therapy (PCIT) (Eyberg 1988), a related yet distinct parent behavior training program, is an evidence-based intensive intervention for preschool children with disruptive behavior disorders. Parents are trained in behavioral management techniques within a play-therapy context; the therapist works with the parent-child dyad and provides "live" interactive coaching and immediate feedback to change interaction patterns within the dyad. A number of studies have reported positive effects of PCIT on outcomes for young children with externalizing problems, reducing hyperactive as well as disruptive behavior and improving compliance with maintenance of gains 6 years later (Hood and Eyberg 2003).

Although PCIT has not been used specifically to treat ADHD in preschoolers, many studies of PCIT included preschool children who met DSM diagnostic criteria for ADHD and reported benefit in parent- and/or teacher-rated ADHD symptoms (Eisenstadt 1993; Eyberg et al. 2001; Nixon 2001).

Child training. There have been a few studies in which behavioral management techniques have been applied within the preschool setting to treat individual preschool children presenting with hyperactive, inattentive and disruptive behaviors. We identified four published case series (Billings and Wasik 1985; Bornstein and Quevillon 1976; Bryant and Budd 1982; McGoey and DuPaul 2000) and two single-case reports (Allen et al. 1967; McCain and Kelley

1993) in preschool children with ADHD symptoms in which child training was conducted within the context of the classroom setting and ADHD outcomes were assessed with direct observation using a within-subject comparison design (Table 6). There was a wide variation in the inclusion criteria and the procedure used for ADHD diagnosis, study design, behavior techniques and outcome measures employed in the studies.

Only one study utilized a combination of a structured diagnostic interview with the parent and dimensional threshold on a rating scale for ADHD (McGoey and DuPaul 2000), one study included children who were given a diagnosis of ADHD prior to their study participation with no confirmation of the diagnosis by the study investigators (McCain and Kelley 1993), and four studies included children based on teacher complaints of hyperactive, inattentive, or disruptive behaviors. The two single-case reports and one case series (McCain and Kelley 1993) employed a reversal design, and three of the case series employed multiple baselines across subjects.

The sample sizes were small ranging from 1–4 children. Behavioral techniques used in the studies included self-instructional training to encourage on-task behavior in three studies, and shaping procedure with contingent reinforcement and/or response cost was employed to decrease hyperactive, disruptive, and impulsive behavior in three studies. Information regarding treatment integrity was reported only in one study (McGoey and DuPaul 2000) Treatment effect on number of activity changes, on-task behavior, and disruptive behavior was assessed through classroom observation (3 studies employed a blinded observer). All studies reported improved task-related attention and ability to delay activities and decreased disruptive behaviors.

Only three studies conducted follow-up assessment beyond the immediate intervention period, two studies reported maintenance of gains 2 weeks (McGoey and DuPaul 2000) and 22.5 weeks later (Bornstein and Quevillon 1976) and one study reported increase in attending behavior immediately following treatment, but gains were not maintained at follow-up 2 weeks later (Billings and Wasik 1985).

Behavioral approaches applied to the whole classroom affect all children in the classroom and reduce the sense of "unfairness" of ADHD children receiving special treatment. Whole classroom approaches reduce the burden of designing individual programs for multiple children with problem behaviors in the classroom. Finally, this approach may benefit whole class environment, producing a more positive climate (Conduct Problems Prevention Research Group 1999). In the classroom treatment group in the Barkley et al. (2000) study, the kindergarteners meeting dimensional threshold for hyperactive, impulsive, inattentive, and aggressive scores randomized to the special behavior treatment classrooms showed improvements over children randomized to the regular, no treatment classrooms. However, the positive effects did not generalize beyond the classroom setting and were not evident at two-year follow-up (Shelton et al. 2000).

Summary of psychosocial interventions. There is evidence for short-term efficacy of psychosocial interventions, especially parent behavior training, in reducing disruptive behaviors in preschool children; evidence is much more limited for ADHD outcomes. Four randomized studies employed parent behavior training in preschool children formally diagnosed with ADHD and one of these studies reported improvement in ADHD symptoms. Evidence for efficacy of child training is limited to case series/case reports that included a total of 16 preschool children, only one of these studies employed a structured diagnostic procedure and blinded classroom observation, and reported improvement in ADHD symptoms.

Since it has been postulated that long-term behavioral improvements require psychosocial interventions (Ialongo et al. 1993), preschool years are an especially opportune time to promote appropriate inhibitory control by teaching positive and consistent parenting skills as well as training children directly (Diamond et al. 2007; Dowsett and Livesey 2000).

Alternative treatments for attention-deficit/ hyperactivy disorder in preschool children

Here we review four alternative treatment options that may be more practical and/or ef-

TABLE 6. PUBLISHED STUDIES OF PSYCHOSOCIAL TREATMENTS IN PRESCHHOOL CHILDREN WITH ATTENTION-DEFICIT/HYPERACTIVITY DISORDER: CHILD TRAINING

Authors	Age in years	N	Procedure for ADHD Diagnosis & Inclusion Criteria	Psychosocial intervention	Study Design/ Duration	Outcome Assessment (for ADHD and disruptive behaviors)	Study Outcome
Allen et al., 1967	4.5	1	No clinical diagnosis of ADHD, preschool classroom teacher complaint of moving constantly from 1 activity to another confirmed by classroom observation	Teacher administered shaping procedure with contingent social reinforcement	Single-subject, prospective, open-label treatment, four-stage design: baseline, reinforcement, reversal and reinstatement/ Forty-seven 50-minute periods	Classroom observation for number of activity changes	Number of activity changes decreased by 50% compared to baseline and reversal conditions.
Bornstein & Quevillon, 1976	4	3	No clinical diagnosis of ADHD, Head Start teacher complaint of highly disruptive classroom behavior, inability to complete standard preschool classroom tasks, short attention span, not attending to tasks, overactivity	Individual 2-hour massed self-instruction training session with verbal modeling, prompts, reinforcement and fading	Case series, prospective, blind, multiple baseline design across subjects and an observer-expectancy control manipulation/40 observation days over 10 weeks	Classroom observation for on-task behavior	On-task behavior increased from an average of 11.7% at baseline to 77% post-treatment and 70.7% at follow-up 22.5 weeks later. Behavioral gains were transferred to the classroom setting. Gains maintained at follow-up 22.5 weeks later
Bryant & Budd, 1982	4–5	3	No clinical diagnosis of ADHD, remedial classroom teacher complaint of low rates of on-task behavior, high distractibility and non-compliance	Nine or more individually administered 10-minute sessions of self-instructional training over 3–8 days followed by classroom intervention with contingent reinforcement by the teacher	Case series, prospective, open-label treatment, multiple baseline design across subjects and sequential administration of self-instructional training and classroom intervention/ 8 days	Classroom observation for on-task and disruptive behaviors, work completion, and work accuracy	On-task behavior increased from an average of 43.8% at baseline to 53.3% after self-instructional training and 67.7% after introduction of the classroom intervention, work accuracy increased with self-instructional training. Rate of work completion increased after the classroom intervention with contingent reinforcement was instituted.

Study	Age	N	Diagnosis/Inclusion Criteria	Intervention	Design/Duration	Measures	Results
Billings & Wasik, 1985	4.2–4.8	4	No clinical diagnosis of ADHD, Head Start teacher complaint of off-task, disruptive and inattentive behavior, and at least 25% off-task behavior on observation	Individual 2-hour massed self-instruction training session with verbal modeling, prompts, reinforcement and fading	Case series, prospective, open-label treatment, multiple baseline design across subjects; one child used as control/ 4 weeks	Blinded classroom observation for on-task behavior and teacher interactions. Self-control Rating Scale completed by the teacher	Increase in attending behavior immediately following treatment phase, but gains were not maintained at follow-up 2 weeks later. Observed high levels of teacher attention to negative behaviors may have maintained the inappropriate behaviors in the children.
McCain & Kelley, 1993[1]	5	1	ADHD diagnosis by the referring pediatrician, teacher complaints of inattentive, impulsive, distractible, and disruptive classroom behavior, Conners' Rating Scale-Teacher (CRS-T) scores >2 SD	Daily school-home notes and home-based positive reinforcement contingency	Single-subject, prospective, open-label treatment. reversal (ABAB) design/ 4 weeks	Blinded classroom observation for on-task, number of activity changes and disruptive behaviors	On-task behaviors increased from an average of 58% in the baseline and reversal conditions to 84.5% in the active treatment conditions. Number of activity changes and disruptive behaviors decreased from an average of 7 and 31% respectively in the baseline and reversal conditions to 2 and 8% in the active treatment conditions.
McGoey & DuPaul, 2000	4.3–5.1	4	ADHD diagnosis on a parent interview using the Diagnostic Interview for Children and Adolescents and parent or teacher rated Early Childhood Inventory; cutoff threshold on the Hyperactivity and the Attention Problems subscales of the Behavioral Assessment System for Children	Teacher administered token reinforcement and response cost	Single-subject, prospective, open-label treatment, reversal design to compare token reinforcement and response cost counterbalanced between participants; a peer comparison child matched for age from each classroom for a measure of expected behavior in the classroom/ 36–40 sessions	Teacher-ratings on the ADHD Rating Scale, Preschool and Kindergarten Behavior Scales, Teacher Acceptability Ratings, blinded classroom observation	Both interventions were associated with reductions in hyperactivity and disruptive behaviors in 3 of the 4 participants to levels commensurate with their matched peers. Reductions in disruptive behaviors observed initially with both interventions for the 4th participant were replicated with reintroduction of response cost but were not replicated with reintroduction of token reinforcement. Gains maintained at 2 week follow up

[1] Parents had previously participated in a group parent training with improvement in the child's behavior at home, but behavioral problems in the preschool had continued.

fective during preschool years than later, may be better justified to try at this age, and may be undertaken in conjunction with standard treatments such as behavioral and pharmacological treatment. As with established treatments, information about alternative treatments is mostly available for school age children.

The quality of evidence ranges from randomized controlled trials to anecdote. In evaluating the evidence, or lack thereof, it is important to consider relative risk, difficulty, and expense. An intervention that is safe, easy, cheap, and sensible (SECS) can be accepted pragmatically on less evidence than one that is risky, difficult, or expensive (in terms of either cost or parental effort and time, which is a resource that should not be squandered on unproven intense treatments).

Of the myriad of alternative treatments advocated for ADHD, four seem especially applicable to preschoolers: elimination diets, vitamin/mineral and other dietary supplementation, vestibular stimulation, and massage. For a review of other popular alternatives, such as EEG and biofeedback that may be more appropriate for older children, see (Arnold 1999; Arnold et al. 2002).

Elimination diets. At the time of the 1982 NIH Consensus Development Conference on Defined Diets and Childhood Hyperactivity (1982) most elimination diets (defined diets) were popularly known as Feingold diets. The Feingold (1975) hypothesis had stated that many children are sensitive to dietary salicylates and artificially added colors, flavors, and preservatives, and that eliminating the offending substances from the diet could ameliorate learning and behavior problems including ADHD. Despite a few positive studies (Swanson and Kinsbourne 1980; Williams et al. 1978), most controlled studies were interpreted by the investigators and reviewers as nonsupportive of the hypothesis (Conners 1980; Kavale and Forness 1983; Mattes 1983). The consensus panel called for more controlled research.

Since the 1982 NIH Consensus Development Conference, a literature search revealed 9 peer-reviewed reports on the use of elimination diets (additive free diet [food colors and/or preservatives] and/or few-foods diet) involv-

ing preschool children who either had a diagnosis of ADHD or displayed ADHD Symptoms (Table 7). Two studies included preschool children only (Bateman et al. 2004; Kaplan et al. 1989); the other 7 studies included both school age and preschool children with children ranging in age from 1.6–15 years (mean age ranging from 7.3–9.7 years). Only three of these seven studies specified the number of preschoolers participating in the studies (Boris and Mandel 1994; Egger et al. 1985; Rowe and Rowe 1994). A DSM diagnosis of ADHD was the required inclusion criteria in only three of the studies (Carter et al. 1993; Egger et al. 1992; Kaplan et al. 1989); one study was a population-based study (Bateman et al. 2004), and the remaining four studies included children with a DSM diagnosis of ADHD or ADHD symptoms.

Many of the studies did not use rigorous diagnostic procedures. Most studies employed a multi-phase design with open elimination diet (additive free diet and/or few-foods diet), open challenge to identify the incriminated food(s) followed by a randomized, placebo-controlled double-blind challenge with food additives (food colors and/or preservatives) in 5 studies (Bateman et al. 2004; Kaplan et al. 1989; Pollock and Warner 1990; Rowe 1988; Rowe and Rowe 1994) and/or the incriminated food in 4 studies (Boris and Mandel 1994; Carter et al. 1993; 1985; 1992).

In order to maintain the blind, food colors and/or food preservatives were administered in a capsule and/or meals were provided to the study participants. The few-foods or oligoantigenic diet most commonly included two meats (e.g., lamb and chicken), two carbohydrates sources (e.g., potatoes and rice), two fruits (e.g., banana and apple), vegetables (any brassica, e.g., cauliflower, cabbage, broccoli, or Brussels sprouts), cucumber, celery, carrots, parsnip, salt, pepper, water, calcium, and vitamins.

All studies demonstrated either significant improvement compared to a placebo condition or deterioration on placebo-controlled challenge of offending substances. The two studies that included preschoolers only are of particular relevance (Bateman et al. 2004; Kaplan et al. 1989). Both studies investigated additive free diet. Kaplan et al. (1989) conducted a within-sub-

TABLE 7. PUBLISHED STUDIES OF ALTERNATIVE TREATMENTS IN PRESCHOOL CHILDREN WITH ATTENTION-DEFICIT/HYPERACTIVITY DISORDER: ELIMINATION DIETS

Authors	Age Range in years (Mean age ± SD in years)	N/n < 6 years	Procedure for ADHD Diagnosis; Inclusion Criteria	Type of intervention	Study Design/ Duration	Outcome Assessment (for ADHD and disruptive behaviors)	Study Outcome
Egger et al., 1985	2–15 years (7.3[1])	76/10	Clinical assessment, dimensional cutoff score on short form of the Conners' Rating Scale; Hyperkinetic syndrome or behavioral disturbance with overactivity	Oligoantigenic (few-foods) diet[2]	Elimination diet followed by challenge, 3-phase design: 4-week open elimination diet (oligoantigenic diet), open weekly reintroduction of foods and synthetic colorings, 4-week or longer double-blind, placebo-controlled crossover challenge trial of one incriminated food/ Information about duration of the open reintroduction phase not provided	Conners' Abbreviated Scale, actometer recording	Improvement on parent ratings on the Conners' scale during placebo compared to the active substance in the double-blind crossover phase. 62/76 (82%) improved in the open elimination phase" no treatment effect on actometer readings. IgE levels were in the atopic range for age in 68% of the responders and 20% of the non-responders
Rowe, 1988	3–15 (7.7 ± 2.9)	55/ n < 6 not specified	Clinical assessment; Suspected hyperactivity	Feingold diet (no synthetic food colorings)	Elimination diet followed by challenge, 3-phase design: 6-week open elimination diet (Feingold diet with no synthetic food colorings), open sequential liberalization of the diet, double-blind. placebo-controlled crossover challenge trial with azo dyes (carmoisine and tartrazine)/ 18 weeks	Daily 8-item parent- and teacher-completed checklist of ADHD and behavioral symptoms	40/55 (72%) improved on open Feingold diet; 26/55 (47%) showed placebo effect as they remained improved after discontinuing the Feingold diet; 14/40 (35%) had an adverse reaction to the open-reintroduction of synthetic additive; 2/8 (25%) children completing the double-blind trial reacted adversely to the dye challenge.
Kaplan et al., 1989	3.5–6 (4.48 ± 1.04)	24/24	Clinical interview, Conners' Parent Rating Scale rating > 1 SD; DSM III criteria for ADDH along with sleep problems and physical complaints	No food dyes. flavors, preservatives, monosodium glutamate, chocolate, caffeine and any suspected food, little sugar	Elimination design: 3-week baseline diet, double-blind, placebo-controlled crossover phase on 3-week placebo control (equivalent) diet and 4-week experimental diet counterbalanced across subjects/ 10 weeks	Conners' Abbreviated Symptom Questionnaire (CASQ), 10-item physical signs and symptoms questionnaire, Visual Attention Span Test	Significantly lower parent scores on the CASQ during experimental diet phase compared to the baseline and placebo diet phases. 14/24 (58%) had behavioral and sleep improvement with negligible placebo effect
Pollock & Warner, 1990	2.8 – 15.3 (8.9[1])	39/ n < 6 not specified	No clinical assessment for a diagnosis of ADHD: History of	Artificial food coloring free elimination diet	Challenge design: Double-blind placebo controlled, crossover challenge with artificial food colors.	Connors' Hyperactivity Index	Mean daily Connors' Hyperactivity Index scores during the 2 active weeks were higher than placebo. However. the changes were small. were not

Authors	Age Range in years (Mean age ± SD in years)	N/n < 6 years	Procedure for ADHD Diagnosis; Inclusion Criteria	Type of intervention	Study Design/ Duration	Outcome Assessment (for ADHD and disruptive behaviors)	Study Outcome
			improvement in ADHD symptoms with a diet free of artificial food colors prior to study entry		Maintenance of food additive elimination diet of each child for the duration of the trial/ 7 weeks		clinically significant and were not detected by parents. Outcome results are reported for 19/39 (48.7%) completers.
Egger et al., 1992	3–15 (9.3[1])	40/ n < 6 not specified	Clinical assessment, cutoff threshold on parent rated short form of Conners' Rating Scale; DSM III-R diagnosis of hyperkinetic syndrome	Oligoantigenic (few-foods diet) water, calcium, magnesium, zinc and vitamins	Desensitization. 4-phase design: Open elimination diet, open sequential reintroduction, double-blind placebo controlled, 2-parallel groups trial of enzyme-potentiated desensitization with 3 intradermal injections of mixed food antigens and food additives (food colors and food preservatives) every 2 months followed by open reintroduction of provoking foods/ 7 or more months	Parent rated short form of Conners' Rating Scale	Conners's scores decreased from a mean of 23 at baseline to 7.5 after open-elimination diet. Significantly more children in the active group (n = 15) were able to continue to eat the previously identified provoking food versus in the placebo group.
Carter et al., 1993	3–12[3]	78/ n < 6 not specified	Standardized psychiatric interview, ratings on the Conners' Rating Scale Parent and Teacher (CRS-P and CRS-T); DSM III criteria for ADHD	Few-foods diet[2] bottled water, sunflower oil. milk-free margarine, and already suspected foods were avoided	Elimination diet followed by challenge, 3-phase design: Open restricted (few foods) diet for 3–4 weeks, open sequential reintroduction of the offending foods, 4-week double-blind, placebo-controlled crossover challenge trial/ 10–12 weeks	CRS-P, global rating of severity of behavior problems by the parent, direct behavior observation for ADHD symptoms	76% (59/78) improved on open restricted diet, 80% (47/59) relapsed with open challenges, 74% (14/19) completers in the double blind trial showed reductions in parent-rated symptoms of hyperactivity and irritability (mean difference between active and placebo CRS-P scores = 5.2), and directly observed ADHD symptoms while on placebo compared to the incriminated food

Study	Age (mean)	N	Diet	Diagnosis	Design	Outcome Measure	Results
Rowe and Rowe, 1994	2–14 (7.1 ± 3.5)[4]	200/25	Synthetic coloring free elimination diet	No clinical assessment for a diagnosis of ADHD; Children referred for suspected hyperactivity in association with diet	Elimination diet followed by challenge. 2-stage study: 6-week open trial of a diet free of synthetic colorings, double-blind, placebo-controlled, crossover randomized trial with 6 different doses of tartrazine/ 9 weeks	Conners' Abbreviated Parent-Teacher Questionnaire (CAPTQ), Behavior Rating Inventory (BRI)	150/200 (75%) improved with elimination diet in the open trial. Worsening of CAPTQ and BRI scores reported during the dye challenge with tartrazine. Younger preschool children were described as restless, disruptive, easily distracted and excited. high as a kite, out of control, and displayed constant crying, tantrums, irritability, and severe sleep disturbance.
Boris and Mandel, 1994	3–11 (7.5 ± 2.2)	16/6	Elimination diet (dairy products, wheat, corn, yeast, soy, citrus, egg, chocolate, and peanuts) and artificial colors and preservatives prohibited	No information provided on the procedure for diagnosing ADHD: DSM III diagnosis of ADHD, cutoff threshold for Conners' Rating Scale-Parent-48 (CRS-P-48)	Elimination diet followed by challenge: 2-week open elimination diet, 1-month open sequential food challenges, 7-day double-blind placebo controlled food challenge (DBPCFC)/ 7 weeks	CRS-P-48	73% (19/26) improved on open elimination diet, 79% (15/19) responders were atopic. During the DBPCFC mean CRS-P-48 Hyperactivity index score on challenge days was 18 ± 7 compared to 8.4 ± 4.9 on placebo days. Atopic subjects were more likely to respond to the elimination diet.
Bateman et al. 2004 challenge	3.2–4 (3.7[1])	277/277	Artificial food coloring and sodium benzoate free diet	Cutoff threshold on the EAS Activity Scale and Weiss-Werry-Peters Activity Scale (WWPAS); 3–4 year old children living on the Isle of Wight	Elimination diet followed by challenge in 4 groups of children with hyperactivity crossed with atopy (Hyperactive [HA]/ Atopic [AT] not-HA/AT, HA/not- AT, and not- HA/ not-AT): 1-week artificial food coloringand sodium benzoate freediet, double-blind, placebo controlled challenge with 1-week of 20 mg of artificial food colorings and 45 mg of sodium benzoate or placebo separated with one week of washout/ 4 weeks	Parent completed daily WWPAS ratings, weekly in-clinic assessments on structured tasks for inattention, activity and impulsivity	Reduction in parent-rated hyperactivity between baseline and end of the week of elimination diet. Greater increase in parent-rated hyperactivity during the dye period compared to the placebo challenge period. No effect detected with direct behavioral observation. No effect of atopy or severity of hyperactivity symptoms.

[1]SD not provided.
[2]Few-Foods diet included two meats (e.g., lamb and chicken), two carbohydrates sources (e.g., potatoes and rice), two fruits (e.g., banana and apple or pear), vegetables (cabbage, sprouts, cauliflower, broccoli, cucumber, celery, carrots, parsnip), salt, pepper, water, calcium, and vitamins.
[3]Mean age not provided.
[4]Mean age reported for the 34 children participating in the double-blind trial.

ject, placebo-controlled double-blind crossover trial of elimination (additive free) diet and placebo control diet in 24 preschool children (3.56 years of age) with a DSM-III diagnosis of ADHD along with sleep problems and/or other symptoms (e.g., stuffy nose, stomach ache) indicative of food sensitivity. Food was provided for every member of the household. Parent Conners' Abbreviated Symptom Questionnaire ratings were significantly lower during the elimination diet phase compared to the placebo control diet phase (p < .01). Bateman et al. (2004) conducted a population-based, randomized, double-blind, placebo-controlled challenge study of elimination diet (additive free) in 277 3-year-old preschoolers (4 groups of preschoolers with hyperactivity crossed with atopy). Preschoolers in all four groups showed a general increase in parent rated hyperactivity symptoms with artificial food colors and benzoate preservatives, with effect size of d = 0.5 compared to placebo challenge. There was no effect of prior levels of hyperactivity or by atopy. Table 7 presents a summary of the available studies on elimination diet that included preschool children with ADHD or ADHD symptoms and monitored ADHD outcome.

A related dietary strategy, simple elimination of sugar or candy, has not garnered convincing scientific support from repeated placebo-controlled acute challenge studies (Ferguson et al. 1986; Krummel et al. 1996; Wender and Solanto 1991; Wolraich et al. 1995) despite a few encouraging reports (Goldman et al. 1986). Even a well-controlled 3-week trial of a sugar-restricted diet found no effect (Wolraich et al.1994). However, Wesnes et al. (2003) did demonstrate in a sample of school children not diagnosed for ADHD that a whole-grain cereal and milk breakfast resulted in fewer inattentive symptoms over the course of the morning than the same number of calories in a glucose drink. It does not appear that sugar or candy restriction alone is a widely applicable treatment for ADHD. On the other hand, sugar is not an essential food group, and there does not appear to be any risk from restriction or elimination of candy and other densely sugared foods.

In summary, there is some evidence for efficacy of elimination diet, especially additive free diet, in preschool children with ADHD. The 4 studies showing efficacy of few-foods diet included a mixed age sample and either did not specify the number of preschoolers or did not report outcome separately for preschoolers, thus making it difficult to assess specific response of the preschoolers to the few-foods diet.

Dietary elimination (additive free diet and/or few-foods diet) may be more practical as well as more effective for preschoolers than for older patients because of better caregiver control of diet, and can be considered when there is a history of formula intolerance, food sensitivity, or general allergic diathesis. It is important to emphasize that an elimination diet trial should be implemented only under the supervision of the child's primary healthcare provider and a nutritionist to ensure that growing preschoolers do not suffer from nutritional deficiencies with the restricted diet. The restricted diet (additive free diet and/or few-foods diet) can be tried for 2 weeks (Egger et al. 1985). If there is no benefit from the restricted diet, it should be discontinued. A stringent elimination diet should not continue for more than 2 weeks without obvious benefit because of the danger of imbalance, especially of calcium and some vitamins. If there is benefit, start adding back the restricted foods weekly (Egger et al. 1985), one food component at a time to identify the problem foods to be excluded from a less restrictive permanent diet.

Vitamin/mineral supplementation. Unfortunately, there is no research on effects of Recommended Daily Allowance/Recommended Dietary Intake (RDA/RDI) of multivitamins/minerals in diagnosed ADHD children even though some reports suggest mild deficiencies in diet and blood levels that might be addressed. However, in a randomly assigned double-blind placebo-controlled trial of RDA vitamin and mineral supplementation in 47 6-year-old children not selected for ADHD, Benton and Cook (1991) found an 7.6 point IQ advantage (p < .001), mainly based on nonverbal ability increases. They also found increased concentration and decreased fidgeting on a frustrating task (p < .05), and advantage on a reaction time task reflecting sustained attention

(Cohen's d = 1.3, p < .05). These data warrant a controlled trial in ADHD, although the benefit may be confined to a subgroup with poor diets (Benton 2001).

Regarding a more specific nutrient, Metallinos-Kasaras et al. (2004) found in 3- and 4-year-old children with anemia (and serum lead levels of <50 ppb) not diagnosed with ADHD that iron supplementation (15 mg/day) yielded significant improvements in selective attention compared to placebo. There were no effects of iron supplementation in preschoolers who were not anemic. As seen in Table 8, there is one case report in a 3-year-old child (Konofal et al. 2005) and one double-blind, randomized, placebo-controlled trial in 5- to 8-year-old non-anemic children with low serum ferritin levels, diagnosed with ADHD, reporting improvement in ADHD symptoms with iron supplementation (Konofal et al. 2008).

Another nutritional consideration is essential fatty acids, especially omega-3 long-chain polyunsaturated fatty acids. Omega-three deficiency in infants impairs visual attention e.g., (Neuringer 1998). There have been 7 placebo-controlled trials of essential fatty acids relevant to ADHD, all in school-age children.

Five of the seven studies were in children diagnosed with ADHD showing equivocal or no effect in three (Aman et al. 1987; Arnold et al. 1989; Voight et al. 1998), and promising results in two (Sinn and Bryan 2007; Stevens et al. 2003). The other two were in children with dyslexia and developmental coordination disorder, both of which have large overlap with ADHD.

Preschoolers, with their rapid growth/metabolism and smaller bulk for storage of nutrients, may have a special need for nutritional attention. Adequate nutrition becomes even more of a concern when the child is given an appetite-suppressing stimulant for ADHD. It is important in evaluating a preschool child with ADHD to take a careful diet history. If history reveals a diet poor in iron sources, a blood test for iron may be advisable (Konofal et al. 2008). Similarly, if the diet appears unbalanced in other ways, one might suspect other nutritional deficiency.

Recommendation of RDA/RDI multivitamin/minerals is well within the purview of conservative medical practice, at least until the child's diet can be balanced. Consumption of wild ocean fish a couple of times a week is recommended by the American Heart Association to protect against omega-3 deficiency (Kris-Etherton et al. 2002).

Vestibular stimulation. Mulligan (1996) reported significant impairment of vestibular processing in 309 children with ADHD compared to 309 matched 4- to 8-year-old children without ADHD (p < 0.01). As seen in Table 9, improvement in Conners' teacher ratings from vestibular stimulation compared to a sham condition was reported in two randomized studies in a mixed-age sample (school-age and preschool age children) with symptoms of ADHD (Arnold et al. 1985; Bhatara et al. 1981). Bhatara et al (1981) mentioned that the largest effect was found in the younger children.

Vestibular stimulation is not a proven treatment, but the SECS rule may apply here. The vestibular stimulation of rocking, spinning, piggyback and horsie rides, and swings is a natural environment for preschoolers and can be augmented by sit-and-spin toys, swivel chairs, and rotational games.

Massage. The tactile and deep pressure stimulation of massage has been reported to elicit several benefits. Of relevance to ADHD, massage increased on-task behaviors of 3- to 6-year-old autistic children (Escalona et al. 2001), and attentiveness/responsivity and increased vagal activity were associated with increased attention span in 22 preschool children with autism (Field et al. 1997). In adults, it improved math performance (Field et al. 1996), which is sometimes used as an objective outcome measure in pharmacological treatment of ADHD.

The only study in diagnosed ADHD was a randomized, controlled trial in 28 adolescent boys with DSM-III-R ADHD. Massage was reported to reduce teacher-rated Conners' 10-item scale scores from 28 at baseline to 11.3 while the relaxation therapy controls deteriorated from 19.6 to 28.5 (Field et al. 1998). There are no studies on effects of massage in preschool children with ADHD.

Massage of the child by the parent appears to be a safe and cheap intervention that at least

TABLE 8. PUBLISHED STUDIES OF ALTERNATIVE TREATMENTS IN PRESCHOOL CHILDREN WITH ATTENTION-DEFICIT/HYPERACTIVITY DISORDER: NUTRITIONAL SUPPORT

Authors	Age in years (Mean age ± SD) in years	N/n < 6 years	Procedure for ADHD Diagnosis; Inclusion Criteria	Type of Intervention	Study Design/ Duration	Outcome Assessment (for ADHD and disruptive behaviors)	Study Outcome
Konofal et al., 2005	3	1/1	Clinical diagnosis, parent and teacher Conners' Rating Scale: DSM-IV diagnosis of ADHD, low serum ferritin level	Iron supplementation (ferrous sulphate 80 mg/day)	Case report/ 8 months	Parent and teacher Conners' Rating Scale	Parent and teacher reports of improvement in impulsivity, hyperactivity and behavior with ferrous sulphate treatment
Konofal et al., 2008	5–8 (6.05 ± 1.05)	23/ n < 6 not specified	Clinical diagnosis; DSM-IV diagnosis of ADHD, normal hemoglobin level, serum ferritin level <30 ng/ml,	Iron supplementation (ferrous sulphate 80 mg/day)	Double-blind, randomized, placebo controlled, parallel groups (ferrous sulphate, placebo)/ 12 weeks	Parent and teacher Conners' Rating Scale, ADHD-RS, CGI	Significant decrease in ADHD-RS and CGI-Severity ratings with ferrous sulphate compared to placebo. Improvement on parent and teacher Conners' Rating Scale with with ferrous sulphate compared to placebo was significant at the trend level ($p = 0.076$)

TABLE 9. PUBLISHED STUDIES OF ALTERNATIVE TREATMENTS IN PRESCHOOL CHILDREN WITH ATTENTION-DEFICIT/HYPERACTIVITY DISORDER: VESTIBULAR STIMULATION

Authors	Age in years	N/ n < 6 years	Procedure for ADHD Diagnosis; Inclusion Criteria	Type of Intervention	Study Design/ Duration	Outcome Assessment (for ADHD and disruptive behaviors)	Study Outcome
Bhatara et al., 1981	4–14 (mean & median = 8)	18/3	Clinical assessment, cutoff threshold on the Davids hyperkinetic scale: clinical DSM II diagnosis of hyperkinetic reaction of childhood	Vestibular and visual stimulation	Crossover design with twice weekly vestibular stimulation with eyes open in a lighted room for 4 weeks and 4 weeks of placebo contact in random order/ 8 weeks	Parent- and teacher-completed Shortened Conners' Rating Scale and Davids Hyperkinetic Scale	Teacher Conners' ratings and psychiatrist's assessment showed significant treatment benefit for children younger than 10 years. Parent ratings showed significant placebo effect from the control sitation. Mild side effects, mostly nausea, were noted from the vestibular stimulation, none with-drew from the study because of side effects. Five children took concomitant psychotropic medication.
Arnold et al., 1985	5–9 (mean & median = 7)	30/ n < 6 years not specified	Teacher-completed rating for DSM III seminal draft criteria for ADDH, cutoff threshold on the Davids Hyperkinetic Scale, Conners' Rating Scale; Nonclinical sample from elementary schools meeting DSM III seminal draft criteria for ADDH	Vestibular and visual stimulation	Crossover design with children randomized to 1 of the 2 series: 4 weeks each of control condition, combined visual and vestibular stimulation and either vesribular stimulation alone or visual stimulation alone/ 12 weeks with follow-up at 1 year	Parent- and teacher-completed Davids Hyperkinetic Scale, Conners' Rating Scale	Improvement on teacher ratings at the end of treatment and at one-year follow-up with comparatively larger effect size for vestibular stimulation alone than for either visual stimulation alone or the tactile-auditory-vestibular control condition

should improve parent-child relationship and fits naturally into the cuddling, roughhousing, and other tactile stimulation appropriate for preschoolers. Massage may be especially helpful at bedtime.

Summary of alternative treatments. Of the four alternative interventions described, only the elimination diet has some convincing evidence at this point, and it is probably applicable to only a minority of children with ADHD (although probably a larger percent of preschoolers than of older children (Dulcan and Benson 1997). However, the other three interventions have some controlled evidence (albeit not conclusive), are safe, easy, cheap, and sensible, seem more widely applicable in preschool children, and can be implemented in conjunction with standard behavioral and/or pharmacological treatment.

CONCLUSIONS

Pharmacological intervention studies outnumber nonpsychopharmacological intervention studies. Pharmacological interventions have been studied in comparatively larger samples of preschool children and have tended to use more rigorous methodology than nonpsychopharmacological interventions.

Specifically, MPH demonstrates efficacy compared to placebo in treating ADHD symptoms in preschool children with DSM diagnosis of ADHD in at least five double blind, randomized, controlled, group treatment trials (Barkley 1988; Conners 1975; Greenhill et al. 2006; Musten et al. 1997; Short et al. 2004). Thus for informing clinical practice, adequacy of MPH efficacy data in preschool children is at Level A. In terms of safety data, preschoolers are reported to be sensitive to the adverse effects of MPH with increased rate of irritability, mood changes, withdrawal, and lethargy (Wigal et al. 2006) and a decreased rate of height and weight velocity (Swanson et al. 2006). Additionally, no information about long-term safety and effects of MPH on brain development of preschool children is available. Hence, caution is needed when considering pharmacological treatments in preschool children with

ADHD. Information about the efficacy and safety of other stimulants and non-stimulants in preschool children is at Level C.

Among nonpsychopharmacological interventions, there are comparatively more studies for parent behavior training than child training, and evidence is sparse for alternative interventions for treating ADHD in preschool children. Adequacy of parent behavior training (PBT) data is at Level B as shown by improvement in ADHD symptoms with PBT (n = 30) compared to a Parent Counseling and Support Group (n = 28) and a Waiting List Control Group (n = 20) in preschool children meeting DSM-IV diagnostic criteria for ADHD (Sonuga-Barke et al. 2001). Efficacy of child training in preschool children with ADHD was supported in one single case design series that included preschool children with a formal diagnosis of ADHD (N = 4) and showed reductions in hyperactivity and disruptive behaviors with both token reinforcement and response cost in a reversal design (McGoey and DuPaul 2000). Hence, adequacy of the child training data is at Level B, the small number of subjects limits the generalizability of the findings.

Adequacy of additive free elimination diet data is at Level B as shown by one double-blind crossover study that included 24 preschool children with a formal diagnosis of ADHD and showed improvement in ADHD symptoms with the elimination diet compared to the placebo diet (Kaplan et al. 1989). The evidence for other alternative treatments is generally at Level C.

In summary, the level of evidence to support short-term treatment of preschool ADHD with MPH is Level A and with parent behavior training, child training and additive-free elimination diet is Level B. It is important to emphasize that the difference between the level of evidence for adequacy of pharmacological and nonpharmacological treatments for preschool ADHD does not necessarily indicate difference in efficacy between these treatments; rather it indicates relative paucity of adequate research with nonpharmacological treatments compared to pharmacological treatments. There is only one study that followed preschoolers, formally diagnosed with ADHD, prospectively for 10 months and reported long-term effectiveness of MPH. There are no studies of comparative and/or combined efficacy or long-term safety of any of the treatment interventions for ADHD in preschoolers.

CLINICAL GUIDELINES

Given the short- and long-term safety concerns and lack of information about effect of psychopharmacological interventions on brain development of preschoolers, there is a strong clinical consensus that psychosocial interventions should be tried first in preschoolers with ADHD (Dulcan and Benson 1997; Gleason et al. 2007; Kollins et al. 2006). A psychosocial intervention plan should address child's behavior problems both at home and at school. Parent behavior training should be offered to the caregivers, and parents should be encouraged to work with their child's preschool or daycare teacher to integrate coordinated behavior management strategies at home and at preschool or daycare. Direct child training in the classroom can be implemented as indicated. Comorbid disorders should be identified and appropriate work-up and interventions (e.g., speech, language, and communication assessment and treatment for preschoolers presenting with language delays) should be included in the treatment plan. It is important to assess and support treatment and social support needs of the caregivers. If the caregivers believe that their child's behavioral symptoms become worse with food additives and/or certain foods, a careful trial of additive free and/or the restricted diet can be implemented under the supervision of a nutritionist and the child's pediatrician, as described previously.

Pharmacological intervention can be considered when psychosocial intervention has been unsuccessful (Dulcan and Benson 1997) or only partially successful. Care and caution should be exercised in selecting medication dosage for preschool children. Practitioners need to consider the unique sensitivity of preschool children to adverse events and should follow the rule of "start low, go slow" allowing sufficient time on a particular dose to estimate adverse effects and efficacy. At the same time care should be taken to avoid undertreatment with

lower doses. Preschoolers should be followed closely for monitoring of possible emergence of adverse effects and dosage adjustment with weekly or biweekly (every other week) visits for the first 1–2 months and then monthly for maintenance visits once the preschooler is on an optimal dose.

Parent and teacher rating scales (e.g., CRS, SNAP, CBCL-1$\frac{1}{2}$, ADHD-RS) should be collected for baseline behaviors and repeated regularly for ongoing monitoring of treatment response during follow-up visits.

As mentioned previously, MPH has the best evidence (Greenhill et al. 2006) and is most frequently started at 2.5 mg BID and increased to 7.5 mg BID or TID over the course of 2–4 weeks depending on the child's response and any side effects. It is important to note that there are a minority of preschoolers who may benefit from 1.25 mg TID of MPH; 15% of the preschoolers in the PATS were reported to be best responding to 1.25 mg TID, and teachers reported improved ADHD symptoms with 1.25 mg TID compared to placebo (Greenhill et al. 2006).

Decision for a BID or TID dose may be based on the child's and family's needs. For example, some parents want their preschooler to take medication only when the child attends school and hence may prefer BID dose instead of the TID dose used in the PATS (Greenhill et al. 2006).

There is no controlled efficacy data for long acting MPH or other psychostimulants or nonstimulants in preschoolers with ADHD. If a preschooler does not respond to MPH, clinicians are left to extrapolate data from older school-age children. Based on school-age ADHD treatment data, if a child does not respond to a trial of one class of stimulants (e.g., MPH), switching to the other class (e.g., amphetamines) is recommended before using another drug class (Arnold et al. 1978; Dulcan and Benson 1997; Elia et al. 1991). There is no empirical data to guide dosing schedules for amphetamines in preschoolers with ADHD; it has been suggested that amphetamines are twice as potent as MPH (Pelham et al. 1999). If a preschooler does not respond to stimulants and/or has unacceptable side effects, a trial of atomoxetine or alpha-agonists is recommended (Gleason et al. 2007). As mentioned previously, there is no controlled efficacy or dose response data for atomoxetine or alpha-agonists in preschoolers with ADHD. Improvement in ADHD symptoms in 22, 5- and 6-year-old children (mean age 6.1 ± 0.58 years) was reported in a prospective open-label trial with 10–40 mg/day or 0.47–1.88 mg/kg/day of atomoxetine (mean dose = 1.25 mg/kg/day ± 0.35 mg/kg/day) administered as a single morning dose or BID (morning and afternoon) (Kratochvil et al. 2007). Adverse effects included mood lability in 54.5% and decreased appetite in 50% of the children. Regarding alpha-agonists, there are only 2 case reports of open-label treatment with clonidine (0.025 mg TID) and guanfacine (0.25 mg BID to 0.5 mg BID) both reporting improvement in ADHD symptoms and side effect of sedation early in treatment.

The limited evidence for efficacious treatment options relative to the frequency with which preschool children are referred for treatment of ADHD is striking. Additionally, it is noteworthy that as noted earlier, nonpharmacological treatment investigations lag behind pharmacological treatment studies in preschoolers formally diagnosed with ADHD. This is especially salient since there are short- and long-term safety concerns and there is little information regarding effect of pharmacological agents on the brain development of preschool children with ADHD. Because of the fewer safety concerns compared to pharmacological treatments, clinicians, caregivers of preschoolers with ADHD, professional organizations making treatment recommendations, and the community at large prefer sychosocial interventions as a first line of treatment for preschool ADHD. This calls for more research to find the best possible treatments matched with parent preferences in order to expand the limited intervention options that are currently available for treating ADHD in preschoolers. There is an urgent need for well-designed, blind, randomized, controlled, between-group treatment trials to study comparative and combined efficacy and safety of psychopharmacological, psychosocial and alternative treatments in well characterized samples of preschool children with ADHD. It is important to study the long-term outcome and safety of treatment interventions and their impact on the developing brain of preschool children with ADHD.

DISCLOSURES

Dr. Ghuman has received research funding from Bristol-Myers-Squibb. Dr. Arnold has research funding from Shire, Neuropharm, and Autism Speaks, consults with Shire, Neuropharm, Novartis, Targacept, and Organon, and is on the speaker's bureau for Shire, Novartis, and McNeil. Dr. Anthony has no conflicts of interest or financial ties to report.

ACKNOWLEDGMENTS

This paper is based in part on a symposium presented at the October 2004 Annual Meeting of the American Academy of Child and Adolescent Psychiatry held in Washington, DC. The authors thank Drs. Harinder Ghuman and Alan Gelenberg for their helpful suggestions, support, and encouragement in writing this paper.

REFERENCES

Achenbach TM, Rescorla LA: Manual for ASEBA Preschool Forms & Profiles. Burlington, VT: University of Vermont, Research Center for Children, Youth, & Families. 2000.

Alessandri SM, Schramm K: Effects of dextroamphetamine on the cognitive and social play of a preschooler with ADHD. J Am Acad Child Adolesc Psychiatry 30:768–772, 1991.

Allen KE, Henke LB, Harris FR, Baer DM, Reynolds NJ: Control of hyperactivity by social reinforcement of attending behavior. J Educ Psych 58:231–237, 1967.

Aman MG, Mitchell EA, Turbott SH: The effects of fatty acid supplementation by Efamol on hyperactive children. J Abnorm Child Pyschol 15:75–90, 1987.

Anastopoulos AD, Shelton TL, DuPaul GJ, Guevremont DC: Parent training for attention deficit hyperactivity disorder: Its impact in parent functioning. J Abnorm Child Psychol 21:581–596, 1993.

Angold A, Egger HL: In: A Handbook of Infant and Toddler Mental Assessement. Edited by Del Carmen-Wiggins R, Carter A. New York, Oxford University Press, 2004, 123–139.

Arnold LE: Treatment alternatives for attention-deficit/hyperactivity disorder (ADHD). J Attention Disorders 3:30–48, 1999.

Arnold LE, Christopher J, Huestis R, Smeltzer DJ: Methylphenidate vs dextroamphetamine vs caffeine in minimal brain dysfunction: Controlled comparison by placebo washout design with Bayes' analysis. Arch Gen Psychiatry 35:463–473, 1978.

Arnold LE, Clark DL, Sachs LA, Jakim S, Smithies C: Vestibular and visual rotational stimulation as treatment for attention deficit and hyperactivity. Amer J Occupational Therapy 39:84–91, 1985.

Arnold LE: Treatment alternatives for attention deficit hyperactivity disorder. In Attention Deficit Hyperactivity Disorder: State of the Science-Best Practices. Edited by Jensen PS, Cooper JR, Kingston, NJ: Civic Research Institute, pp.13-1, 2002.

Arnold LE, Kleykamp D, Votolato NA, Taylor WA, Kontras SB, Tobin K: Gamma-linolenic acid for attention-deficit hyperactivity disorder: Placebo-controlled comparison to D-amphetamine. Biol Psychiatry 25:222–228, 1989.

Barkley RA: The effects of methylphenidate on the interactions of preschool ADHD children with their mothers. J Am Acad Child Adolesc Psychiatry 27:336–341, 1988.

Barkley RA: Behavioral inhibition, sustained attention, and executive functions: Constructing a unifying theory of ADHD. Psychol Bull 121: 65–94, 1997.

Barkley RA: How should attention deficit disorder be described? Harv Ment Health Lett 14:8, 1998.

Barkley RA: Issues in the diagnosis of attention-deficit/hyperactivity disorder in children. Brain Dev 25:77–83, 2003.

Barkley RA, Fischer M, Newby RF, Breen MJ: Development of a multimethod clinical protocol for assessing stimulant drug response in children with attention deficit disorder. J Clin Child Psychology 17:14–24, 1988.

Barkley RA, Karlsson J, Pollard S: Effects of age on the mother-child interactions of ADD-H and normal boys. J Abnorm Child Psychol 13:631–637, 1985.

Barkley RA, Karlsson J, Strzelecki E, Murphy JV: Effects of age and Ritalin dosage on the mother-child interactions of hyperactive children. J Consult Clin Psychol 52:750–758, 1984.

Barkley RA, Shelton TL, Crosswait C, Moorehouse M, Fletcher K, Barrett S, Jenkins L, Metevia L: Multimethod psycho-educational intervention for preschool children with disruptive behavior: Preliminary results at post-treatment. J Child Psychol Psychiatry 41:319–332, 2000.

Bateman B, Warner JO, Hutchinson E, Dean T, Rowlandson P, Gant C, Grundy J, Fitzgerald C, Stevenson J: The effects of a double blind, placebo controlled, artificial food colourings and benzoate preservative challenge on hyperactivity in a general population sample of preschool children.[erratum appears in Arch Dis Child. 2005 Aug;90(8):875; PMID: 16040891]. Archives of Disease in Childhood 89:506–511, 2004.

Beckwith L: Prevention science and prevention programs. In Handbook of Infant Mental Health. Edited by Zeanah CH. New York, Gulford Press, pp. 439–456, 2000.

Benton D: Micro-nutrient supplementation and the intelligence of children. Neurosci Biobehav Rev 25:297–309, 2001.

Benton D, Cook R: Vitamin and mineral supplements improve the intelligence scores and concentration of six-year-old children. Personality and Individual Differences 12:1151–1158, 1991.

Bhatara V, Clark DL, Arnold LE, Gunsett R, Smeltzer DJ: Hyperkinesis treated by vestibular stimulation: An exploratory study. Biol Psychiatry 16: 269–79, 1981.

Bierman KL, Coie JD, Dodge KA, Foster EM, Greenberg MT, Lochman JE, McMahon RJ, Pinderhughes EE: Fast track randomized controlled trial to prevent externalizing psychiatric disorders: Findings from grades 3 to 9. J Am Acad Child Adolesc Psychiatry 46:1250–1262, 2007.

Billings DC, Wasik BH: Self-instructional training with preschoolers: An attempt to replicate. J Appl Behav Anal 18:61–67, 1985.

Blackman JA: Attention-deficit/hyperactivity disorder in preschoolers. Does it exist and should we treat it? Pediatr Clin North Am 46:1011–1025, 1999.

Bor W, Sanders MR, Markie-Dadds C: The effects of the Triple P-Positive Parenting Program on preschool children with co-occurring disruptive behavior and attentional/hyperactive difficulties. J Abnorm Child Psychol 30:571–587, 2002.

Boris M, Mandel FS: Foods and additives are common causes of the attention deficit hyperactive disorder in children. Ann Allergy 72:462–468, 1994.

Bornstein PH, Quevillon RP: The effects of a self-instructional package on overactive preschool boys. J Appl Behav Anal 9:179–188, 1976.

Bryant D, Vizzard LH, Willoughby M, Kuperschmidt J: A review of interventions for preschoolers with aggressive and disruptive behavior. Early Educ Dev 10:17–68, 1999.

Bryant LE, Budd KS: Self-instructional training to increase independent work performance in preschoolers. J Appl Behav Anal 15:259–271, 1982.

Byrne JM, Bawden HN, DeWolfe NA, Beattie TL: Clinical assessment of psychopharmacological treatment of preschoolers with ADHD. J Clin Exp Neuropsychol 20:613–627, 1998.

Campbell NB, Tamburrino MB, Evans CL, Franco KN: Fluoxetine for ADHD in a young child. J Am Acad Child Adolesc Psychiatry 34:1259–1260, 1995.

Campbell SB. Behavior problems in preschool children: Clinical and developmental issues (2nd ed.). New York, Guilford Press, 2002.

Campbell SB, Ewing LJ: Follow-up of hard-to-manage preschoolers: adjustment at age 9 and predictors of continuing symptoms. J Child Psychol Psychiatry 31:871–889, 1990.

Campbell SB, Shaw DS, Gilliom M: Early externalizing behavior problems: toddlers and preschoolers at risk for later maladjustment. Dev Psychopathol 12:467–488, 2000.

Capage LC, Foote R, McNeil CB, Eyberg SM: Parent-child interaction therapy: An effective treatment for young children with conduct problems. Behavior Therapist 21:137–138, 1998.

Carter AS, Briggs-Gowan MJ, Davis NO: Assessment of young children's social-emotional development and psychopathology: Recent advances and recommendations for practice. J Child Psychol Psychiatry 45: 109–134, 2004.

Carter CM, Urbanowicz M, Hemsley R, Mantilla L, Strobel S, Graham PJ, Taylor E: Effects of a few food diet in attention deficit disorder. Arch Dis Child 69:564–568, 1993.

Cesena M, Lee DO, Cebollero AM, Steingard RJ: Case study: Behavioral symptoms of pediatric HIV-1 encephalopathy successfully treated with clonidine. J Am Acad Child Adolesc Psychiatry 34:302–306, 1995.

Chacko A, Pelham WE, Gnagy EM, Greiner A, Vallano G, Bukstein O, Rancurello M: Stimulant medication effects in a summer treatment program among young children with attention-deficit/hyperactivity disorder. J Am Acad Child Adolesc Psychiatry 44:249–257, 2005.

Chang CC, Tsou KS, Shen WW, Wong CC, Chao CC: A social skills training program for preschool children with attention-deficit/hyperactivity disorder. Chang Gung Med J 27:918–23, 2004.

Chorpita BF, Daleiden EL: Tripartite dimensions of emotion in a child clinical sample: Measurement strategies and implications for clinical utility. J Consult Clin Psychol 70:1150-1160, 2002.

Chorpita BF, Yim LM, Donkervoet JC, Arensdorf A, Amundsen MJ, McGee C, Serrano A, Yates A, Burns JA, Morelli P: Toward large-scale implementation of empirically supported treatments for children: A review and observations by the Hawaii Empirical Basis to Services Task Force. Clin Psychol 9:165–190, 2002.

Chugani HT: Positron emission tomography: Principles and applications in pediatrics. Mead Johnson Symposium on Perinatal & Developmental Medicine: 15–18, 1987.

Cohen NJ, Sullivan J, Minde K, Novak C, Helwig C: Evaluation of the relative effectiveness of methylphenidate and cognitive behavior modification in the treatment of kindergarten-aged hyperactive children. J Abnorm Child Psychol 9:43–54, 1981.

Coie JD, Dodge KA. Aggression and antisocial behavior. In Handbook of Child Psychology Third Edition. Edited by Damon W (editor in chief), Eisenberg N (volume editor). New York, John Wiley, pp. 779-862, 1998.

Conduct Problems Prevention Research Group: Initial impact of the fast track prevention trial for conduct problems: II. Classroom effects. J Consult Clin Psych 67: 648-657, 1999.

Conduct Problems Prevention Research Group: Evaluation of the first 3 years of the fast track prevention trial with children at high risk for adolescent conduct problems. J Abnorm Child Psychol 30:19–35, 2002.

Conners CK: Controlled trial of methylphenidate in preschool children with minimal brain dysfunction. Int J Ment Health 4:61–74, 1975.

Conners CK. Food Additives and Hyperactive Children. New York, Plenum Press,1980.

Conners CK. Conners' Rating Scales–Revised (CRS-R): Technical Manual. North Tonawanda, New York: Multi-Health Systems, 2001.

Connor DF: Preschool attention deficit hyperactivity disorder: A review of prevalence, diagnosis, neurobiology, and stimulant treatment. J Dev Behav Pediatr 23:S1–S9, 2002.

Corrin EG. Child group training versus parent and child group training for young children with ADHD. In Fairleigh Dickinson U., ProQuest Information & Learning 2004:3516–3516.

Coyle J. Biochemical development of the brain: Neurotransmitters and child psychiatry. Psych Pharmacosci Child Adolesc:3–25, 1997.

Cunningham CE, Siegel LS, Offord DR: A developmental dose-response analysis of the effects of methylphenidate on the peer interactions of attention deficit disordered boys. J Child Psychol Psychiatry 26:955–971, 1985.

Danforth J: The outcome of parent training using the behavior management flow chart with a mother and her twin boys with oppositional defiant disorder and attention-deficit hyperactivity disorder. Child Fam Behav Therapy 21:59–80, 1999.

Davidson MC, Amso D, Anderson LC, Diamond A: Development of cognitive control and executive functions from 4 to 13 years: Evidence from manipulations of memory, inhibition, and task switching. Neuropsychologia 44:2037–2078, 2006.

Diamond A, Barnett WS, Thomas J, Munro S: Preschool program improves cognitive control. Science 318:1387–1388, 2007.

Diamond A, Taylor C: Development of an aspect of executive control: Development of the abilities to remember what I said and to "Do as I say, not as I do." Develop Psychobiol 29:315–334, 1996.

Dishion TJ, McMahon RJ: Parental monitoring and the prevention of child and adolescent problem behavior: A conceptual and empirical formulation. Clin Child Fam Psychol Rev 1:61–75, 1998.

Dowsett SM, Livesey DJ: The development of inhibitory control in preschool children: Effects of "executive skills" training. Develop Psychobiol 36:161–174, 2000.

Drash P, Solomon E, Long K, Stolberg A. Hyperactivity in preschool children as non-compliance: A new conceptual basis for treatment. Florida Psychological Association Twenty-Ninth Annual Meeting; 1976.

Dulcan MK, Benson RS: AACAP Official Action. Summary of the practice parameters for the assessment and treatment of children, adolescents, and adults with ADHD. J Am Acad Child Adolesc Psychiatry 36:1311–1317, 1997.

DuPaul GJ. ADHD Rating Scale-IV: Checklists, Norms, and Clinical Interpretation. New York, Guilford Press, 1998.

DuPaul GJ, McGoey KE, Eckert TL, VanBrakle J: Preschool children with attention-deficit/hyperactivity disorder: Impairments in behavioral, social, and school functioning. J Am Acad Child Adolesc Psychiatry 40:508–515, 2001.

Egeland B, Kalkoske M, Gottesman N, Erickson MF: Preschool behavior problems: Stability and factors accounting for change. J Child Psychol Psychiatry 31:891–909, 1990.

Egger HL, Erkanli A, G Keeler, Potts E, Walter BK, Angold A: Test-retest reliability of the preschool age psychiatric assessment (PAPA). J Am Acad Child Adolesc Psychiatry 45:538–549, 2006.

Egger HL, Angold A: Common emotional and behavioral disorders in preschool children: Presentation, nosology, and epidemiology. J Child Psychol Psychiatry 47:313–337, 2006.

Egger J, Carter CM, Graham PJ, Gumley D, Soothill JF: Controlled trial of oligoantigenic treatment in the hyperkinetic syndrome. Lancet 1:540–545, 1985.

Egger J, Stolla A, McEwen LM: Controlled trial of hyposensitisation in children with food-induced hyperkinetic syndrome. Lancet 339:1150–1153, 1992.

Eisenstadt TH, Eyberg S, McNiel CB, Newcomb K, Funderburk B: Parent-child interaction therapy with behavior problem children: Relative effectiveness of two stages and overall treatment outcome. J Clin Child Psychol 22:42–51, 1993.

Elia J, Borcherding BG, Rapoport JL, Keysor CS: Methylphenidate and dextroamphetamine treatments of hyperactivity: Are there true nonresponders? Psychiatry Res 36:141-155, 1991.

Elliot J, Prior M, Merrigan C, Ballinger K: Evaluation of a community intervention programme for preschool behavior problems. J Paediatrics Child Health 38:41–50, 2002.

Emde RN, Bingham RD, Harmon RJ, Zeanah CH, Jr. Classification and the diagnostic process in infancy. In Handbook of Infant Mental Health. Edited by Zeanah CH. New York, John Wiley, pp. 225–235, 1993.

Erhardt D, Baker BL: The effects of behavioral parent training on families with young hyperactive children. J Behav Ther Exp Psychiatry 21:121–132, 1990.

Escalona A, Field T, Singer-Strunck R, Cullen C, Hartshorn K: Brief report: Improvements in the behavior of children with autism following massage therapy. J Autism Develop Disorders 31:513–516, 2001.

Espy KA, Kaufmann PM, McDiarmid MD, Glisky ML: Executive functioning in preschool children: Performance on A-not-B and other delayed response format tasks. Brain Cogn 41:178–199, 1999.

Eyberg S: Parent-child interaction therapy: Integration of traditional and behavioral concerns. Child Family Behav Ther 10:33–46, 1988.

Eyberg SM, Boggs SR, Algina J: Parent-child interaction therapy: a psychosocial model for the treatment of young children with conduct problem behavior and their families. Psychopharmacol Bull 31:83–91, 1995.

Eyberg SM, Funderburk BW, Hembree-Kigin TL, McNeil CB, Querido JG, Hood KK: Parent-child interaction therapy with behavior problem children: One and two year maintenance of treatment effects in the family. Child Family Behav Ther 23:1–20, 2001.

Feingold BF: Hyperkinesis and learning disabilities linked to artificial food flavors and colors. Amer J Nursing 75:797–803, 1975.

Ferguson HB, Stoddart C, Simeon JG: Double-blind challenge studies of behavioral and cognitive effects of sucrose-aspartame ingestion in normal children. Nutrition Rev 44 Suppl:144–150, 1986.

Field T, Ironson G, Scafidi F, Nawrocki T, Goncalves A, Burman I, Pickens J, Fox N, Schanberg S, Kuhn C: Massage therapy reduces anxiety and enhances EEG pattern of alertness and math computations. Int J Neurosci 86:197–205, 1996.

Field T, Lasko D, Mundy P, Henteleff T, Kabat S, Talpins S, Dowling M: Brief report: Autistic children's attentiveness and responsivity improve after touch therapy. J Autism Develop Disorders 27:333–338, 1997.

Field TM, Quintino O, Hernandez-Reif M, Koslovsky G: Adolescents with attention deficit hyperactivity disorder benefit from massage therapy. Adolescence 33:103–108, 1998.

Firestone P, Musten LM, Pisterman S, Mercer J, Bennett S: Short-term side effects of stimulant medication are increased in preschool children with attention-deficit/hyperactivity disorder: A double-blind placebo-controlled study. J Child Adolesc Psychopharmacol 8:13–25, 1998.

Fischer M, Newby RF: Assessment of stimulant response in ADHD children using a refined multimethod clinical protocol. J Clin Child Psychol 20:232–244, 1991.

Fischer M, Rolf JE, Hasazi JE, Cummings L: Follow-up of a preschool epidemiological sample: Cross-age continuities and predictions of later adjustment with internalizing and externalizing dimensions of behavior. Child Dev 55:137–150, 1984.

Funderburk BW, Eyberg SM, Newcomb K, McNeil CB, Hembree-Kigin T, Capage L: Parent-child interaction therapy with behavior problem children: Maintenance of treatment effects in the school setting. Child Family Behav Ther 20:17–38, 1998.

Garon N, Bryson SE, Smith IM: Executive function in preschoolers: A review using an integrative framework. Psychological Bull 134: 31–60, 2008.

Ghuman JK, Ginsburg GS, Subramaniam G, Ghuman HS, Kau AS, Riddle MA: Psychostimulants in preschool children with attention-deficit/hyperactivity disorder: Clinical evidence from a developmental disorders institution. J Am Acad Child Adolesc Psychiatry 40:516–24, 2001.

Ghuman JK, Riddle MA, Vitiello B, Greenhill LL, Chuang SZ, Wigal SB, Kollins SH, Abikoff HB, McCracken JT, Kastelic E: Comorbidity moderates response to methylphenidate in the Preschoolers with Attention-Deficit/Hyperactivity Disorder Treatment Study (PATS). J Child Adolesc Psychopharmacol 17: 2007.

Gimpel GA, Kuhn BR: Maternal report of attention deficit hyperactivity disorder symptoms in preschool children. Child Care Health Develop 26:163–176, 2000.

Gleason MM, Egger HL, Emslie GJ, Greenhill LL, Kowatch RA, Lieberman AF, Luby JL, Owens J, Scahill LD, Scheeringa MS: Psychopharmacological treatment for very young children: Contexts and guidelines. J Am Acad Child Adolesc Psychiatry 46:1532–1572, 2007.

Goldman JA, Lerman RH, Contois JH, Udall JN, Jr.: Behavioral effects of sucrose on preschool children. J Abnorm Child Psychol 14:565–577, 1986.

Graham YP, Heim C, Goodman SH, Miller AH, Nemeroff CB: The effects of neonatal stress on brain development: Implications for psychopathology. Develop Psychopathol 11:545–565, 1999.

Greenhill L, Kollins S, Abikoff H, McCracken J, Riddle M, Swanson J, McGough J, Wigal S, Wigal T, Vitiello B, Skrobala A, Posner K, Ghuman J, Cunningham C, Davies M, Chuang S, Cooper T: Efficacy and safety of immediate-release methylphenidate treatment for preschoolers with ADHD. J Am Acad Child Adolesc Psychiatry 45:1284–1293, 2006.

Handen BL, Feldman HM, Lurier A, Murray PJ: Efficacy of methylphenidate among preschool children with developmental disabilities and ADHD. J Am Acad Child Adolesc Psychiatry 38:805–812, 1999.

Hembree-Kigin TL, McNeil CB. Parent-Child Interaction Therapy. New York, Plenum Press,1995.

Henry GK: Symbolic modeling and parent behavioral training: Effects on noncompliance of hyperactive children. J Behav Ther Exp Psychiatry 18:105–113, 1987.

Hood KK, Eyberg SM: Outcomes of parent-child interaction therapy: Mothers' reports of maintenance three to six years after treatment. J Clin Child and Adolesc Psychol 32:419–429, 2003.

Huang HL, Chao CC, Tu CC, Yang PC: Behavioral parent training for Taiwanese parents of children with attention-deficit/hyperactivity disorder. Psychiatry Clin Neurosci 57:275–281, 2003.

Huttenlocher PR: Morphometric study of human cerebral cortex development. Neuropsychologia 28:517–527, 1990.

Ialongo NS, Horn WF, Pascoe JM, Greenberg G, Packard T, Lopez M, Wagner A, Puttler L: The effects of a multimodal intervention with attention-deficit hyperactivity disorder children: A 9-month follow-up. J Am Acad Child Adolesc Psychiatry 32:182–189, 1993.

Jensen PS, Kettle L, Roper MT, Sloan MT, Dulcan MK, Hoven C, Bird HR, Bauermeister JJ, Payne JD: Are stimulants overprescribed? Treatment of ADHD in four U.S. communities. J Am Acad Child Adolesc Psychiatry 38:797–804, 1999.

Jobson KO, Potter WZ: International Psychopharmacology Algorithm Project Report. Psychopharmacol Bull 31:457–459, 491–500, 1995.

Jones K, Daley D, Hutchings J, Bywater T, Eames C: Efficacy of the Incredible Years basic parent training programme as an early intervention for children with conduct problems and ADHD. Child Care Health Dev 33:749–756, 2007.

Jones LB, Rothbart MK, Posner MI: Development of executive attention in preschool children. Dev Sci 6:498–504, 2003.

Judice SL, Mayes LC. Psychopharmacological treatment of preschoolers. In Pediatric Psychopharmacology: Principles and Practice. Edited by Martin A, Scahill L, Charney DS, Leckman JF. New York, Oxford University Press, pp. 654–667, 2003.

Kaplan BJ, McNicol J, Conte RA, Moghadam HK: Dietary replacement in preschool-aged hyperactive boys. Pediatrics 83:7–17, 1989.

Kavale KA, Forness SR: Hyperactivity and diet treatment: A meta-analysis of the Feingold hypothesis. J Learn Disabil 16:324–330, 1983.

Kellam SG, Ling X, Merisca R, Brown CH, Ialongo N: The effect of the level of aggression in the first grade classroom on the course and malleability of aggressive behavior into middle school.[erratum appears in 2000 Winter;12(1):107]. Dev Psychopathol 10:165–185, 1998.

Kollins S, Greenhill L, Swanson J, Wigal S, Abikoff H, McCracken J, Riddle M, McGough J, Vitiello B, Wigal T, Skrobala A, Posner K, Ghuman J, Davies M, Cunningham C, Bauzo A: Rationale, design, and methods of the Preschool ADHD Treatment Study (PATS). J Am Acad Child Adolesc Psychiatry 45:1275–1283, 2006.

Konofal E, Cortese S, Lecendreux M, Arnulf I, Mouren MC: Effectiveness of iron supplementation in a young child with attention-deficit/hyperactivity disorder. Pediatrics 116:e732–734, 2005.

Konofal E, Lecendreux M, Deron J, Marchand M, Cortese S, Zaïm M, Mouren MC, Arnulf I: Effects of iron supplementation on attention deficit hyperactivity disorder in children. Pediatric Neurol 38:20–26, 2008.

Kratochvil CJ, Greenhill LL, March JS, Burke WJ, Vaughan BS: The role of stimulants in the treatment of preschool children with attention-deficit hyperactivity disorder. CNS Drugs 18:957–966, 2004.

Kratochvil CJ, Vaughan BS, Mayfield-Jorgensen ML, March JS, Kollins SH, Murray DW, Ravi H, Greenhill LL, Kotler LA, Paykina N: A pilot study of atomoxetine in young children with attention-deficit/hyperactivity disorder. J Child Adolesc Psychopharmacol 17:175–186, 2007.

Kris-Etherton PM, Harris WS, Appel LJ. Fish consumption, fish oil, omega-3 fatty acids, and cardiovascular disease. Circulation 106:2747–2757, 2002.

Krummel DA, Seligson FH, Guthrie HA: Hyperactivity: Is candy causal? Crit Rev Food Sci Nutr 36:3147, 1996.

Lahey BB, Pelham WE, Loney J, Kipp H, Ehrhardt A, Lee SS, Willcutt EG, Hartung CM, Chronis A, Massetti G: Three-year predictive validity of DSM-IV attention deficit hyperactivity disorder in children diagnosed at 4-6 years of age. Am J Psychiatry 161:2014–2020, 2004.

Lavigne JV, Arend R, Rosenbaum D, Binns HJ, Christoffel KK, Gibbons RD: Psychiatric disorders with onset in the preschool years: I. Stability of diagnoses. J Am Acad Child Adolesc Psychiatry 37:1246–1254, 1998.

Lee BJ: Clinical experience with guanfacine in 2- and 3-year-old children with attention deficit hyperactivity disorder. Infant Mental Health 18:300-305, 1997.

Marshall E: Planned ritalin trial for tots heads into uncharted waters. Science 290:1280, 2000.

Mattes JA: The Feingold diet: A current reappraisal. J Learn Disabil 16:319–323, 1983.

Matthews SG: Early programming of the hypothalamo-pituitary-adrenal axis. Trends Endocrinol Metabol 13:373–380, 2002.

Mayes SD, Crites DL, Bixler EO, Humphrey FJ, 2nd, Mattison RE: Methylphenidate and ADHD: Influence of age, IQ and neurodevelopmental status. Dev Med Child Neurol 36:1099–1107, 1994.

McCain A, Kelley M: Managing the classroom behavior of an ADHD preschooler: The efficacy of a school-home note intervention. Child Family Behav Ther 15:33–44, 1993.

McGee R, Partridge F, Williams S, Silva PA: A twelve-year follow-up of preschool hyperactive children. J Am Acad Child Adolesc Psychiatry 30:224–32, 1991.

McGoey K, DuPaul G: Token reinforcement and response cost procedures: Reducing the disruptive behavior of preschool children with ADHD. Sch Psychol Q 15:330–343, 2000.

McGoey K, DuPaul G, Eckert T, Volpe R, Van Brackle J: Outcomes of a multi-component intervention for preschool children at-risk for attention-deficit/ hyperactivity disorder. Child Family Behav Ther 27:33–56, 2005.

McGoey K, Eckert T, GJ. D: Early intervention for preeschool-age children with ADHD: A literature review. J Emot Behav Disorder 10:14–28, 2002. Metallinos-Katsaras E, Valassi-Adam E, Dewey KG, Lonnerdal B, Stamoulakatou A, Pollitt E: Effect of iron supplementation on cognition in Greek preschoolers. Eur J Clin Nutr 58:1532–1542, 2004.

Michelson D, Faries D, Wernicke J, Kelsey D, Kendrick K, Sallee FR, Spencer T: Atomoxetine in the treatment of children and adolescents with attention-deficit/hyperactivity disorder: A randomized, placebo-controlled, dose-response study. Pediatrics 108:E83, 2001.

Minde K: The use of psychotropic medication in preschoolers: Some recent developments. Can J Psychiatry 43:571–575, 1998.

Mulligan S: An analysis of score patterns of children with attention disorders on the Sensory Integration and Praxis Tests. Am J Occup Ther 50:47–54, 1996.

Musten LM, Firestone P, Pisterman S, Bennett S, Mercer J: Effects of methylphenidate on preschool children with ADHD: Cognitive and behavioral functions. J Am Acad Child Adolesc Psychiatry 36:1407–1415, 1997.

National Institutes of Health. Developmental Psychopharmacology. Washington, DC, National Institutes of Health, 2000.

Nemeroff CB: Neurobiological consequences of childhood trauma. J Clin Psychiatry 65(Suppl 1):18–28, 2004.

Neuringer M: Overview of omega-3 fatty acids in infant development: Visual, cognitive, and behavioral outcomes. NIH Workshop on Omega-3 Essential Fatty Acids and Psychiatric Disorders, September 2–3, 1998.

Nigg JT: Is ADHD a disinhibitory disorder? Psychol Bull 127:571–578, 2001.

Nigg JT: Response inhibition and disruptive behaviors: Toward a multiprocess conception of etiological heterogeneity for ADHD combined type and conduct disorder early-onset type. Ann N Y Acad Sci 1008:170–182, 2003.

NIH Consensus Development Conference on Defined Diets and Childhood Hyperactivity: JAMA 248:290–292, 1982.

Nixon RDV: Changes in hyperactivity and temperament in behaviourally disturbed preschoolers after parent-child interaction therapy (PCIT). Behav Change 18:168–176, 2001.

Pear R. White House seeks to curb pills to calm the young. New York Times:1–4, 2000.

Pelham WE, Gnagy EM, Chronis AM, Burrows-MacLean L, Fabiano GA, Onyango AN, Meichenbaum DL, Williams A, Aronoff HR, Steiner RL: A comparison of morning-only and morning/late afternoon Adderall to morning-only, twice-daily, and three times-daily methylphenidate in children with attention-deficit/hyperactivity disorder. Pediatrics 104:1300–1311, 1999.

Pelham WE Jr, Wheeler T, Chronis A: Empirically supported psychosocial treatments for attention deficit hyperactivity disorder. J Clin Child Psychol 27:190–205, 1998.

Petras H, Kellam SG, Brown CH, Muthen BO, Ialongo NS, Poduska JM: Developmental epidemiological courses leading to antisocial personality disorder and violent and criminal behavior: Effects by young adulthood of a universal preventive intervention in first- and second-grade classrooms. Drug Alcohol Depend 95S1:S45–S59, 2008.

Pisterman S, Firestone P, McGrath P: The effects of parent training on parenting stress and sense competence. Can J Behav Sci 24:41–58, 1992.

Pisterman S, McGrath P, Firestone P, Goodman JT, Webster I, Mallory R: Outcome of parent-mediated treatment of preschoolers with attention deficit disorder with hyperactivity. J Consult Clin Psychol 57:628–635, 1989.

Pollock I, Warner JO: Effect of artificial food colours on childhood behaviour. Arch Dis Child 65:74–7, 1990.

Quay HC: Inhibition and attention deficit hyperactivity disorder. J Abnorm Child Psychol 25:7–13,1997.

Rappley MD, Eneli IU, Mullan PB, Alvarez FJ, Wang J, Luo Z, Gardiner JC: Patterns of psychotropic medication use in very young children with attention-deficit hyperactivity disorder. J Dev Behav Pediatr 23:23–30, 2002.

Rappley MD, Mullan PB, Alvarez FJ, Eneli IU, Wang J, Gardiner JC: Diagnosis of attention-deficit/hyperactivity disorder and use of psychotropic medication in very young children. Arch Pediatr Adolesc Med 153:1039–1045, 1999.

Richman N, Stevenson J, Graham P. Pre-School to School: A Behavioural Study. London: Academic Press,1982.

Rowe KS: Synthetic food colourings and "hyperactivity": A double-blind crossover study. Aust Paediatr J 24:143–147, 1988.

Rowe KS, Rowe KJ: Synthetic food coloring and behavior: A dose response effect in a double-blind, placebo-controlled, repeated-measures study. J Pediatr 125:691–698, 1994.

Rubin KH, Bukowski WM, Parker JG, Eisenberg N, Damon W, Lerner RM. Peer interactions, relationships, and groups. In Handbook of Child Psychology, Vol. 3, Social, Emotional, and Personality Development, Sixth Ed. Edited by Damon W, Lerner RM, Eisenberg, N. New York, John Wiley, pp. 571–645, 2006.

Rueda MR, Posner MI, Rothbart MK: The development of executive attention: Contributions to the emergence of self-regulation. Dev Neuropsychol 28:573–594, 2005.

Schleifer M, Weiss G, Cohen N, Elman M, Cvejic H, Kruger E: Hyperactivity in preschoolers and effect of methylphenidate. Am J Orthopsychiatry 45:38–50, 1975.

Shelton TL, Barkley RA, Crosswait C, Moorehouse M, Fletcher K, Barrett S, Jenkins L, Metevia L: Multimethod psychoeducational intervention for preschool children with disruptive behavior: Two-year posttreatment follow-up. J Abnorm Child Psychol 28:253–266, 2000.

Short EJ, Manos MJ, Findling RL, Schubel EA: A prospective study of stimulant response in preschool children: Insights from ROC analyses. J Am Acad Child Adolesc Psychiatry 43:251–259, 2004.

Shure MB, Bohart AC, Stipek DJ. How to think, not what to think: A problem-solving approach to prevention of early high-risk behaviors. In Constructive and Destructive Behavior: Implications for Family, School, and Society.Edited by Bohart AC, Stipek DJ, Washington DC, American Psychological Association, pp. 271–290, 2001.

Sinn N, Bryan J: Effect of supplementation with polyunsaturated fatty acids and micronutrients on learning and behavior problems associated with Child ADHD. J Dev Behav Pediatrics 28:82–91, 2007.

Sonuga-Barke EJ, Daley D, Thompson M, Laver-Bradbury C, Weeks A: Parent-based therapies for preschool attention-deficit/hyperactivity disorder: A randomized, controlled trial with a community sample. J Am Acad Child Adolesc Psychiatry 40:402–408, 2001.

Speltz ML, Varley CK, Peterson K, Beilke RL: Effects of dextroamphetamine and contingency management on a preschooler with ADHD and oppositional defiant disorder. J Am Acad Child Adolesc Psychiatry 27:175–178, 1988.

Stanley P, Stanley L: Prevention through parent training: Making more of a difference. Kairaranga: 47-54, 2005.

Stevens L, Zhang W, Peck L, Kuczek T, Grevstad N, Mahon A, Zentall S, Arnold L, Burgess J: Polyunsaturated fatty acid supplementation in children with inattention, hyperactivity and other disruptive behaviors. Lipids 38:1007–1021, 2003.

Stiefel I, Dossetor D: The synergistic effects of stimulants and parental psychotherapy in the treatment of attention deficit hyperactivity disorder. J Paediatr Child Health 34:391–394, 1998.

Strayhorn JM, Weidman CS: Reduction of attention deficit and internalizing symptoms in preschoolers through parent-child interaction training. J Am Acad Child Adolesc Psychiatry 28:888–896, 1989.

Strayhorn JM, Weidman CS: Follow-up one year after parent-child interaction training: Effects on behavior of preschool children. J Am Acad Child Adolesc Psychiatry 30:138–143, 1991.

Swanson J, Greenhill L, Wigal T, Kollins S, Stehli A, Davies M, Chuang S, Vitiello B, Skrobala A, Posner K, Abikoff H, Oatis M, McCracken J, McGough J, Riddle M, Ghuman J, Cunningham C, Wigal S: Stimulant-related reductions of growth rates in the PATS. J Am Acad Child Adolesc Psychiatry 45:1304–1313, 2006.

Swanson JM. School-Based Assessments and Interventions for ADD Students. Irvine, CA, KC Publishing, 1992.

Swanson JM, Kinsbourne M: Food dyes impair performance of hyperactive children on a laboratory learning test. Science 207:1485–1487, 1980.

Task Force on Psychological Intervention Guidelines: Template for developing guidelines: Interventions for mental disorders and psychological aspects of physical disorders. Washington DC, American Psychological Association, 1995.

Task Force on Research Diagnostic Criteria: Infancy and preschool: Research diagnostic criteria for infants and preschool children: The process and empirical support. J Am Acad Child Adolesc Psychiatry 42:1504–1512, 2003.

US Food and Drug Administration: Regulations requiring manufacturers to assess the safety and effectiveness of new drugs and biological products in pediatric patients. Federal Register 62:43899-43916, 1997.

US Public Health Service. Report of Surgeon General's Conference on Children's Mental Health: A National Action Agenda. Washington, DC: US Department of Health and Human Services, 2000.

Vitiello B, Abikoff HB, Chuang SZ, Kollins SH, McCracken JT, Riddle MA, Swanson JM, Wigal T, McGough JJ, Ghuman JK: Effectiveness of methylphenidate in the 10-month continuation phase of the Preschoolers with Attention-Deficit/Hyperactivity Disorders Treatment Study (PATS). J Child Adolesc Psychopharmacol 17:593–604, 2007.

Voight R, Llorente A, Jensen C, Berretta M, Boutte C, Heird W. Effect of dietary docosohexaenoic acid supplementation on children with ADHD: Preliminary unpublished data. NIH workshop on Omega-3 Essential Fatty Acids and Psychiatric Disorders, September 2–3, 1998.

Webster-Stratton C, Reid J, Hammond M: Social skills and problem-solving training for children with early-onset conduct problems: Who benefits? J Child Psychol Psychiatry 42:943–952, 2001.

Wender EH, Solanto MV: Effects of sugar on aggressive and inattentive behavior in children with attention deficit disorder with hyperactivity and normal children. Pediatrics 88:960–966, 1991.

Wesnes KA, Pincock C, Richardson D, Helm G, Hails S: Breakfast reduces declines in attention and memory over the morning in schoolchildren. Appetite 41:329–331, 2003.

Wigal T, Greenhill L, Chuang S, McGough J, Vitiello B, Skrobala A, Swanson J, Wigal S, Abikoff H, Kollins S, McCracken J, Riddle M, Posner K, Ghuman J, Davies M, Thorp B, Stehli A: Safety and tolerability of methylphenidate in preschool children with ADHD. J Am Acad Child Adolesc Psychiatry 45: 1294–1303, 2006.

Wilens TE, Biederman J, Brown S, Monuteaux M, Prince J, Spencer TJ: Patterns of psychopathology and dysfunction in clinically referred preschoolers. J Dev Behav Pediatr 23:S31–S36, 2002.

Wilens TE, Biederman J, Spencer TJ: Attention deficit/hyperactivity disorder across the lifespan. Annu Rev Med 53:113–131, 2002.

Williams JI, Cram DM, Tausig FT, Webster E: Relative effects of drugs and diet on hyperactive behaviors: An experimental study. Pediatrics 61:811–817, 1978.

Wilson SJ, Lipsey MW: School-based interventions for aggressive and disruptive behavior update of a meta-analysis. Am J Prevent Med 33:130–143, 2007.

Wolraich ML, Lindgren SD, Stumbo PJ, Stegink LD, Appelbaum MI, Kiritsy MC: Effects of diets high in sucrose or aspartame on the behavior and cognitive performance of children. N Engl J Med 330:301–307, 1994.

Wolraich ML, Wilson DB, White JW: The effect of sugar on behavior or cognition in children. A metaanalysis. JAMA 274:1617–1621, 1995.

Zito JM, Safer DJ, dosReis S, Gardner JF, Boles M, Lynch F: Trends in the prescribing of psychotropic medications to preschoolers. JAMA 283:1025–1030, 2000.

Zito JM, Safer DJ, Valluri S: Psychotherapeutic medication prevalence in Medicaid-insured preschoolers. J Child Adolesc Psychopharmacol 17:195, 2007.

Address reprint requests to:
Jaswinder K Ghuman, M.D.
University of Arizona
Room AHSC 7304
1501 N. Campbell Ave.
Tucson, Arizona 85724-5002

E-mail: jkghuman@email.arizona.edu

Index